QUALITY BY DESIGN

QUALITY BY DESIGN

A Clinical Microsystems Approach

Second Edition

Edited by

Marjorie M. Godfrey
Tina C. Foster
Julie K. Johnson
Eugene C. Nelson
Paul B. Batalden

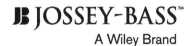

A Wiley Brand

Published by John Wiley & Sons, Inc., Hoboken, New Jersey.
Published simultaneously in Canada.

For general information on our other products and services or for technical support, please contact our Customer Care Department within the United States at (800) 762-2974, outside the United States at (317) 572-3993 or fax (317) 572-4002.

Wiley also publishes its books in a variety of electronic formats. Some content that appears in print may not be available in electronic formats. For more information about Wiley products, visit our web site at www.wiley.com.

Library of Congress Cataloging-in-Publication Data applied for:

Paperback ISBN: 9781119218692

Cover Design: Wiley
Cover Image: © marigold_88/Getty Images

Set in 10/13pt NewBaskerVilleStd by Straive, Chennai, India

Printed and bound by CPI Group (UK) Ltd, Croydon, CR0 4YY

C9781119218692_080125

The manufacturer's authorized representative according to the EU General Product Safety Regulation is Wiley-VCH GmbH, Boschstr. 12, 69469 Weinheim, Germany, e-mail: Product_Safety@wiley.com.

We dedicate this book to

Our teachers – *we are grateful to have learned from the pioneers/luminaries in the fields of improvement and learning.*

We have been fortunate to learn directly from several of these thought leaders: James Brian Quinn, the "father" of micro-meso-macrosystem thinking, Parker Palmer, Karl Weick, Don Berwick, Staffan Lindblad, Maureen Bisognano, Atul Gawande, Brenda Zimmerman, Trish Greenhalgh, Jody Hoffer Gittell, and Edgar Schein. Through their writings, we have benefited from other thought leaders such as W. Edwards Deming, Florence Nightingale, Avedis Donabedian, and Donald Schön.

We are also grateful to the members of the clinical microsystem, including members of the communities who coproduce care and help us co-design systems that will provide the right care, at the right time, at the right place, every time.

Our families Our loved ones who support our passion and pursuit for excellence in health care.

CONTENTS

TABLES, FIGURES, AND EXHIBITS

Tables

Figures

Exhibits

FOREWORD

Paul B. Batalden, MD; Eugene C. Nelson, DSc, MPH

Introduction

The meeting was about making real change in U.S. healthcare services. Professor Diane Meier, Director of the Center to Advance Palliative care and expert on palliative medicine, presented the story of the development of palliative care. As she reflected on the progress made in the quality of health care, she identified at least seven contributing levers for change:

1. The "business" case
2. The "quality" case
3. Social marketing to create specific audience awareness
4. Clinician training
5. Payment
6. Regulation, accreditation, certification
7. Policy change

Quality by Design, second edition, helps with each of these levers. It offers insights that can help you build the "quality" case, and it offers the basic information that can form necessary clinician education and training. It indirectly contributes to each of the other levers by bringing the basic unit where professionals and individual patients, families and communities meet (the clinical microsystem) into sharp focus.

Context and Importance of Clinical Microsystems

This book describes how the real work of healthcare services gets done and how that work can be improved. It begins with the recognition that healthcare service today is not "soloist" work. Clinical microsystems are groups of professionals and patients who regularly use information and technology to help them work together to realize shared aims. Effective clinical microsystems are based on trust and communication that builds a positive patient-professional relationship. Together, the microsystem groups can work to help patients flourish and minimize the burden of illness. Microsystems form the basic building blocks for modern healthcare service.

When the first edition of this book was written, we had the deep belief that healthcare service professionals actually have two jobs: to do their work and to improve their work. The addition of practical improvement "know-how" ensures that the healthcare professionals of today and tomorrow will be ready to lead the changes needed. We believe that this second edition has benefitted significantly from the reflections and experiences of hundreds of people and can help practitioners learn and master the basics of improvement as they put them to use for the benefit of the patients they serve.

The Clinical Microsystem: A Perspective and an Approach to Improvement

Clinical microsystems do not need to be "installed" or "implemented" – they already exist. However, their performance and functional effectiveness vary substantially. The first edition of this book suggested several ways that clinical microsystems might be recognized and improved. Since that book, many have engaged in the job of improving these small systems, and much has been written and spoken about their efforts. New insights, new frames, and new data have emerged. This version brings together these new insights and combines them with the introductions found in the first edition. This book provides today's healthcare leaders, practicing clinicians, and clinical learners with what they need to get started on the road to measurably improve healthcare services in a way that can be sustained and further improved upon.

The first part of the book offers a panoramic and refreshed view of quality improvement and includes useful theoretical frameworks, important principles, practical tools, and powerful techniques, often in the context of real-world cases. It covers fundamentals such as patient-centered care, patient safety, and quality measurement, and introduces emerging issues such as the co-production of health and healthcare services, integration of care across different levels of the system, and building rich information environments enabled by information technology.

The second part of the book provides specific guidance and a "path-forward" curriculum. Of particular note is the advancement of clinical microsystems to mesosystems of care since people usually receive care in more than one microsystem during episodes of care. Leaders at all levels of the healthcare system can use it to successfully integrate quality improvement into the daily work of clinical professionals and support staff who serve all kinds of patients with all kinds of health-related needs.

Editors and Authors

This second edition of *Quality by Design* was directed by three editors who are known for leading, teaching, and writing about quality improvement in the frontlines of care. Marjorie M. Godfrey (PhD, MS, BSN, FAAN) and Tina C. Foster (MD, MPH, MS) began working in the 1990s as quality improvement leaders and teachers at Dartmouth, which continues to be their professional home. Julie K. Johnson (MSPH, PhD) received her doctorate degree from Dartmouth and enjoys a distinguished career in quality and safety working as a professor and researcher. She is currently based at the Feinberg School of Medicine in Chicago, Illinois. We have had the privilege of working very closely with the editors and believe they have produced a wonderful book.

They have enlisted the aid of a diverse group of authors with wide-ranging, real-world experience and strong credentials in healthcare service improvement and innovation. The authors have brought their firsthand knowledge and worldwide experience about healthcare service and its improvement into each of the book's chapters.

Conclusion

Today, we recognize the need to build quality improvement "know-how" into the education of tomorrow's healthcare professionals – the doctors and nurses and allied health professionals of the future. We also recognize the need to build this same quality improvement "know-how" into the work of busy clinicians. This work and the knowledge of clinical microsystems make it possible for everyday medical practices and clinical units to be improved from "the inside out." Those are the improvements likely to last. Go for it.

PREFACE

Marjorie M. Godfrey, PhD, MS, BSN, FAAN; Tina C. Foster, MD, MPH, MS; Julie K. Johnson, MSPH, PhD

This second edition of *Quality by Design* is about both clinical microsystems – the place where patients, families, and care teams meet – *and* other systems in health care, primarily mesosystems, which comprise multiple microsystems that (ideally) work together for a common aim. It is about what leaders at all levels need to know and do to create the conditions for excellent care at the front line. Is the care correct? Timely? Caring? Desired? Efficient? Is the care coproduced with patients and families in a way all parties can support? These questions are answered millions of times a day as real patients and families interact with real teams in real clinical microsystems and mesosystems. The experience by people in these interactions can range from "perfect" to "dreadful" (and everything in between).

In reading and using this book, we hope you will make discoveries about microsystems *and* mesosystems. We sincerely hope you will use the tools and processes and apply the lessons in your actual care settings; discuss the concepts with colleagues, patients, and families; and learn from your experiments.

What is a Clinical Microsystem?

A clinical microsystem is many things serving many purposes to many people.

A locus of professional formation: The place where people learn how to become competent healthcare professionals who work together and continue to develop over time. At the heart of the development of the caring and competent healthcare professional is the integration of the learning of "the head, the hands, and the heart" with the ability to take action to values.

A living system laboratory: A place to test changes in care design and delivery and to observe and work with complexity. Clinical micro- and mesosystems are living, complex adaptive systems that have simple rules, autonomous but interdependent agents, patterns of ordered relationships, and processes. Micro- and mesosystems offer opportunities to understand the work of small delivery systems in their natural context. While some problems they face are simple, many are complicated and complex.

A source of workforce motivation or alienation: The place where pride in work flourishes or flounders. Clinical microsystems are the locus of most workforce dissatisfiers and many genuine motivators for pride and joy in work. The hygiene factors in work, identified long ago by Herzberg (1987), such as work policy, administration, supervision, interpersonal relations, and working conditions, are often mandated by the macrosystem, yet are largely made manifest in the microsystems. So too are the motivating factors, such as the work itself, responsibility, recognition, and sense of achievement.

A building block of health care: The place that connects with other microsystems to form a continuum of care (mesosystem). In primary, secondary, and tertiary care settings, these small systems connect the core competencies of health professionals to the needs of patients, families, and communities. In isolation or in concert with other microsystems, the clinical microsystem makes it easy or difficult to do the right thing. Microsystems exist – not because we have installed them – but because they are where real healthcare work gets done. The idea that patients and providers are members of the same system is not new. In the 1930s, the famed physiological biochemist L. J. Henderson noted that patients and their caregivers were best thought of as members of the same system (Henderson, 1935).

The home of clinical policy in use: The place where policies are enacted and used in actual care. Much has been made of formal guidance for caregivers from the aphorisms of Hippocrates to today's guidelines, protocols, pathways, and evidence syntheses. Often, however, this formal guidance is the guidance we espouse but do not practice. Clinical microsystems have policies in use about access, about the use of information and telecommunication technologies to offer care, about the daily use of science and evidence, about staffing and the continuing development of people, and more. Sometimes a policy-in-use is written, sometimes not. Debates often rage about the espoused policies, whereas the policies in use often remain misunderstood and unexamined.

A maker of healthcare value and safety: The place where costs are incurred and reliability and safety succeed or fail. Clinical microsystems, like other systems, can make it easy to do the right thing. Microsystems that work as high-reliability organizations, similar to those described by Weick and colleagues, are "mindful" of their interdependent interactions (Weick, 2002; Weick and Sutcliffe, 2001).

The facilitator of patient satisfaction: The place where patients and families coproduce care with staff and experience that care as meeting or not meeting their needs. Clinical microsystems are the locus of control for many, if not most, of the variables that account for patient satisfaction with health care. Ensuring that patients get access when they want and need it should be a goal of the scheduling processes of the microsystem. Making needed information readily available should be a priority of the microsystem. A culture that reflects genuine respect for the patient and careful listening to what patients have to say results in social learning for the microsystem. The patterns of staff behavior that the patients perceive and interpret as meeting their unique needs (or not) are generated at the level of the microsystem (Schein, 1999).

Microsystems and mesosystems are critically important to patients, families, healthcare professionals, and the communities they serve. However, they are often not recognized in daily practice and improvement, and we felt it was therefore imperative to write a second edition of this book, updating it with new considerations about mesosystems and ways of working together. In doing so, we hope that the reality and the power of systems thinking in general – and clinical microsystem thinking in particular – can be unleashed and popularized, so that outcomes and value can be improved continuously (from the inside out and from the bottom up) and health professionals at all organizational levels will have a better chance of having their everyday work in sync with their core values and their strong desire to do the right thing well.

References

Henderson, L. J. "Physician and Patient as a Social System." *New England Journal of Medicine*, 1935, 212, 819-823.

Herzberg, F. "One More Time: How Do You Motivate Employees?" *Harvard Business Review*, September–October 1987, p. 109-120.

Schein, E. H. *The Corporate Culture Survival Guide: Sense and Nonsense About Culture Change*. San Francisco: Jossey-Bass, 1999.

Weick, K. E. "The Reduction of Medical Errors Through Mindful Interdependence." In M. M. Rosenthal and K. M. Sutcliffe (eds), *Medical Error: What Do We Know? What Do We Do?* San Francisco: Jossey-Bass, 2002, 177-199.

Weick, K. E., and Sutcliffe, K. M. *Managing the Unexpected: Assuring High Performance in an Age of Complexity*. San Francisco: Jossey-Bass, 2001.

ACKNOWLEDGMENTS

We are indebted to many wonderful people and outstanding organizations in the United States and around the world who helped make the original book and this second edition possible. Although it is impossible to recognize everyone who contributed to this endeavor, we would like to mention some individuals and organizations that merit special attention, and we ask forgiveness from those whom we should have mentioned and somehow overlooked.

First, we acknowledge and thank our mentors, Paul B. Batalden, Gene Nelson, and Edgar H. Schein, who have guided our individual and collective learning experiences in the world of healthcare improvement. We are fortunate to have had the opportunity to stand on the shoulders of these giants.

We offer a reminder that this book was inspired by the groundbreaking scholarship of James Brian Quinn, Professor Emeritus at Dartmouth's Tuck School of Business Administration. His friendship and insights were incredibly supportive and encouraged our own studies. The original 20 clinical microsystems that we studied taught us much about the possibilities to provide superior care to patients and communities and inspire our continued efforts.

We acknowledge the support of The Dartmouth Institute for Health Policy and Clinical Practice for the original research and the work of translating research into practice. A primary partner in the translation to practice has been the Cystic Fibrosis Foundation. Bruce Marshall, executive vice president and chief medical officer, has provided never-ending support and encouragement to adapt microsystem thinking to improve care systems for people with cystic fibrosis. We are grateful for this practice laboratory for the advancement of testing and knowledge to improve care and develop frontline interprofessional staff.

Quality by Design, second edition, is the product of decades of work and applied research nationally and globally. We are grateful to the Jönköping Academy (JA), Jönköping University, and Qulturum at Region Jönköping County, Jönköping, Sweden, for showing us how interactive research and practice coexist to cocreate learning health systems with the people they serve. Their vision of "live a good life in a good place" serves as a reminder that the health system does not work alone and that multiple systems must work together in support of communities to achieve the ultimate goal of health. Dozens of graduate and doctoral students research a variety of topics on microsystems in health care to advance the field of knowledge. JA offers a clinical microsystem graduate-level course based on The Dartmouth Institute graduate course. Qulturum provides guidance and support to regional, national, and international leaders and interprofessional colleagues to improve care guided by clinical microsystem principles. We want to thank Göran Henriks and his team at Qulturum for hosting the annual International Clinical Microsystem Festival during the last week of February. Since its beginnings in 2003, the festival has grown to include participants from 20 countries who have created a learning network, adapting and learning about the microsystem approach from each other at the festival and throughout the year. Of special note are the Region Jönköping County leaders who include microsystem principles in their work and support the festival and our ongoing collaboration. We offer deep appreciation and admiration to Mats Boestig, chief medical officer and director of health care, Region Jönköping County, and Anette Nilsson, development strategist. Boel Andersson-Gäre, professor at Jönköping Academy for Improvement of Health and Welfare, has inspired us with the leadership, research, and academic rigor that she provides in continued knowledge development in clinical microsystems.

We are grateful that Agneta Jansmyr, chief executive officer, Region Jönköping County, always encouraged and supported our collaboration. Her passing in March 2020 left us reflecting on the memory of her as an exemplar of reflective practice with clear, yet gentle leadership.

We gratefully acknowledge the first Microsystem Coaching Academy (MCA) established outside of Dartmouth at Sheffield Teaching Hospitals in Sheffield, UK. The MCA partnership under the leadership of Tom Downes, clinical lead for quality improvement at Sheffield Teaching Hospitals, and Steve Harrison, deputy director of organizational development at Sheffield Teaching Hospitals NHS Foundation Trust, has provided a new context to explore adaptation of these materials in the UK, Scotland, and Ireland. This generative relationship has resulted in advancement of practice in the approach of clinical microsystems and new learning and sharing opportunities. The MCA has graciously hosted the annual Microsystem Academy EXPO each June since 2015 to connect colleagues from the UK and around the world who are adapting and learning about the microsystem approach.

Many of our colleagues who contributed to the case examples and writing went above and beyond our expectations in storytelling and collaboration. In this respect, we wish to thank Boel Andersson-Gäre, professor at Jönköping Academy for Improvement of Health and Welfare (Jönköping, Sweden), and Susanne Kvarnström, senior human resource officer, head of HR-Academy (Region Östergötland, Sweden), and Department of Health, Medicine, and Caring Sciences, Linköping University (Linköping, Sweden), for the research and academic rigor they provide in continued knowledge development in clinical microsystems.

Martin J. Wildman and Steve Harrison (Sheffield, UK) provided the case example focused on cystic fibrosis care in the UK; Don Caruso, chief executive officer at Dartmouth-Hitchcock (Keene, NH) offered a view of leadership from multiple levels of the organization; Gay L. Landstrom, system vice-president and chief nursing officer at Trinity Health (Livonia, MI); and Joan Clifford, medical center director and chief executive officer at Edith Nourse Rogers Memorial Veterans Hospital (Bedford, MA), provided case examples of leading and helping frontline leaders and staff to be successful in creating a joyful work environment. Randy Messier, Health Care Quality Improvement Consultant (Fairfield, VT), an internationally-known team coach on quality based in the microsystem approach, shared an example of achieving patient-centered medical home certification while developing sustainable improvement capabilities. Maren Batalden, associate chief quality officer at Cambridge Health Alliance (Boston, MA); Cristin Lind, freelance facilitator and consultant of co-creation and patient partnership (Stockholm, Sweden); and Helena Hvitfeldt, chief scientific officer of TioHundra AB Hospital and Health Care (Norrtälje, Sweden) – all shared their experiences in coproduction and partnership with patients and families. Paul R. Barach, clinical professor, Wayne State University School of Medicine (Chicago, IL); Gautham K. Suresh, section head and service chief, neonatology, Texas Children's Hospital (Houston, TX); and Tanya Lord, director, Patient Family Engagement at Foundation for Healthy Communities (Nashua, NH) contributed knowledge and a personal story about safety in health care to emphasize the issues to consider in micro- and mesosystems of care. Brant J. Oliver, improvement scientist, Dartmouth-Hitchcock (Lebanon, NH); John N. Mecchella, assistant professor, Dartmouth-Hitchcock (Lebanon, NH); and Ann Marie Hess, primary care redesign consultant (Portland, ME) – all demonstrated masterful application of micro-, meso-, and macrosystem measurement techniques and models in the case examples they offered. Paul N. Uhlig, associate professor, University of Kansas School of Medicine (Witchita, KS), joined colleagues in the professional education chapter to contribute social fields perspectives in education design. Tom Downes and Steve Harrison shared their evolving knowledge and processes of mesosystem improvement through their FLOW efforts in the UK with an emphasis on "The Big Room," adapted from Toyota production.

We wish to express our appreciation for the extensive contributions and tireless efforts of our writing, designing, and proofing teams. We have special appreciation for Coua Early, for reviewing, proofing, and updating materials and graphics based on her knowledge and insight in the original clinical microsystem research to ensure our accuracy.

We deeply appreciate Cherie Caviness, who has tirelessly worked on this manuscript for months on end, always with an eye for accuracy and proper formatting.

We will always be grateful to the Robert Wood Johnson Foundation for its generous support of the Clinical Microsystem Research Program, RWJ Grant Number 036103, and to our project officer and colleague at the foundation, Susan Hassmiller, who has always been deeply interested in supporting and promoting this body of work.

We deeply appreciate the editorial skills and long-time support from our publisher Jossey-Bass, who has provided support and assisted us in important and tangible ways.

THE EDITORS

Marjorie M. Godfrey PhD, MS, BSN, FAAN is Founding Executive Director, the Institute for Excellence in Health and Social Systems, Research Professor, Department of Nursing, University of New Hampshire. Affiliate Professor Jönköping University, Jönköping, Sweden. Previously Founding Co-Director Dartmouth Institute Microsystem Academy, Geisel School of Medicine, Dartmouth College.

She is a practitioner-researcher of improvement in health care who has a keen interest in helping frontline staff be the best they can be to provide the best care they can through applied clinical microsystem theory, team coaching, and leadership development. Godfrey's primary interest is engaging interprofessional healthcare teams in learning about and improving local healthcare delivery systems with a focus on patients, professionals, and outcomes.

Dr. Godfrey has served on national panels including the McColl University/Robert Wood Johnson Foundation, the National Institutes of Health, National Cancer Institute, and the American Association of Colleges of Nursing (AACN) providing expert guidance based in system thinking, interprofessional team practice, and team coaching. Her career has included collaboration with leaders at all levels of health systems and interprofessional improvement teams to extensively coach and adapt clinical microsystem theory in the United States, Sweden, Canada, Norway, France, Switzerland, Kosovo, Tunisia, Chile, Ireland, Australia, Saudi Arabia and the United Kingdom.

In Sweden she has collaborated with senior leaders at Karolinksa Institutet, the Quality Registry Center, the Jönköping Academy, Jönköping County, and Qulturum to support innovation and transformation at all levels of their healthcare systems teaching clinical microsystem processes and team coaching frameworks to interprofessionals.

In England, Dr. Godfrey has collaborated with Dr. Tom Downes and Steve Harrison to adapt, design, implement, and evaluate the first Dartmouth Institute affiliated Microsystem Coaching Academy at Sheffield Teaching Hospitals. The formal partnership is active in the study of team coaching, research, and evaluation to advance the field of team coaching and healthcare improvement using the clinical microsystem framework.

For the past 20 years, Marjorie has provided leadership and guidance to the Cystic Fibrosis Foundation, Bethesda, Maryland to support the mission to partner with the CF community. In partnership with CF senior leaders and frontline interprofessional improvement teams including people with CF and their families in North America, she has adapted and taught clinical microsystem applied theory, leadership development, and team coaching through the improvement fundamentals and CF Lung Transplant Learning and Leadership Improvement Collaboratives

She has advised, led, and coached national programs at the American Thrombosis and Hemostasis Network, Vermont Oxford Network, Traumatic Brain Injury Foundation, Quality Improvement Organizations (QIOs), Cincinnati Children's Hospital Medical Center, Exempla Health System, UC Davis, Maine Medical Center, University of Virginia Health System, and the Geisinger Health System. In addition, Marjorie has served as faculty member for national meetings and technical advisor to the Idealized Design of Clinical Office Practices initiative at the Institute for Healthcare Improvement.

Marjorie is a certified relational coordination facilitator and a board member of the Relational Coordination Research Collaborative led by Jody Hoffer Gittell based at The Heller School for Social Policy and Management, Brandeis University in Waltham, Massachusetts. She has partnered with the American Association of Colleges of Nursing (AACN) to integrate the clinical microsystem framework in the Clinical Nurse Leader Program and served as visiting faculty at several schools of nursing.

Dr. Godfrey is co-author of the best-selling textbooks, *Quality by Design*, 2007 and *Value by Design*, 2011 (Jossey-Bass) and the lead author and architect of the Clinical Microsystems "A Path to Healthcare Excellence" series. She also created the Clinical Microsystem website, www.clinicalmicrosystem.org, which serves as a vehicle for information sharing and networking for the community of microsystem thinkers and designers. Dr. Godfrey's PhD dissertation from Jönköping University in Sweden "Improvement Capability at the Front Lines of Healthcare: Helping through Leading and Coaching" is the culmination of a career of helping frontline teams accomplish healthcare improvement and led to the development of the Team Coaching Model.

She speaks regularly at national and international meetings to share practical application stories and provide instruction on microsystem concepts and team coaching. She is a strong advocate for young professionals and students in health care, identifying opportunities to support their professional development and their integration into healthcare systems.

Marjorie M. Godfrey has a Doctor of Philosophy in Nursing with a focus on healthcare improvement innovation and leadership from Jönköping University, School of Health Sciences, Jönköping, Sweden; an MS degree in outcomes, health policy, and healthcare improvement from the Center for the Evaluative Clinical Sciences at Dartmouth; a BSN degree from Vermont College at Norwich University; and a nursing diploma from Concord Hospital School of Nursing.

Tina C. Foster is Professor of Obstetrics and Gynecology and Community and Family Medicine at the Geisel School of Medicine at Dartmouth and The Dartmouth Institute. She practices at Dartmouth-Hitchcock Medical Center (DHMC) in Lebanon, NH and serves as Vice-Chair for Education in the Dept. of Ob-Gyn. She is board certified in Ob-Gyn and Preventive Medicine. A graduate of UC San Francisco medical school, she obtained her MPH (1998) at the Harvard School of Public Health and MS (2001) at Dartmouth's Center for Evaluative Clinical Sciences while she was a fellow in the VA Quality Scholars national fellowship program in White River Junction, VT. She is former Program Director for the Dartmouth-Hitchcock Leadership Preventive Medicine Residency (DHLPMR), a unique residency focused on the improvement of health and healthcare services. From 2003-2013 she was Associate Director of Graduate Medical Education at DHMC. From 2013-14 she served as national director for the VA Quality Scholars and Chief Resident in Quality and Safety programs. At The Dartmouth Institute (TDI), she co-directed the Microsystems Academy with Marjorie M. Godfrey and co-led two courses in TDI's residential MPH program as well as the Practicum course for the online MPH program and a course in TDI's online certificate program. She is a member of TDI's COproduction Laboratory and active in the ongoing development of the International Coproduction of Health Network (ICoHN), focusing her work on building Communities of Practice.

Julie K. Johnson is a Professor in the Department of Surgery and the Center for Healthcare Studies at Northwestern University in Chicago, Illinois. Julie's career interests involve building a series of collaborative relationships to improve the quality and safety of health care through teaching, research, and clinical quality improvement. She has a master's degree in public health from the University of North Carolina and a PhD in evaluative clinical sciences from Dartmouth College in Hanover, New Hampshire. Johnson's PhD dissertation, "Forming, Operating, and Improving Microsystems of Health Care", was an exploratory, descriptive study of clinical microsystems and helped shape early thinking of success characteristics of high performing microsystems. Since completing her PhD in 2000, Julie has focused her research on activities related to quality and safety of patient care. Regardless of the area of research that engages her time, the clinical microsystem has been the organizing framework for how she thinks about research and practice. She has extensive experience conducting qualitative research as part of implementation research studies and has used qualitative evaluation methods to study errors in ambulatory pediatric settings, to conduct observations in pediatric cardiac surgery, to observe how clinical teams function on inpatient medicine rounds, and to improve transitions of patient care. In her current role as the Associate Director of Evaluation for the Illinois Surgical Quality Improvement Collaborative (ISQIC) at Northwestern University, Julie aligns her experience and expertise in implementation science, improvement science, and qualitative research studies to evaluate a large 56-hospital surgical improvement collaborative. Julie works with front line clinical teams at Northwestern Memorial Hospital to design, implement, and evaluate activities to improve VTE prophylaxis and Enhanced Recovery after Surgery (ERAS) protocols, to assess local QI readiness and local contextual adaptations, and to create patient and provider tools to facilitate implementation and rapid cycle learning. Furthermore, she has extensive experience evaluating learning collaboratives and coaching collaborative participants such as the Cystic Fibrosis Foundation's Leading and Learning Collaborative on Transition to Lung Transplant. As a teacher, she has a special interest in developing and using serious games as a way to engage learners with important concepts related to understanding and improving the quality and safety of healthcare.

Paul B. Batalden is an Active Emeritus Professor of Pediatrics, Community and Family Medicine and the Dartmouth Institute for Health Policy and Clinical Practice at The Geisel School of Medicine at Dartmouth College and Guest Professor of Quality Improvement and Leadership at Jönköping University in Sweden.

He is the Project Director of the International CoProduction of Health Network; a member of the Dartmouth/Karolinska/Cincinnati Children's Hospital and Medical Center design team for the new Cystic Fibrosis and Adult Inflammatory Bowel Disease care model; the Hennepin County Medical Center Congestive Heart Failure Services Improvement team; the Robert Wood Johnson Foundation sponsored international comparison of social support for chronic illness; and Co-director of the CHA-Gold Innovation Fellowship program at Cambridge Health Alliance, Boston, MA.

He teaches about the leadership of improvement of health care quality, safety and value at Dartmouth, the Institute for Healthcare Improvement and the Jönköping Academy for the Improvement of Health and Welfare in Sweden.

He chairs the Leadership Preventive Medicine Residency Advisory Committee at Dartmouth. He is a member of the Board of Advisors of the Anderson Center, Cincinnati Children's Hospital and Medical Center.

Previously he founded, created or helped develop the Institute for Healthcare Improvement (IHI), the U.S. Veteran Administration National Quality Scholars program, the IHI Health Professions Educational Collaborative, the General Competencies of the Accreditation Council for Graduate Medical Education, the Center for Leadership and Improvement at Dartmouth, the Dartmouth Hitchcock Leadership Preventive Medicine Residency, the annual Health Professional Educator's Summer Symposium (aka "Summer Camp") at Dartmouth, the SQUIRE publication guidelines for the improvement of healthcare service, the Improvement Science Fellowship Program of The Health Foundation in the UK and the Vinnvård Improvement Science Fellowships in Sweden. He is a member of the Minnesota Academy of Medicine and the National Academy of Medicine of the U.S. National Academy of Sciences.

He is currently interested in improving the value of the contribution that healthcare services make to better health. He and his colleagues are launching an International Coproduction Network with multiple communities of practice to further develop the idea of the coproduction of healthcare service, based at Dartmouth and Jönköping University.

Eugene C. Nelson is director of Population Health Measurement at The Dartmouth Institute for Health Policy and Clinical Practice and professor of Community and Family Medicine at the Geisel School of Medicine at Dartmouth. He is an international leader in health care improvement and the development and application of measures of system performance, health outcomes, and patient experience. He is the recipient of the Joint Commission on Accreditation of Healthcare Organizations' Ernest A. Codman lifetime achievement award for his work on outcomes measurement in health care.

For over twenty years, Nelson has been one of the nation's leaders in developing and using measures of health care delivery system performance for the improvement of care. His success in developing the clinical value compass and instrument panels to measure health care system performance has made him one of the premier quality and value measurement experts in the country.

During this same time period, Nelson was doing pioneering work in bringing modern quality improvement thinking into the mainstream of health care. Working with friends and colleagues – Paul B. Batalden, Donald Berwick, James Roberts, and others – he helped launch the Institute for Healthcare Improvement and served as a founding board member. In the early 1990s, Nelson and his colleagues at Dartmouth began to develop clinical microsystem thinking, and he started to use these ideas in his work as a professor (in Dartmouth Medical School's graduate program in the

Center for Clinical and Evaluative Sciences), as a health system leader at DHMC, and as an adviser to innovative health care systems in North America and Europe.

Although based at Dartmouth, Nelson works with many organizations in the United States and abroad and is the author of more than one hundred and fifty articles, books, and monographs.

He received his AB degree from Dartmouth College, his MPH degree from Yale Medical School, and his DSc degree from the Harvard School of Public Health. He is married to Sandra Nelson, who practices law, and has three children – Lucas, Alexis, and Zach.

THE CONTRIBUTORS

Boel Andersson-Gäre, MD, PhD, Professor, Jönköping Academy, School of Health and Welfare, Jönköping University; Director Futurum, Region Jönköping County.

Paul R. Barach, MD, MPH, clinical professor, Wayne State University School of Medicine.

Maren Batalden, MD, MPH, associate chief quality officer; associate director of graduate medical education; senior medical director of medical management of the accountable care organization, Cambridge Health Alliance, Boston, Massachusetts.

Don Caruso, MD, MPH, Chief Executive Officer, President, Cheshire Medical Center – Dartmouth Hitchcock.

Joan Clifford, DNP, RN, FACHE, NEA-BC, medical center director-CEO, Edith Nourse Rogers Memorial Veterans Hospital, Bedford, Massachusetts.

Tom Downes, MB BS, MRCP, MBA, MPH (Harvard), Consultant Physician and Clinical Lead for Quality Improvement, Sheffield Teaching Hospitals, UK.

Coua Early, MS, quality specialist, The Microsystem Academy, Lebanon, NH, USA.

Steve Harrison, BSc, MA, deputy director of organisational development, Sheffield Teaching Hospitals NHS Foundation Trust, Sheffield, UK.

Göran Henriks, Psychologist, MBA, chief executive of Learning and Innovation, Qulturum, Region Jönköping County, Sweden.

AnnMarie R. Hess, NP, MSN, MS, primary care redesign consultant, Clinical Performance Management, Inc.

Helena Hvitfeldt, PhD, researcher, Karolinska Institute, Department of LIME (Learning, Informatics, Management and Ethics) Medical Management Center; Stockholm County Council, Quality Register Center (QRC) and Chief Scientific Officer, TioHundra AB Hospital and Health Care, Norrätlje, Sweden.

Susanne Kvarnström, RN, PhD, Senior Human Resource Officer, Head of HR-Academy, Region Östergötland, Sweden, and Department of Health, Medicine, and Caring Sciences, Linköping University, Linköping, Sweden.

Gay L. Landstrom, PhD, RN, NEA-BC, system vice president and chief nursing officer, Trinity Health, Livonia, Michigan.

Cristin Lind, BA, freelance facilitator and consultant, Co-creation and Patient Partnership, QRC Stockholm, Stockholm County Council, Sweden.

Tanya Lord, PhD, MPH, director, patient and family engagement, Foundation for Healthy Communities, Nashua, New Hampshire.

John N. Mecchella, DO, MPH, assistant professor of medicine, Dartmouth-Hitchcock Medical Center and The Dartmouth Institute for Health Policy & Clinical Practice; associate chief health information officer, Dartmouth-Hitchcock Medical Center.

Randy Messier, MT, MSA, PCMH-CCE, principal, Randy Messier LLC, Fairfield, VT; senior associate, The Dartmouth Institute Microsystem Academy; Senior Associate, The Tupelo Group.

Brant J. Oliver, PhD, MS, MPH, APRN-BC, assistant professor, The Dartmouth Institute and Geisel School of Medicine at Dartmouth (Departments of Community & Family Medicine & Psychiatry), Hanover, New Hampshire; adjunct associate professor, MGH Institute of Health Professions, Boston, Massachusetts; faculty senior scholar, White River Junction VAMC, White River Junction, Vermont; healthcare improvement scientist, Dartmouth-Hitchcock Research Collaboratory, Lebanon, New Hampshire.

Edgar H. Schein, PhD, Sloan Fellows professor of management emeritus, MIT Sloan School of Management.

Gautham K. Suresh, MD, DM, MS, FAAP, professor of pediatrics, Texas Children's Hospital; section head and service chief, neonatology, Baylor College of Medicine.

Paul N. Uhlig, MD, MPA, associate professor, University of Kansas School of Medicine-Wichita.

Martin J. Wildman, PhD, MPH, DEBH, MRCP, DTM&H, MBChB, BSc, honorary senior clinical lecturer, Health Services Research, ScHARR, University Sheffield; consultant physician in respiratory medicine and adult CF, Sheffield Teaching Hospitals, NHS Foundation Trust.

INTRODUCTION

Marjorie M. Godfrey, Tina C. Foster, Julie K. Johnson

Batalden and Nelson note in the foreword that practical improvement "know-how" ensures that the healthcare professionals of today and tomorrow will be ready to lead the changes needed to adapt to an ever-changing world. This could not be more evident than during the COVID-19 pandemic. Our colleagues around the world who have learned and now practice microsystem thinking report daily how their practical improvement "know-how" has provided them with the fundamental knowledge and skills they need to effectively assess, diagnose, and treat their changing healthcare environment. They have a framework, a disciplined scientific approach to improvement, and the ability to lead interprofessional teams strategically and with confidence. They have a deeply ingrained habit of engaging everyone in problem-solving, regardless of position in the hierarchy, using effective communication skills. Dynamic and generative relationships have been possible as a result of their study of practical improvement.

Our vision is threefold. Healthcare systems work well for patients and families each and every time a patient needs help. Healthcare systems work for the professionals each and every day, so the professionals can be proud of the services they coproduce with patients and families. Healthcare systems are capable of continually improving, incorporating new discoveries and caring for new and changing health needs. The assumption underlying this vision is that patients and families, clinicians and staff are all part of the same system, and they all want the same thing. They want the system to work the way it needs to work 100 percent of the time.

We all know that sometimes the system works perfectly and lives are saved; we celebrate these events and are thankful. We also recognize that sometimes the system fails and lives are lost; we deplore these events and are remorseful. We need to recognize these failures as learning opportunities and the fundamental question we can ask is "What can healthcare professionals and staff do in concert with patients and families to improve care, transform the system, and create perfect care?"

Need

The serious gaps and flaws in healthcare systems are even more evident in the COVID-19 pandemic. Dr. Anthony Fauci, director of the National Institute of Allergy and Infectious Diseases addressed the House Oversight and Reform Committee hearing March 11, 2020, and reported, "The system is not really geared to what we need right now. . . for [coronavirus testing]." "That [system] is a failing. It is a failing. Let's admit it" (Hellmann, 2020).

Although specific to the pandemic, Dr. Fauci's comment was not news to those working at the front lines of patient care. Patients and families often experience both the best of care and the worst of care in a single illness episode. Sometimes the system does too much (overuse); sometimes too little (underuse); sometimes the system does it wrong (misuse; IOM, 2001). The healthcare system must be transformed to be safe, timely, effective, efficient, equitable, and most important, patient-centered. The need for change is clear, but the pathway to affordable, durable, attractive system change often lies hidden.

Purpose

This book aims to improve healthcare systems by providing a new, clear pathway for improving care *from the inside out*. It is a microsystem approach; and it is both complex and simple. It is complex because it requires a deep understanding of patients, families, and professionals and the changing environments that they meet in. It is simple because, at the end of the day, the goal is just this: to achieve the best outcomes by developing reliable, efficient, and responsive systems that have the capability of coproducing care in a way that meets the needs of "this" patient while continually improving care for the "next" patient.

The microsystem approach requires a clear focus on the *front lines* of care, the small clinical systems where quality, value, and safety are made. We recognize that this change will not take place without leadership to promote change *from the outside in.* The microsystem approach invites senior, midlevel, and frontline leaders to align policy – mission, vision, and values – with strategy, operations, and people to create what Quinn (1992) has referred to as an "intelligent enterprise," an organization that is smart and is able to get smarter (Bossidy, Charan, and Burck, 2004; Liker, 2004). The organization's intelligent activity results in:

- *Doing and improving:* realizing the synergy between proactive work to improve care at all levels of the system and the business of coproducing care with patients and families.
- *Refining operations and learning:* blending a constant drive for operational excellence with organizational learning by relentless reflection on actual performance compared to the patients' needs and by never-ending trials of new ways to improve performance to meet patients' needs, with conscious learning from each attempt.

Scope

The scope of this book is broad. The ideas and methods are of interest to leaders at all levels and those at the front lines including patients and families. It describes research on high-performing clinical microsystems, case studies, guiding principles, and specific tools, techniques, and methods that can be adapted to diverse clinical practices and teams. Of necessity, it has not only wide scope but considerable depth. In short, this book aims to provide a comprehensive and detailed understanding of what it will take for healthcare professionals to transform the healthcare systems that they are part of.

Health care is the concern of both small units and large health systems: microsystems, mesosystems, macrosystems and metasystems. Our primary focus is on the *sharp end* of care – the places where care is actually coproduced. We call these small frontline systems of care *clinical microsystems.* Whether we recognize it or not, clinical microsystems (such as medical practices, emergency response teams, emergency departments, open-heart surgery teams, intensive care units, inpatient care units, nursing home units, home health teams, and palliative care teams) are the basic building blocks of all healthcare systems.

Although care is *coproduced* in the frontline units (the clinical micro- and mesosystems), most of these small systems are not freestanding; they are usually part of a larger organization (macrosystem). In addition, many macrosystems are increasingly part of an even larger organization (metasystem) where there are multiple macrosystems and an overarching structure to oversee the business of healthcare delivery.

Therefore, it is essential to draw out the relationships *within and between* the small frontline systems that actually provide care and the macrosystems, such as hospitals, group practices, integrated health systems, extended care facilities, and home health agencies. A top-performing health system (at the macro- and metasystem level) will successfully knit together mission, vision, strategy, and operations from the top to the bottom of the organization in a way that makes sense and gives the organization the capability of providing high-quality and high-value care, of improving care, and of competing under challenging market conditions.

Overview of the Contents

This book is divided into three parts. The chapters in Part One explore the many facets of microsystems. In this second edition, we have added considerations for exploring and learning about mesosystems. Part One provides research, frameworks, new international case studies, principles, and practical examples. At the end of each chapter, we include mesosystem considerations, review and discussion questions, and additional learning activities. Part Two is an appendix including the new "Accelerating Improvement in Clinical Mesosystems Action Guide." Based on the original Microsystem workbooks, this new Action Guide provides a practical framework for evaluation, understanding and enhancing mesosystems that support care delivery. Part Three is available online at www.clinicalmicrosystem.org and includes the original first edition Chapters 11-24 with fundamental tools, advice and the Dartmouth Microsystem Improvement Curriculum. Here is a brief preview of what we cover in Part One.

- *Chapter One* highlights the original clinical microsystem research, the success characteristics of high-performing microsystems, and adds a new focus on microsystem research around the world.
- *Chapter Two* provides insights into the development of high-performing clinical microsystems and adds a new case study from Sheffield, UK, describing how to assess, diagnose, and treat a microsystem by exploring the 5Ps and using the Dartmouth Microsystem Improvement Curriculum.
- *Chapter Three* explores the essence of leadership from the top down and the bottom up in organizations. The new case study describes in detail how leadership at the macro-, meso-, and microsystem can help an organization develop into a value-based healthcare system from a pay-for-performance system. Emphasis is placed on vertical and horizontal integration of micro- and mesosystems.
- *Chapter Four* shifts attention to enabling high performance of everyone at the front lines of microsystems. Two case studies show how leaders at all levels of the organization can create the conditions for frontline microsystem leaders and staff to be the best they can be every day.

- *Chapter Five* provides a clear focus on why understanding the context of improvement is important. The 5Ps provide guidance and a structure to deeply understand local context while engaging the front line in this assessment.
- *Chapter Six* turns the spotlight on the role of coproduction of healthcare services and includes a framework to help guide coproduction of services at the level of micro-, meso-, and macrosystems, and how these concepts can be integrated into the Dartmouth Microsystem Improvement Ramp.
- *Chapter Seven* delves into the issue of safety and reliability in the microsystem. The case study provides a personal and emotional story of error in health care, which helps outline key principles needed to provide safe and reliable care.
- *Chapter Eight* describes the vital role that data play in creating a rich information environment that supports care both in real time and systemic improvement over time. Examples of registries, data tracking dashboards and cascading measures highlight how health systems can become learning health systems guided by data.
- *Chapter Nine* is a new chapter exploring microsystems' unique opportunities for interprofessional learning by both students and interprofessional staff. The case studies demonstrate how microsystem thinking can inform educational program design.
- *Chapter Ten* introduces the mesosystem. Two case studies demonstrate the use of basic clinical microsystem principles assessing, diagnosing, and treating in the context of a mesosystem and add new concepts important for multiple microsystems that must work together.
- The *Afterword* is written by Göran Henriks, chief executive of Learning and Innovation at Qulturum in Region Jönköping County, Sweden. As a strategic collaborator, colleague, friend of the Dartmouth clinical microsystem research and practical application and an internationally recognized leader of healthcare improvement, Göran challenges us to have courage to "take into perspective" and to reflect in our fast-changing world as we leverage micro-, meso-, and macrosystems to provide health to the populations we serve.

Part Two

The appendix includes a new mesosystem action guide, focused on assessing, analyzing, and improving mesosystems of care. The Dartmouth Microsystem Improvement Curriculum (DMIC) framework is adapted to address mesosystems of care in this new workbook. The worksheets are easily adaptable to any mesosystem, pathway, or continuum of care and help provide an organized and disciplined approach to improving care.

The scientific approach to improvement requires data and information supplemented by intuitive knowledge of your micro- and mesosystem to enable the best decision-making for improvement. The collection of worksheets complements the work in this book and are necessary to gain deep insight into information and data not commonly explored by all members of the clinical micro- and mesosystem. We recommend reviewing the suggested data and information list to identify whether your healthcare system can provide *current* micro- and mesosystem-level data and information. If you cannot find *current* data and information that is from the correct level of care you aim to improve, the worksheets are helpful tools to aid your collection of data and information to inform your improvement selection and decision-making.

For more information related to microsystem and mesosystem workbooks, DMIC action-learning programs as well as information on what organizations are doing with these techniques, visit our microsystem website: http://www.clinicalmicrosystem.org.

Part Three

This section includes practical tools and advice that can help propel organization-wide transformation by applying improvement concepts and enhancing team dynamics, communication, and relationships. This is a condensed version of the first edition's Part Two: Chapters Eleven through Twenty-four.

M3 Matrix. You will also find an overview of the path to making durable improvements in a health system: the M3 Matrix. This matrix suggests actions that should be taken by leaders at three levels of the health system (micro-, meso-, and macrosystem) to begin the transformation journey.

Dartmouth Microsystem Improvement Curriculum (DMIC). Part Three also includes a core curriculum to be used over time with frontline staff in microsystems to build their capability to provide excellent care, promote a positive work environment, and contribute to the larger organization in essential ways. This curriculum details an action-learning program that can be adapted for use in many different ways and in virtually any healthcare delivery system. The topics covered sequentially in this action-learning program are:

- An introduction to microsystem thinking
- Organizing an interdisciplinary improvement team to learn and use effective meeting skills
- Assessing your microsystem by using the 5Ps
- Using the PDSA↔SDSA model for improvement

- Selecting themes for improvement based on the 5Ps and other relevant data and information
- Narrowing the improvement focus with a global aim statement to guide improvement
- Creating process maps
- Creating a specific aim statement based on the process map findings
- Using cause and effect diagrams to understand possible causes of some of the findings
- Adding brainstorming and multi-voting to effective meeting skills
- Exploring change concepts, evidence-based and best practice
- Measuring and monitoring improvement
- Using action plans and Gantt charts to help keep improvement on track and organized
- Following up on improvement with storyboards, data walls, and playbooks

The final section recaps the main ideas presented in Part Two and suggests ways to continue on the path to excellence. It also includes a case study.

How to Use This Book

This book complements and builds on *Quality by Design*, first edition, with the hope of stimulating deeper thinking into leading and improving systems in health care based on clinical microsystem research. *Quality by Design*, second edition, can be used in several ways and is intended to provide guidance, information, and resources depending on what the reader's improvement needs may be. Readers are invited to return to the book repeatedly to explore the different parts of the book, chapters, case studies, and the mesosystem workbook.

- Part One features cases and principles; it provides a comprehensive understanding of microsystem thinking, principles, and approaches with real life examples and stories. It should be read by anyone who wishes to gain a wide and deep understanding of microsystem thinking.
- Part Two provides a hands-on guide to exploring mesosystems in health care. The worksheets can help you arrange and take action in an organized fashion to assess the mesosystem's current state. New questions and perspectives in viewing multiple microsystems as a mesosystem help to see the possibilities for improvement and excellence.

- Part Three offers suggestions for leaders at all levels of the organization about practical actions they can take to build effective performance capability. The M3 Matrix and an action-learning program complete with tools, methods, techniques, and a real-life example of application in a primary care setting can help anyone anywhere interested in improving performance. We offer very specific information that can be used to assess, diagnose, and improve health care, medical practices, and microsystem units of many types. Part Three should be read and put into practice by anyone who wishes to improve health care and to lead large and small systems to achieve peak performance in their frontline microsystems – the places where patients and families and care teams meet.

References

Bossidy, L., Charan, R., and Burck, C. *Confronting Reality: Doing What Matters to Get Things Right.* New York, NY: Crown Business, 2004.

Hellmann, J. "Top health official Fauci: People in US not easily getting coronavirus testing 'is afailing'." [https://thehill.com/policy/healthcare/487230-fauci-it-is-a-failing-that-people-cant-easily-get-tested-for-coronavirus-in]. Mar. 2020.

Institute of Medicine (U.S.), Committee on Quality of Health Care in America... *Crossing the Quality Chasm: A New Health System for the 21st Century.* Washington, DC: National Academies Press, 2001.

Liker, J. K. *The Toyota Way: 14 Management Principles from the World's Greatest Manufacturer.* New York, NY: McGraw-Hill, 2004.

Nelson, E. C., Batalden, P. B., and Godfrey, M. M. *Quality by design: A Clinical Mcrosystems approach.* San Francisco, CA: Jossey-Bass, 2007.

Quinn, J. B. *Intelligent Enterprise: A Knowledge and Service Based Paradigm for Industry.* New York, NY: Free Press, 1992.

CHAPTER ONE

CLINICAL MICROSYSTEMS

Success Characteristics of High-Performing Microsystems

Julie K. Johnson, Marjorie M. Godfrey, Boel Andersson-Gäre, Susanne Kvarnström, Tina C. Foster

AIM

The aim of this chapter is to introduce the concept of clinical microsystems, summarize the foundational research on clinical microsystems, and highlight the strategic and practical importance of healthcare system improvement work, focusing specifically on the design and redesign of small, functional clinical units.

LEARNING OBJECTIVES

By the end of this chapter the reader will be able to:

1. Discuss the theory and contexts for microsystems in health care.
2. Describe ways microsystems function in a healthcare system.
3. Summarize important research on microsystems in health care.
4. List concepts and mechanisms for improving quality and value in clinical practice.

Quality by Design: A Clinical Microsystems Approach, Second Edition. Edited by Marjorie M. Godfrey, Tina C. Foster, Julie K. Johnson, Eugene C. Nelson and Paul B. Batalden.
© 2025 John Wiley & Sons, Inc. Published 2025 by John Wiley & Sons, Inc.

Introduction

Clinical microsystems are the small, functional, frontline units that provide health-care services to most people. They are the essential building blocks of larger organizations and of the health system. They are the place where patients, families, and care teams meet. The quality and value of care produced by a large healthcare system can be no better than the services generated by the small systems of which it is composed. This chapter begins with a sharp focus on clinical microsystems in health care and then expands its focus to explore contexts for microsystems within the overall healthcare system. After summarizing some important research on microsystems, the chapter concludes with a discussion on essential elements for making sustainable improvements in the quality and value of health care.

Background

There was a time when health care was a simpler affair. Omniscient clinicians delivered care in patients' homes or in a solo office. Unhurried nurses met every clinical need in hospital settings. Health care was embodied in an intimate one-to-one relationship that joined patient with doctor or nurse and was supported by relatively little medical science. We developed and maintained a romantic view that health care was a professional activity for heroic soloists (Batalden, Ogrinc, and Batalden, 2006; Morse, 2010).

Today, however, that activity, those participants and relationships, and indeed the very goals of health care are much more complex. An *interdisciplinary* team of clinicians and staff, backed up by ancillary services and information technology, work in partnership with patient and family members to promote health and care for health problems. Participants draw upon medical science and biomedical technology, which expands at an astonishing (and sometimes overwhelming) rate. Clinical settings are diverse and have specialized resources as well as unique safety hazards. Regulators, payers, and consumers all have vested interests in quality performance data that are increasingly available for public review. Health care today has grown, for the most part, into a many-to-one relationship, where "many" refers to health-care professionals and "one" refers to the patient, and in some cases into a many-to-many relationship when family and caregivers are included. Health care is now supported by rapidly proliferating biomedical knowledge, expensive technology, and administrative infrastructure.

And yet, if we look again at the "sharp end" of the healthcare system, at the place where each patient is in direct contact with healthcare professionals, we can discern the fundamental building block that remains the foundation of all healthcare systems. We call this building block the clinical microsystem. The clinical microsystem is the place where patients, families, and caregivers meet. It is the locus of value creation in health care. Although our healthcare system generally works well, all too often it fails to provide what is needed.

True Structure of the System, Embedded Systems, and the Need to Transform Frontline Systems

The true structure of the healthcare system patients' experiences varies widely. Patients in need of care may find:

- Clinical staff working together – or against each other.
- Smooth-running frontline healthcare units – or units in tangles.
- Information readily available, flowing easily, and in a timely fashion – or not.
- Healthcare units that are embedded in helpful larger organizations – or cruel Byzantine bureaucracies.
- Healthcare units that are seamlessly linked together – or totally disjointed.
- High-quality, sensitive, efficient services – or care that is wasteful, expensive, and at times harmful or even lethal.

The system that provides healthcare services is composed of a few basic parts – frontline clinical microsystems, *mesosystems*, and overarching *macrosystems*. These systems have a clinical aim and are composed of patients and families, staff, information, and *information technology*, which are interrelated to meet the needs of patient subpopulations needing care.

Here are four fundamental assumptions about the structure of the healthcare system:

1. Smaller systems are embedded within larger systems.
2. These smaller systems (microsystems) produce quality, safety, and cost outcomes at the front line of care.
3. Interactions between microsystems (mesosystems) provide comprehensive care.
4. Ultimately, the outcomes of a macrosystem can be no better than the outcomes of the microsystems and mesosystems of which it is composed.

Donald Berwick's "chain of effect in improving health care quality" (Berwick, 2001; see Figure 1.1) shows the major elements that need to work well, and work well

FIGURE 1.1 CHAIN OF EFFECT IN IMPROVING HEALTHCARE QUALITY.

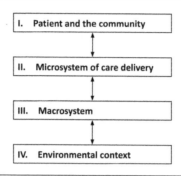

Source: Donald M. Berwick. In Nelson, E. C. and others, 2007, p. 6. Used with permission.

together, for high-quality care, highlighting the pivotal role played by the microsystems of care delivery. Clinical microsystems are the places where patients and families and healthcare teams meet, and consequently they are positioned at the sharp end of the healthcare system, where care is provided, medical miracles happen, and tragic mistakes are made. Our approach in the first edition of this book focused primarily on the microsystem level, where frontline clinical teams interact with patients and produce outcomes. In this edition of the book, we include a focus on the mesosystems and networks of care where multiple microsystems come together with patients and families to coproduce care and services (see Figure 1.2).

Describing Clinical Microsystems

Microsystems involve people in varying roles, such as patients and clinicians; they also involve processes and recurring patterns – cultural patterns, information flow patterns, and patterns of results. A clinical microsystem is defined as a small group of people (including health professionals and care-receiving patients and their families) who work together in a defined setting on a regular basis (or as needed) to create care for discrete subpopulations of patients. As a functioning unit, it has clinical and business aims, linked processes, a shared information and technology environment, and provides care and services that can be measured as performance outcomes. The clinical microsystem evolves over time and is often embedded in larger systems or organizations. As a living, *complex adaptive system,* the microsystem has many functions, which include (1) to do the work associated with core aims; (2) to meet member needs; and (3) to maintain itself over time as a functioning clinical unit (Nelson and others, 2007, p. 7).

Microsystems, the essential building blocks of the health system, can be found everywhere and vary widely in terms of quality, safety outcomes, and cost performance.

FIGURE 1.2 NETWORK OF CARE.

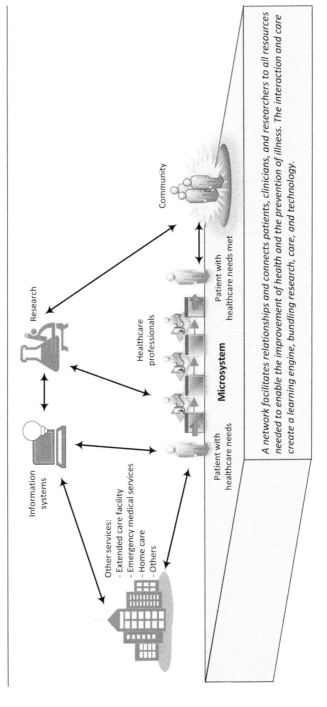

A network facilitates relationships and connects patients, clinicians, and researchers to all resources needed to enable the improvement of health and the prevention of illness. The interaction and care create a learning engine, bundling research, care, and technology.

A microsystem is the local milieu in which patients, family members, providers, support staff, information, and processes converge for the purpose of providing care to individual people to meet their health needs. If a person were to explore his or her local health system, he or she would discover myriad clinical microsystems, including a family practice, a renal dialysis team, an orthopedic practice, an in vitro fertilization center, a cardiac surgery operating room, a neonatal intensive care unit, a home healthcare service, an emergency department, an inpatient maternity unit, a rapid response team, and an extended care facility. Clinical microsystems are living units that change over time and always have patients (persons with a health need) at their center. They come together to meet patients' needs – and they may disperse once a need is met (for example, a rapid response team or Emergency Medical Services (EMS) team forms quickly, comes together around the patient for a short period of time, and disperses after the patient has stabilized or has been transported).

Individual microsystems can be tightly or loosely connected with one another and perform better or worse under different operating conditions. Our ability to see them as functional, interdependent systems is often challenged by our conventions of compartmentalizing and departmentalizing health care: considering separately, for example, human resources, accounting, and information technology. Our commitment to professional disciplines and specialties as an organizing principle often creates barriers that impede the daily work of clinical microsystems.

One way to visually depict clinical microsystems is with a high-level diagram that portrays a typical microsystem's anatomy – the set of elements that come together, like biological structures that work together toward a common goal, to form the microsystem organism. Figure 1.3 illustrates the anatomy of a typical internal medicine practice. This clinical microsystem, like all others, has a mission, or core purpose – in this case, to achieve the best possible outcomes for patients. It is composed of patients who form different subpopulations, such as healthy, chronic, and high-risk, and professionals, including clinicians and support staff, who interact with patients and perform distinct roles, such as physicians, nurses, nurse practitioners, medical assistants, and so on. The patients and staff work together to meet patients' needs by engaging in direct care processes, such as providing access, assessing needs, diagnosing problems, establishing treatment plans, and following up over time. These direct care processes are assisted by supporting microsystems and their distinct tools and resources, such as medical records, scheduling, diagnostic tests, pharmacy, and billing. The results of the interactions between patients and staff and between clinical and support processes produce patterns of critical results, such as biological and safety outcomes, functional status and risk outcomes, patient perceptions of goodness of care, and cost outcomes that combine to represent the *value* of care. The patterns of results also include the elements of practice culture, such as what it feels like to work in the microsystem, as well as elements important to business success, such as direct costs, operating revenues, and productivity.

FIGURE 1.3 ANATOMY OF A CLINICAL MICROSYSTEM.

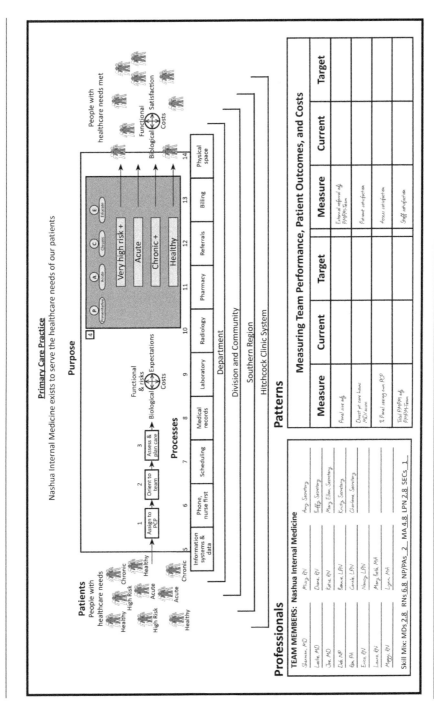

Source: Nelson, E. C. and Batalden, P. B., unpublished document, 1998. In Nelson, E. C. and others, 2007, p. 11. Used with permission.

Another important feature of the clinical microsystem is that it has a semipermeable boundary that mediates relationships with patients and families and with many support services and other microsystems. Furthermore, the clinical microsystem is embedded in, influences, and is influenced by a larger organization that itself is embedded in particular environments: payment, regulatory, cultural, social, and political. Thus, the clinical microsystem, although a comparatively simple concept, is in fact a complex, adaptive system that evolves over time.

Complex adaptive systems are found in nature and in human groups. They can be contrasted with mechanical systems, which tend to be more predictable and not subject to emergent behavior. Fritjof Capra, a noted physicist and author, suggests that a useful way to analyze complex adaptive systems arising in nature is to use a framework that addresses structure, process, and patterns (Capra, 1996; Nelson and others, 1998), an interesting parallel to Donabedian's "structure, process, outcomes" model (Donabedian, 1966). Patterns can be seen as the consistent behaviors, sentiments, and results that emerge from the relationships and activities of the parts involved in a complex adaptive system (Zimmerman, Lindberg, and Plsek, 1999; Plsek, 2001a; Plsek and Greenhalgh, 2001b).

Previous Research on Microsystems, Organizational Performance, and Quality

The clinical microsystem research described in this chapter represents an extension of the authors' earlier work on improvement in health care. In 1996, the authors wrote a four-part series on clinical improvement, which was published in the *Joint Commission Journal on Quality Improvement* (Batalden and others, 1996; Mohr and others, 1996; Nelson and others, 1996a; Nelson and others, 1996b). That series described concepts and methods for improving the quality and value of care provided for specific subpopulations of patients.

The more recent body of work builds on the earlier work in several ways. The primary emphasis of the authors' initial work was on the clinical processes that generate outcomes – quality and costs – for patients served by clinical systems. The newer body of work retains a strong emphasis on clinical processes and patient-based outcomes but expands the frame to include:

- An explicit focus on the local context – the distinctive features of a particular microsystem.
- Consideration of the information environment that supports or undermines care delivery.
- The interactions and relationships among people within microsystems and the interactions between clinical microsystems (the mesosystem) that work together to provide comprehensive care.

- The relationships between clinical microsystems and the larger systems in which they are embedded: mesosystems, macrosystem, and community.

The research on microsystems described in this chapter generally builds on ideas developed by Deming (1986), Senge (1990), Wheatley (1992), and others who have applied systems thinking to organizational development, leadership, and improvement. The fields of chaos theory, complexity science, and complex adaptive systems have also influenced our thinking (Peters, 1987; Wheatley, 1992; Kelly, 1994; Arrow, McGrath, and Berdahl, 2000; Plsek, 2001a; Plsek and Greenhalgh, 2001b; Hock, 2005; Zimmerman, Lindberg, and Plsek, 2008).

The seminal idea for the microsystem in healthcare stems from the work of James Brian Quinn, summarized in his book *Intelligent Enterprise* (Quinn, 1992). He reported on primary research conducted on the world's best-of-the-best service organizations, including FedEx, Mary Kay Inc., McDonald's, Intel, SAS, and Nordstrom. His aim was to determine what these extraordinary organizations were doing to enjoy such explosive growth, high margins, and wonderful reputations with customers. He found that these service sector leaders organized around, and continually engineered, the frontline interface that connected the organization's core competency with the needs of the individual customer. Quinn called this frontline interface the *smallest replicable unit*, or the minimum replicable unit, that embedded the service delivery process. The smallest replicable unit idea – or the microsystem idea, as we call it – has critical implications for strategy, information technology, and other key aspects of creating intelligent enterprise. Two excerpts from Quinn's book convey the power and scope of this organizing principle and the need for senior leaders to focus their attention on creating the conditions to continually improve the performance of frontline delivery units:

- On core strategy: "Critical to relevant effective system design is conceptualizing the smallest replicable unit and its potential use in strategy as early as possible in the design process" (Quinn, 1992, p. 104).
- On informatics and improvement: "Through careful work design and iterative learning processes, they reengineered their processes to use this knowledge and also developed databases and feedback systems to capture and update needed information at the micro levels desired" (Quinn, 1992, p. 105).

In 1998, as part of the Institute of Medicine's (IOM) Committee on Quality of Health Care in America, Dartmouth was tasked with identifying and studying a sampling of the best-quality, best-value small clinical units in North America. After a national search for the highest-quality clinical microsystems, Donaldson and Mohr (2000) interviewed the leaders from 43 high-performing clinical microsystems and analyzed the transcripts to determine the characteristics that seemed to be most responsible for enabling these high-quality microsystems to be successful. Eight dimensions were associated with high quality:

- Constancy of purpose
- Investment in improvement
- Alignment of role and training for efficiency and staff satisfaction
- Interdependence of care team to meet patient needs
- Integration of information and technology into workflows
- Ongoing measurement of outcomes
- Supportiveness of the larger organization
- Connection to the community to enhance care delivery and extend influence.

Ultimately, this initial research into clinical microsystems provided important background material for the IOM Committee's *Crossing the Quality Chasm* (IOM, 2001).

In 2000, the Robert Wood Johnson Foundation funded Dartmouth to conduct a more comprehensive study of 20 microsystems representing component parts of a health system (ambulatory, inpatient, home health, nursing home, and hospice care). Investigators screened more than 150 potential sites, conducted preliminary interviews at more than 50 sites, and ultimately selected 20 microsystems. The selection of sites was based on a multi-method approach for identifying the best-of-the-best clinical sites: literature review, identification of sites that had won quality awards, interviews with national experts to identify exemplary microsystems, prior research, demonstration projects conducted by the IOM and the Institute for Healthcare Improvement (IHI), respectively, and interviews with leaders of some of the leading healthcare systems in the United States and Canada, asking them to identify the best-of-the-best microsystems within their large healthcare systems. The investigators then conducted multiday site visits to the 20 top-performing sites to conduct in-depth, semi-structured interviews, observations of clinical work, review of financial documents, and medical record review. Figure 1.4 displays an overview of the research design. (See Appendix 1.1 at the end of this chapter for a complete list of the sites included in the study.)

For each microsystem site, complete data included the screening survey; screening interview; personal, in-depth interviews; and medical and financial records. All 20 sites were exemplary in many ways. Nevertheless, each site was to some extent unique and had its own set of particular strengths and further improvement opportunities with respect to quality and efficiency.

The study of these 20 high-performing sites generated many best-practice ideas that microsystems use to accomplish their goals. Thematic analysis of the transcripts

FIGURE 1.4 RESEARCH DESIGN FOR STUDY OF 20 CLINICAL MICROSYSTEMS.

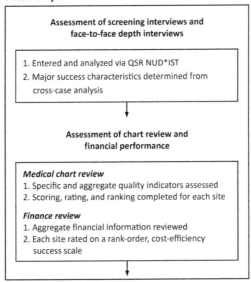

Sampling

Selecting high-performing clinical microsystems via a multitiered search pattern

1. Award winners and measured high performance
2. Literature citations
3. Prior research and field experience
4. Expert opinion
5. Best within best

Choosing 20 clinical microsystems for study

1. Assess outcomes of search pattern
2. Create table of sites by search pattern
3. Conduct survey and telephone interview
4. Choose and invite sites to participate

Data Collection

Two data collection instruments

Self-administered microsystem survey
Self-assessment of performance based on key characteristics

Telephone interview
Examination of delivery processes, the quality of care and services, and cost-efficiency and waste reduction

Two-day site visit for interviews and direct observation

In-depth interviews
Microsystem staff and larger organization staff

Medical chart review
Assessment of technical clinical quality of care

Finance review
Assessment of operational performance and cost efficiency

Data Analysis

Assessment of screening interviews and face-to-face depth interviews

1. Entered and analyzed via QSR NUD*IST
2. Major success characteristics determined from cross-case analysis

Assessment of chart review and financial performance

Medical chart review
1. Specific and aggregate quality indicators assessed
2. Scoring, rating, and ranking completed for each site

Finance review
1. Aggregate financial information reviewed
2. Each site rated on a rank-order, cost-efficiency success scale

Source: Nelson, E. C. and others, 2007, p. 15. Used with permission.

and documents was used to identify the principles, processes, and examples to describe what these exemplary microsystems were doing to achieve superior performance.

The interview information was analyzed with the assistance of content analysis software using the method known as cross-case analysis (Miles and Huberman, 1994). Two members of the research team (T.P.H. and J.J.M.) independently analyzed all the verbatim content and placed the content into affinity groups (coding categories). The coding results from the two analysts were compared, discrepancies between the two were discussed, and consensus was reached to resolve differences.

After all the data were analyzed, some sites displayed evidence of superior performance across the board. That is to say, internal trend data on technical quality, health outcomes, costs, and revenues, in addition to the results from the site interviews and the medical record reviews, provided extremely strong evidence of stellar performance. We used these sites somewhat more heavily in identifying the best-of-the-best processes and methods within the set of 20 high-performing clinical units. We relied especially on several clinical microsystems that had extraordinary results. The members of this select group shared many common methods and processes even though they were in different regions of the country and had little knowledge of one another. For example, all these units made extensive use of daily interdisciplinary huddles; monthly performance review sessions; data displays showing results over time; home-grown, real-time informatics solutions; and annual, all-staff retreats for establishing improvement themes and monitoring performance in mission-critical areas.

Success Characteristics of High-Performing Sites

Analysis of the results suggested that each of the 20 high-performing clinical units was indeed a complex, dynamic system with interacting elements that came together to produce superior performance. No single feature or success characteristic stood alone, and importantly, our research revealed that different clinical units in different contexts serving different types of patients may possess these success characteristics in greater or lesser degrees. That being said, these microsystems shared a set of primary success characteristics which interacted with one another to produce highly favorable systemic outcomes:

- Leadership of microsystem
- Macrosystem support of microsystem
- Patient focus

- Staff focus
- Interdependence of care team
- Information and information technology
- Process improvement
- Performance results.

These primary success characteristics fall into five main groups and interact dynamically with one another. Figure 1.5 displays these groupings. It also shows two additional success characteristics related to health professional education and

FIGURE 1.5 SUCCESS CHARACTERISTICS OF HIGH-PERFORMING CLINICAL MICROSYSTEMS.

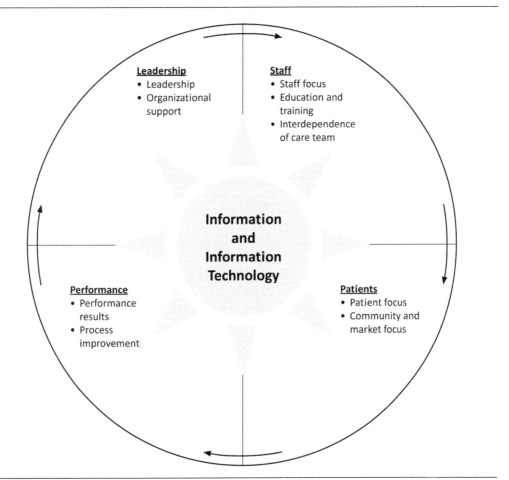

Source: Nelson, E. C. and others, 2007, p. 21. Used with permission.

training and community and market focus (including the financial, regulatory, policy, and market environments) in which the microsystem was embedded. These themes were often mentioned in our research, although not as frequently as the primary ones we had identified.

Principles Associated with Success Characteristics

Each of the primary success characteristics reflects a broad range of features and also reflects underlying principles, as shown in Table 1.1. For example, patient focus reflects a primary concern with meeting all patient needs – caring, listening, educating, responding to special requests, innovating in light of needs, providing a smooth service flow, and establishing a relationship with community and other resources – and can be encapsulated by a simple principle: We are all here for the same reason – the patient.

Specific Examples of Success Characteristics

The site interviews provided many varied and rich examples of the ways that the primary success characteristics manifest themselves in these clinical microsystems. Table 1.2 provides some examples from the original interview notes for each of the primary success characteristics.

Best Practices: Processes and Methods Associated with High Performance

The study of the high-performing sites generated many *best practice* ideas that microsystems can use to accomplish their goals. Some of these noteworthy practices are discussed in *The Clinical Microsystem Action Guide* (Godfrey and others, 2002). Although a complete list of all these noteworthy practices is beyond the scope of this chapter, Table 1.3 provides a sampling of them across the major themes. For example, one process used in many sites to ensure patient focus was to hold a daily case conference to discuss the status of each patient and develop an optimal treatment plan that best matched the patient's changing needs.

The results showed that the top-performing clinical units were vibrant, vital, dynamic, self-aware, and interdependent small-scale clinical organizations led with intelligence and staffed by skilled, caring, self-critical staff.

The success characteristics were generally consistent with the findings of the IOM's 2001 *Crossing the Quality Chasm,* with one important difference. This was the emergence of leadership as a key success factor at the microsystem level. Careful review of the IOM report reveals that leadership threaded through many of the eight dimensions discussed and was strongly present in the high-performing

TABLE 1.1 SCOPE OF PRIMARY SUCCESS CHARACTERISTICS AND ILLUSTRATIVE UNDERLYING PRINCIPLES.

Scope of Success Characteristic	Illustrative Underlying Principle
Leadership. The role of leadership for the microsystem is to maintain constancy of purpose, establish clear goals and expectations, foster positive culture, and advocate for the microsystem in the larger organization. There may be several types of leaders in the microsystem, including formal leaders, informal leaders, and on-the-spot leaders.	The leader balances setting and reaching collective goals with empowering individual autonomy and accountability.
Organizational support. The larger organization provides recognition, information, and resources to enhance and legitimize the work of the microsystem.	The larger organization looks for ways to connect to and facilitate the work of the microsystem. The larger organization facilitates coordination and handoffs between microsystems.
Patient focus. The primary concern is to meet all patient needs—caring, listening, educating, responding to special requests, innovating in light of needs, providing a smooth service flow, and establishing a relationship with community and other resources.	We are all here for the same reason – the patient.
Staff focus. The microsystem does selective hiring of the right kind of people, integrates new staff into culture and work roles, and aligns daily work roles with training competencies. Staff have high expectations for performance, continuing education, professional growth, and networking.	A human resource value chain links the microsystem's vision with real people on the specifics of staff hiring, orienting, and retaining and of providing continuing education and incentives for staff.
Education and training. Expectations are high regarding performance, continuing education, professional growth, and networking.	Intentional training and development of all staff is key to professional formation and optimal contributions to the microsystem.
Interdependence of care team. The interaction of staff is characterized by trust, collaboration, willingness to help each other, appreciation of complementary roles, and recognition that all contribute individually to a shared purpose.	A multidisciplinary team provides care. Every staff person is respected for the vital role he or she plays in achieving the mission.

(continued)

TABLE 1.1 (*Continued*)

Scope of Success Characteristic	Illustrative Underlying Principle
Information and information technology. Information is essential; technology smoothes the linkages between information and patient care by providing access to the rich information environment. Technology facilitates effective communication, and multiple formal and informal channels are used to keep everyone informed all the time, help everyone listen to everyone else's ideas, and ensure that everyone is connected on important topics.	Information is the connector – staff to patients, staff to staff, needs with actions to meet needs.
	The information environment is designed to support the work of the clinical micro system. Everyone gets the right information at the right time to do his or her work.
Process improvement. An atmosphere for learning and redesign is supported by the continuous monitoring of care, the use of benchmarking, frequent tests of change, and a staff empowered to innovate.	Studying, measuring, and improving care is an essential part of our daily work.
Performance results. Performance focuses on patient outcomes, avoidable costs, streamlining delivery, using data feedback, promoting positive competition, and frank discussions about performance, leader balances setting and reaching collective goals with empowering individual autonomy and accountability.	Outcomes are routinely measured, data is fed back to the microsystem, and changes are made based on the data.

Source: Nelson, E. C. and others, 2007, p. 22-23. Used with permission.

microsystems that were studied. Thus, some of the difference between our findings and the IOM findings arose from the use of different systems of classification when examining study results.

The results from our study also differ from Quinn's findings reported in *Intelligent Enterprise* (Quinn, 1992), which were derived from a study on world-class service organizations outside the healthcare sector. The senior leaders Quinn studied had a laser-like strategic and tactical focus on the smallest replicable units within their organizations. They viewed those units as the micro-engines that generated quality and value for their customers, and as vital organs that linked customers with the organization's core competency through actions taken by frontline service providers. Given the importance that Quinn's leaders placed on these units, they iteratively designed, improved, provided incentives, monitored, and replicated units

TABLE 1.2 SPECIFIC EXAMPLES OF THE PRIMARY SUCCESS CHARACTERISTICS.

Success Characteristic	Specific Example
Leadership	• "Leadership here is fantastic, they outline the picture for us and provide a frame, then hand us the paint brushes to paint the picture." • "I have been here for 25 years and it has allowed me to create a system that allows me the freedom to interact and manage the staff like human beings. I get to interact with them as real people and being highly organized allows that flexibility."
Organizational support	• "We are not one of the top priorities so we have been left alone; I support think that's been one of the advantages. We have a good reputation, and when we need something we get it. The larger organization is very supportive in that we get what we want, mostly in terms of resources." • "One of the things that we do fight quite often is the ability to create the protocols that fit our unit, the larger organization protocols don't work. We need to tweak them – and so we do."
Patient focus	• "At first you think you would miss the big cases that you had at a general hospital, and you do at first, but then after a while you realize they were just cases. Here you get to interact with the patient and the patient is not just a case but instead is a person." • "I think medicine had really come away from listening to the patient. People can come in here for a heart disease appointment and all of a sudden they will start to cry. You think, okay, let's see what else is going on. I'd like to think our clinical team is real sensitive to that... . 'My wife left me, I don't see my kids anymore, my job is going down hill.' Jeez and you're feeling tired? I wonder why... . Our purpose is to set an example to those who have forgotten about what it means to be in medicine, which is to help people. It's not about what is the most expensive test you can order." • "We created the unit for patients first. For instance, when we designed the new [unit], we didn't give up family room space."
Staff focus	• "We have high expectations about skills and how we hire new staff... . When we hire new staff we look for interpersonal skills, and a good mesh with values and the mission. We can teach skills but we need them to have the right attitude."
Education and training	• "I like molding people into positions... . I would rather take some one training with no experience and mold them than take someone who thinks they already know everything. We have a way of doing things here for a reason, because it works, so we want people to work here that can grasp this and be part of the organization." • "They allow you here to spread your wings and fly. There are great safety nets as well. You can pursue initiatives. There are always opportunities. They encourage autonomy and responsibility."

(continued)

TABLE 1.2 (*Continued*)

Success Characteristic	Specific Example
Interdependence of care team	• "Together, the team works. When you take any part away, things fall of care team apart. It's really the team that makes this a great place to work."
	• "We decided as a team that our patients needed flu vaccinations, so we all volunteered on a Saturday, opened the practice and had several hundred patients come through. We ended up doing quite a bit more than flu shots including lab work, diabetic foot checks and basic checkups."
	• "Here it's a real team atmosphere. Nobody gets an attitude that is disruptive. People get past the point of acting as individuals and instead work as a real team. It seems that people respect each other. For instance, when I get a new prescription, I go to the residents first. I don't try to bypass them by going to other staff alone. I will sometimes ask the residents to come with me to talk to other staff to make sure we are doing the right thing for the patient."
Information and information technology	• "We use face-to-face, e-mail, and telephone. All of us try to get to the information five different clinics. We have about 250 people in our staff. I know all technology of them, and [the executive director] and [the director of disease care] know most of them. It's about staying in touch... and there is good documentation."
	• "We have a system of electronic discharge. The computer is great. The physician anywhere in a satellite clinic has instantaneous access."
	• "We have good information systems on labs, outpatient notes, immunization, pharmacy.... For instance, the immunization record here is linked to the state database. So they can get that information directly."
Process improvement	• "It goes back to our processes. When we talk about how we do some-improvement thing in our office, we create a flow sheet. We get out the yellow stickies and we talk about every step in the process. And as a group we come up with this. Then we step back and we look at all this extra work that we make for ourselves, and then we streamline it."
	• "Buried treasure. We are constantly on the lookout for tiny things that will improve care for our patients or our own lives, whether it's financial, a system component that needs improvement, or a process change."
	• "I can tell you when I was practicing by myself it was painful at times, to say, 'Here you've got to do this,' and you know we're going to shut down the practice for half a day to get people really up to speed in these principles. But I would say, if you look at industry, they've learned that"It goes back to our processes. When we talk about how we do some-improvement thing in our office, we create a flow sheet. We get out the yellow stickies and we talk about every step in the process. And as a group we come up with this. Then we step back and we look at all this extra work that we make for ourselves, and then we streamline it."
	• "Buried treasure. We are constantly on the lookout for tiny things that will improve care for our patients or our own lives, whether it's financial, a system component that needs improvement, or a process change."

TABLE 1.2 (*Continued*)

Success Characteristic	Specific Example
	• "I can tell you when I was practicing by myself it was painful at times, to say, 'Here you've got to do this,' and you know we're going to shut down the practice for half a day to get people really up to speed in these principles. But I would say, if you look at industry, they've learned that"It goes back to our processes. When we talk about how we do some-improvement thing in our office, we create a flow sheet. We get out the yellow stickies and we talk about every step in the process. And as a group we come up with this. Then we step back and we look at all this extra work that we make for ourselves, and then we streamline it."
	• "Buried treasure. We are constantly on the lookout for tiny things that will improve care for our patients or our own lives, whether it's financial, a system component that needs improvement, or a process change."
	• "I can tell you when I was practicing by myself it was painful at times, to say, 'Here you've got to do this,' and you know we're going to shut down the practice for half a day to get people really up to speed in these principles. But I would say, if you look at industry, they've learned that … you have to do that. The Toyota plant out in Fremont, California, being one of the more prominent examples. The GM executives asked just exactly that. 'How can you afford to shut down the production line?' and they say, 'Well how can you afford not to shut down the production line?'"
	• you have to do that. The Toyota plant out in Fremont, California, being one of the more prominent examples. The GM executives asked just exactly that. 'How can you afford to shut down the production line?' and they say, 'Well how can you afford not to shut down the production line?'"
	• you have to do that. The Toyota plant out in Fremont, California, being one of the more prominent examples. The GM executives asked just exactly that. 'How can you afford to shut down the production line?' and they say, 'Well how can you afford not to shut down the production line?'"
Performance results	• "It takes a little over a minute for us to turn around an operating results room. Since we do the same surgery and we know how many cases there will be in each room, we have shelves with operating packs that after a surgery can be replaced very fast with all the appropriate tools."
	• "We have a very low disposable cost per case, around \$17–\$ 18, compared to an average hospital that has \$250–\$500 for a similar case."
	• "We have the lowest accounts receivable in the entire system. We are very proud of this. What we did was basically look at every category of expense and worked through each detail to get to the most efficient care, for instance, scheduled drugs via the pharmacy."

Source: Nelson, E. C. and others, 2007, p. 24-26. Used with permission.

TABLE 1.3 ILLUSTRATIVE BEST PRACTICES USED BY HIGH-PERFORMING CLINICAL MICROSYSTEMS.

Best Practice Category	Description of Noteworthy Practice
Leading organizations	• Annual retreat to promote mission, vision, planning, and deployment throughout microsystem • Open-door policy among microsystem leaders • Shared leadership within the microsystem (for example, among physician, nurse, and manager) • Use of storytelling to highlight improvements needed and improvements made • Promotion of culture to value reflective practice and learning • Intentional discussions related to mission, vision, values
Staff	• Daily huddles to enhance communication among staff • Daily case conferences to focus on patient status and treatment plans • Monthly all staff (town hall) meetings • Continuing education designed into staff plans for professional growth • Screening of potential hires for attitude, values, and skill alignment • Training and orientation of new staff into work of microsystem
Information and information technology	• Tracking of data over time at microsystem level • Use of feed forward data to match care plan with changing patient needs • Information systems linked to care processes • Inclusion of information technology (IT) staff on microsystem team
Performance and improvement	• Use of benchmarking information on processes and outcomes • Use of data walls and displays of key measures for staff to view and use to assess microsystem performance • Extensive use of protocols and guidelines for core processes • Encouragement of innovative thinking and tests of change

Source: Nelson, E. C. and others, 2007, p. 22-23. Used with permission.

throughout the organization. In contrast, the senior leaders of the larger health systems in which our 20 high-performing healthcare microsystems were embedded were for the most part not focused on supporting excellence in frontline clinical units. These health system leaders showed some recognition of outstanding performance and some degree of special assistance for outstanding units, but they lacked a strategic focus on creating the conditions that would generate excellent interdependent performance in *all* microsystems that constituted their health system. In short, they did not make the attainment of microsystem excellence a basic pillar of their management strategy.

Finally, the clinical microsystem study conducted at Dartmouth has some important limitations briefly summarized in the following list:

1. Reality and reductionism. The reality of clinical microsystems and the health systems in which they are embedded is immensely complex. To study it and learn about it, we inevitably had to reduce enormously the actual reality to a relatively small number of features, dimensions, and interactions. Much is lost in this reduction.
2. Methods. The case study approach adopted for this study gave us scope and depth of analysis but also tended to produce bias in several ways. For example, in case studies, the point of view of the investigator creates insights in some areas and causes blind spots in others. Some of the staff interviewed may be inclined to place their organization in a somewhat more favorable light than warranted by actual conditions and may direct the investigators to learn more about its strengths than its weaknesses.
3. Sample. The observations are based on a small sample of just 20 microsystems that were drawn purposefully from a universe of tens of thousands of microsystems.
4. Data. The data used in the study were primarily subjective and qualitative. Only limited amounts of objective data were gathered and used in the research.
5. Analysis. The method of qualitative data analysis, although it is a conventional and time-honored research tool, requires classification of the raw data – in this case, the text units from the interviews – by the researchers. A different research team analyzing the same raw interview content might arrive at different conclusions.
6. Time-limited findings. The observations are cross-sectional and time limited. Although the microsystems themselves are likely to be changing in small and large ways over time and although each has its own development history and staging, the study "sliced" into the world of each microsystem and "biopsied" its structure, content, processes, outcomes, and patterns at a single point in time.

Despite the limitations in our initial research on clinical microsystems, we gained knowledge and identified success characteristics that fueled our future research and improvement of frontline clinical units.

Building off this original research, the concept of clinical microsystems is increasingly visible in many national and international programs. For example, application of the clinical microsystem framework in Malaysia has focused on the implications of the high-performing characteristics on improving the implementation of

Electronic Medical Records in government hospitals (Ariffin and others, 2008). In Australia, a study published in 2018 reported 22 high-performing general practices and found that interviewees most frequently attributed success to the interdependence of the team members, patient-focused care, and leadership of the practice (Dunham and others, 2018). This is a call-to-action for mesosystem leaders to build support for leadership and team-building.

The case study presented in the next section illustrates the impressive level of research conducted in Sweden to better understand how to apply clinical microsystems concepts with the context of the Swedish healthcare system.

Case Study: International Research on Clinical Microsystems

The Swedish healthcare system has universal coverage for its citizens and is regulated by a healthcare law that states that every citizen has an equal right to health care, information, decision-making, and ought to be treated with dignity. Health care is financed by taxes and is owned and managed by 21 regions. One of the regions, Region Jönköping County, situated in southern Sweden and serving 355,000 inhabitants, has been developing system-wide quality improvement for more than two decades. An important leverage point along this improvement journey was when the county joined the Pursuing Perfection initiative launched by the IHI in 2002 (Andersson-Gäre and Neuhauser, 2007). Many models and theories formed the basis for this effort, such as Deming's quality theories, systems thinking, understanding the crucial role of clinical microsystems, and new roles of leadership at micro-, meso-, and macro levels. At the same time, a close collaboration with The Dartmouth Institute around the practical use of research aimed at a deeper understanding of clinical microsystems was initiated. A large part of this Swedish research is directed toward exploring and cultivating the capability developed through quality improvement collaboratives (QICs) in clinical microsystems. Some of the research efforts are connected to the use of Swedish National Quality Registries (NQR; Peterson, 2015) and similar registries in the United States (Godfrey, 2013) for measurement and feedback. Another recurrent theme in the research addresses the understanding and redesign of person-centered individualized care in clinical microsystem contexts; indeed, a law introduced by the Swedish parliament in 2014 states that patients have the right to access care, information, participation, shared decision-making, and safety (Patient Law 2014:821; Sveriges Riksdag, 2014). Learning dimensions also permeate Swedish microsystem research and some researchers have focused specifically on pedagogical processes and learning design. Brief summaries of some of this large body of ongoing research are presented in the following sections.

Bridging the Gaps

In 2006 a national research program, Vinnvård, was launched in Sweden to test novel approaches to bridge research and practice and to increase knowledge on how to lead, manage, and develop knowledge-based practices to improve quality in health and social care. Supported by a grant from Vinnvård, a unique collaborative effort, "Bridging the Gaps," started between Region Jönköping County (at that time Jönköping County Council), and four academic centers: Jönköping University, Linnaeus University, Uppsala Clinical Research Center, and Helix Vinn Excellence Center, Linköping. Table 1.4 summarizes the research performed within the *Bridging*

TABLE 1.4 NATIONAL AND INTERNATIONAL RESEARCH AND IMPROVEMENT PROGRAMS.

Organization	Program
Institute for Healthcare Improvement (IHI)	Idealized Design of Clinical Office Practice *(Kabcenell, 2002)*
	Pursuing Perfection *(Kabcenell, 2002)*
	Transforming Care at the Bedside *(Rutherford, 2004)*
Cystic Fibrosis Foundation (CFF)	Accelerating Improvement in CF Care Collaborative *(Godfrey, 2014)*
Vermont Oxford Network of Neonatal Intensive Care Units	Your Ideal NICU (https://public.vtoxford.org/)
Florida County Health Department	Improving Wait Times and Patient Satisfaction in Primary Care *(Michael, 2013)*
The Health Foundation, UK	The Improvement Journey (https://www.health.org.uk/publications/reports/the-improvement-journey)
Sheffield Teaching Hospitals	Microsystem Coaching Academy (https://www.sheffieldmca.org.uk)
Jönköping County, Sweden	Bridging the Gaps *(Andersson-Gäre, 2007)*
Masaka, Uganda	Improving Routine Immunizations *(Bazos, 2015)*
Danish Surgical Ward	Improving Interprofessional Team Performance *(Paltved, 2016)*
French Cystic Fibrosis Center	Rare Diseases of Nantes-Roscoff Microsystem Adaptation and Translation to Improve Cystic Fibrosis *(Sabadosa, 2018)*
Norwegian Study	High-performing Teams in Microsystems and Mesosystems *(Brandrud, 2015; 2017)*
Malaysia's Public Hospitals	Improving Electronic Medical Records (EMRS) Practices Through a Clinical Microsystem in the Malaysian Government Hospitals *(Ariffin, 2008)*

the Gaps research program, divided along the themes of QICs, person-centered individualized care, and pedagogical processes and learning design (Andersson-Gäre and Neuhauser, 2007).

The aim in *Bridging the Gaps* was to learn from the ongoing improvement work in the Jönköping healthcare system to tease out and understand more about mechanisms and design principles for successful improvement: "how to improve improvement." Gaps to be "bridged" included those between intended and received quality; knowledge and practice; professionals themselves within multiprofessional organizations; professionals, patients and families, and different levels and groups within the larger healthcare system. The interplay of the following three main perspectives informed this work: (1) actor network theory; (2) systems theory; and (3) sustainability; as did several thematic perspectives – the multiprofessional organization; service quality theory; theories of learning organizations and knowledge management; as well as information logistics. This interplay was used in the process of illuminating research questions, designing subprojects, and analyzing and interpreting empirical findings.

The research program was further characterized by three approaches:

- The empirical focus was in the clinical microsystem to create a firm link to core processes and quality performance in actual healthcare practice.
- As shown in Figure 1.6, the collaborative, interactive, research model involves two interacting systems – the research system and the practice system (Ellström, 2007). In this model both systems are depicted as cyclical, dynamic, and driven by problems/issues originating in research or practice. The basic activities in both systems, that is, research activities (for example, data collection and analyses) and different kinds of organizational actions within the change program are assumed to be informed by explicit or implicit theories based on previous research and/or practical experiences. The process of collaborative research is assumed to produce joint learning between practice and research through common conceptualizations and interpretations of the ongoing change process that becomes "cognitive input" not only into the next cycle of the change process, but also into the next cycle of the research process.
- A commitment to interdisciplinary research with each subproject including different scientific perspectives.

We believe these all are important cornerstones in the emerging field of improvement science.

FIGURE 1.6 A MODEL OF KNOWLEDGE CREATION THROUGH INTERACTIVE RESEARCH.

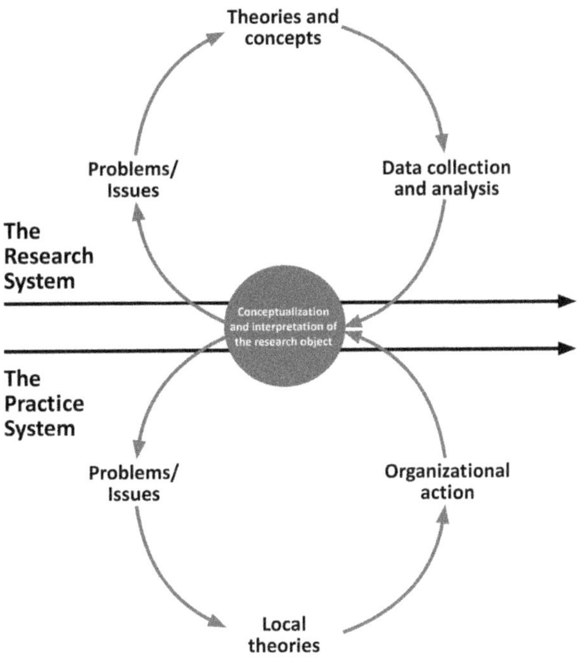

Source: Adapted from Ellstrém, P., 2007, p. 5. Used with permission.

Research on Quality Improvement Collaboratives (QICs) in Clinical Microsystems

Godfrey (2013) explored high-performing clinical microsystems involving a total of 495 health professionals from a variety of healthcare contexts in the United States and Sweden and evaluated interventions to cultivate the improvement capabilities of frontline *interprofessional* teams. For example, an intervention using the *Team Coaching Model* was tested in Sweden and showed increased acquisition of improvement knowledge in the intervention teams compared to teams who were not exposed to the model. The findings showed that leaders can help cultivate healthcare improvement capability by (1) designing structures, processes, and outcomes of their organizational systems to support health improvement activities; (2) setting clear improvement expectations of all staff; (3) developing every staff member's knowledge of their processes and systems to promote action learning in their daily work; and (4) providing a coach and using the structured Team Coaching Model.

Peterson (2015) showed how the NQR can be used in combination with systematic improvement efforts to produce better clinical results. The QICs studied were supported by the Swedish NQR with the intent to help teams close a number of gaps between ordinary clinical practice and evidence-based guidelines. The Team Coaching Model (Godfrey 2013) was added into the study of a QIC in pediatric diabetes care (Peterson, 2015). All 12 clinics included (one-third of pediatric diabetes clinics in Sweden) improved the average HbA1c in their patient populations. An additional success factor in that particular QIC was that patients and parents were included in the redesign of the care processes.

Nordin's (2017) findings illuminate how expressions of shared interpretations in QICs can generate momentum to engage in forthcoming PDSA cycles. *Sensemaking* emerges as a central activity. The thesis suggests that the use of improvement tools must be coupled with inquiry, that thoughtful dialogue is essential, and that leaders play an important role as inquirers. To support this approach, the widely used *Model for Improvement* (Langley and others, 2009) is complemented with a fourth question: "What are our assumptions?" The question pinpoints the need to be thoughtful at every step of improvement, not just in the analysis of the problem at hand.

Johansson and others (2012) developed evidence-based guidelines for the clinical treatment of urinary retention to minimize bladder damage and hospital-acquired urinary tract infections. The urinary retention guidelines were implemented using quality improvement methods (Andersson and others, 2017). The guidelines were interactively constructed by consensus with researchers and frontline clinical experts from various healthcare professions.

Research has also been conducted in welfare arenas such as social care. Neubeck (2016) examined the transfer of quality improvement methods from health care to nonprofit social services, offering insights into what enables and constrains systematic quality improvement in that context. Neubeck concludes that if organizations integrate quality improvement as a part of everyday practice in the microsystem, they develop context-specific knowledge about their services. This context-specific knowledge can be adapted and further developed through dedicated management and understanding of variation.

Research on Person-Centered Individualized Care in Clinical Microsystem Contexts

Interactions among staff and persons living with inflammatory bowel disease, together with elements of the care provided, were analyzed by Rejler (2012) by applying the model of clinical microsystems. The prevalence of anemia, a risk factor for hospitalization, in the population was six percent. The quality improvement intervention to address anemia led to fewer hospitalizations compared to national data and better access to care. The main components in the redesign of the microsystem, described as "patient- and demand-directed care," were:

- A specialist nurse staffed the outpatient clinic full time and could offer patients who contacted the clinic an acute visit at the outpatient clinic within two days.
- Yearly checkups with either the nurse or physician were offered, either as telephone calls or as traditional visits to the clinic.
- A letter sent prior to the checkup included a Quality of Life questionnaire and instructions for laboratory testing of hemoglobin.

Nygårdh's research (2013) focused on quality improvement and patient/family empowerment in a microsystem for care of people with chronic kidney disease. The healthcare professionals in collaboration with researchers attempted to improve the quality of care based on patients' and family members' experiences of empowerment in their encounters with healthcare professionals. The research both explored empowerment from the patients' and family members' perspectives and provided a base for the clinical improvement work, including evaluation and exploration of the improvement process. Significantly higher scores were found for the individualized care in the intervention group compared to the comparison group. When exploring the process, the main themes of "moving spirit" and "encouragement" were facilitators, while the main theme that represented barriers was "limitations of the organization."

Person-centered participation, collaboration, and coproduction in health and social care interprofessional microsystems were also addressed by Kvarnström (2011). The findings show that the various conceptions of participation by the individual actors in the clinical microsystem include themes of togetherness, understanding, and interaction within interprofessional practice. Furthermore, the interprofessional dimensions were mainly understood in terms of increased opportunities for collaboration among patients, families, and professionals and to equalize professionals' expert roles. For frontline professionals, one practical implication of the findings is to acknowledge both the uniqueness of each person and the existing limitations and power structures in health and social care systems.

Research on Pedagogical Processes and Learning Design

Norman (2015) analyzed and explained the pedagogical conditions in QICs in the healthcare system – how contextual conditions influenced learning about specific improvement practices where communication is foundational for learning. The findings showed how staff, in practical improvement work, balance economic values on the one hand against meaningful solutions for the patient on the other. Moreover, the research also showed that market logic and short-term profits superseded goals of a more profound development of knowledge.

Learning is essential for improving the quality of healthcare practice. Thörne's research (2018) on learning processes employs a practice-theory perspective focusing on how learning processes are framed, designed, and redesigned in clinical microsystems with a specific focus on physicians' training. For example, physicians' learning and learning support were interconnected with the mobility of physicians across different contexts and their participation in multiple communities of collaboration and through tensions between responsibilities in healthcare mesosystems (Thörne and others, 2014).

Research conducted with an explicit focus on the clinical microsystem has grown since the first edition of *Quality by Design*, which is a sign of the staying power of the concept as an organizing framework. However, we still see limited practical advice based on empirical evidence about how complex organizational structures can apply microsystem concepts to better manage risk, induce a safer culture, and produce better performance across key performance indicators (Johnson, 2010). Furthermore, macrosystems struggle with how to construct safety interventions and policies that are more resonant and compelling for their multiple microsystems. Similarly, more work is needed to push the boundaries of the application of microsystem research to the mesosystem – an opportunity for all researchers and practitioners in clinical microsystems and mesosystems.

Conclusion

Our healthcare system is immense, complex, and able to deliver delightful and dreadful care. Change must contend with both a linked chain and a network of effects that connects individual patients, families, communities, and clinicians with small, naturally occurring frontline units, which in turn connect with countless large and small host organizations, all of which exist in a modulating policy, legal, social, financial, and regulatory environment. Oversimplification of the health system is as common as it is foolhardy.

Yet with this caution in mind, we believe that the critical role of these naturally occurring, small clinical units, has been largely ignored. For the most part, fundamental changes in the health system have been directed elsewhere – at clinicians, consumers, purchasers, large managed care organizations, policymakers, and so on – and have for the most part ignored the system's essential building blocks.

The domino effect cannot ripple through the system if some of the dominoes are absent. Clinical microsystem thinking has largely been absent in health system reform in the United States. Once again, we are reminded of Quinn's observation, "Critical to relevant effective system design is conceptualizing the smallest replicable unit and its potential use in strategy as early as possible in the design process" (Quinn, 1992, p. 104).

Mesosystem Considerations

This chapter has defined the clinical microsystem and situated it within both meso- and macrosystems. As noted earlier, the mesosystem can only be as good as the microsystems it includes. Important implications for mesosystems are called out in the recurrent themes of leadership and context that pervade the research on microsystems. It can be helpful to consider the mesosystem in two dimensions, horizontal and vertical. The horizontal dimension reflects a patient's journey through multiple microsystems. Consider someone who presents to the internal medicine clinic described earlier in this chapter with cough and fever. As part of the evaluation, supporting microsystems (radiology and lab) are called upon, and perhaps admission to an inpatient microsystem is required for treatment of pneumonia. Ideally the journey through these multiple microsystems is seamless: information shared and readily available, clear and consistent communication, and a clear focus on patient needs. In the vertical dimension, a mesosystem often serves as the connector between the macrosystem and the microsystem. It is often at the mesosystem level (a clinical department within a health system, for example) that high-level organizational goals are translated into discipline- or profession-specific terms, and it is from the mesosystem level that much "managing up" occurs. We will continue to call out implications for mesosystems throughout this book, given the importance of the mesosystem as both "container" and "context" for multiple linked microsystems.

Summary

Clinical microsystems are the smallest replicable units in the healthcare system. Health system redesign can succeed only with leaders who take action to transform these small clinical units to optimize performance, meet and exceed patient needs and expectations, and perfect the linkages between the units. A seamless, patient-centered, high-quality, safe, and efficient healthcare system cannot be realized without the transformation of the essential building blocks that combine to form the care continuum.

The remaining chapters in this book on clinical microsystems will provide useful theories and models, practical ideas, and helpful tools that readers can use to:

- Plan individual patient care and efficient services.
- Create rich information environments.
- Promote the strategic spread of high-performing clinical microsystems that excel at meeting patients' needs and remain stimulating work environments.
- Advance the principles and practice of microsystems to evaluation, improvement, and redesign of mesosystems of care.

Review Questions

1. What are the different levels of a healthcare system? Can you describe an existing healthcare system and point out micro-, meso-, and macrosystem levels?
2. Examine the success characteristics in Figure 1.4. What are the important dimensions of a high-performing clinical microsystem and how might these interact with one another?
3. What are some research findings and implications of the research for healthcare improvement?

Discussion Questions

1. What is meant by the term "value of health care"? What can be done to improve the value of care?
2. Is it possible to have a system in the absence of a common aim or purpose? What is the aim of a healthcare system? Do patients and clinicians and health administrators have a shared aim?
3. What is meant by the statement that most healthcare systems are organized vertically but patients experience care horizontally? How might a healthcare system be organized to enhance the patient's horizontal flow while improving outcomes and decreasing costs?

Additional Activities

1. Think about the healthcare journey of someone with a serious injury or illness – this can be your own experience or the experience of someone you know well. What clinical microsystems did she or he enter as a patient? What ancillary and supporting systems also contributed to the care of the patient as his or her journey progressed?

References

Andersson, A., Johansson, R., Elg, M., and others. "Using Quality Improvement Methods to Implement Guidelines to Decrease the Proportion of Urinary Retention in Orthopaedic Care." *International Archives of Nursing and Health Care*, 2017, 3(65), 1-8. doi.org/10.23937/2469-5823/1510065

Andersson-Gäre, B., and Neuhauser, D. B. "The Health Care Quality Journey of Jönköping County Council, Sweden." *Quality Management in Health Care*, 2007, 16(1), 2-9. doi: 10.1097/00019514-200701000-00002

Ariffin, N. A. N., Yunus, A. M., and Embi, Z. C. "Improving Electronic Medical Records (EMRS) Practices Through a Clinical Microsystem in the Malaysian Government Hospitals." *Communications of the IBIMA*, 2008, 5, 5064.

Arrow, H., McGrath, J., and Berdahl, J. *Small Groups as Complex Systems*. Thousand Oaks, CA: Sage, 2000.

Batalden, P. B., Mohr, J. J., Nelson, E. C., and Plume, S. K. "Improving Health Care: Part 4. Concepts for Improving Any Clinical Process." *Joint Commission Journal on Quality Improvement*, 1996, 22(10), 651-659.

Batalden, P., Ogrinc, G., and Batalden, M. "From One to Many." *Journal of Interprofessional Care*, 2006, 20, 549-551.

Bazos, D. A., Ayers LaFave, L. R., Suresh, G., and others. "The Gas Cylinder, the Motorcycle and the Village Health Team Member: A Proof-Of-Concept Study for the Use of the Microsystems Quality Improvement Approach to Strengthen the Routine Immunization System in Uganda." *Implementation Science*, 2015, 10(30), 1-18. doi 10.1186/s13012-015-0215-3

Berwick, D. "Which Hat is On?" Plenary Address at the Institute for Healthcare Improvement's 12th Annual National Forum, Orlando, FL, 2001.

Brandrud, A. S., Haldorsen, G. S. H., Nyen, B., and others. "Development and Validation of the CPO-Scale, a New Instrument for Evaluation of Healthcare Improvement Efforts." *Quality Management of Health Care*, 2015, 24(3), 109-120.

Brandrud, A. S., Nyen, B., Hjortdahl, P., and others. "Domains Associated with Successful Quality Improvement in Healthcare – A Nationwide Case Study." *BMC Health Service Research*, Sep. 13, 2017, 17, 648. doi: 10.1186/s12913-017-2454-2

Capra, F. *The Web of Life: A New Scientific Understanding of Living Systems*. New York: Anchor Books, 1996.

Deming, W. E. *Out of the Crisis*. Cambridge, MA: MIT Center for Advanced Engineering Study, 1986.

Donabedian, A. "Evaluating the Quality of Medical Care." *Milbank Memorial Fund Quarterly*, 1966, 44(part 2), 166-206.

Donaldson, M., and Mohr, J. *Exploring Innovation and Quality Improvement in Health Care Microsystems: A Cross-Case Analysis. Technical Report for the Institute of Medicine Committee on Quality of Health Care in America.* Washington, DC: Institute of Medicine, 2000.

Dunham, A. H., Dunbar, J. A., Johnson, J. K., and others. "What Attributions Do Australian High Performing General Practices Make for Their Success? Applying the Clinical Microsystems Framework." *BMJ Open*, 2018, 8, e020552. doi: 10.1136/bmjopen-2017-020552

Ellström, P. E. "Knowledge Creation Through Interactive Research: A Learning Perspective." Paper presented at the HSS-07 Conference, Jönköping University, Jönköping, Sweden, 2007.

Godfrey, M. M., Batalden, P. B., Wasson, J. H., and Nelson, E. C. *Clinical Microsystem Action Guide*, Version 2.1. Hanover, NH: Dartmouth Medical School, 2002.

Godfrey, M. M. "Improvement Capability at the Front Lines of Healthcare Helping Through Leading and Coaching." School of Health Sciences, Jönköping University. Dissertation Series No. 46, 2013.

Godfrey, M. M., and Oliver, B. J. "Accelerating the Rate of Improvement in Cystic Fibrosis: Contributions and Insights of the Learning and Leadership Collaborative." *BMJ Quality & Safety*, 2014, 23, i23-i32. doi: 10.1136/bmjqs-2014-002804

Hock, D. *One From Many: VISA and the Rise of Chaordic Organization.* San Francisco, CA: Berrett-Koehler, 2005.

Institute of Medicine (U.S.) Committee on Quality of Health Care in America. *Crossing the Quality Chasm: A New Health System for the 21st Century.* Washington, DC: National Academies Press, 2001.

Johansson, R. M., Malmvall, B. E., Andersson-Gäre, B., and others. "Guidelines for Preventing Urinary Retention and Bladder Damage During Hospital Care." *Journal of Clinical Nursing*, 2012, 22, 347-355.

Johnson, J. K. "The State of Science Surrounding the Clinical Microsystem: A Hedgehog or a Fox?" *BMJ Quality & Safety*, 2010, 19, 473-474. doi: 10.1136/qshc.2010.048819

Kabcenell, A. "Pursuing Perfection: An Interview with Don Berwick and Michael Rothman." *Joint Commission Journal on Quality Improvement*, 2002, 28, 268-278.

Kelly, K. *Out of Control: The Rise of Neo-Biological Civilization.* Reading, MA: Addison-Wesley, 1994.

Kvarnström, S. "Collaboration in Health and Social Care: Service User Participation and Teamwork in Interprofessional Clinical Microsystems." School of Health Sciences, Jönköping University. Dissertation Series No. 15, 2011.

Langley, G. L., Moen, R., Nolan, K. M., and others. *The Improvement Guide: A Practical Approach to Enhancing Organizational Performance*, 2nd edition. San Francisco: Jossey-Bass Publishers, 2009.

Michael, M., Schaffer, S. D., Egan, P. L., and others. "Improving Wait Times and Patient Satisfaction in Primary Care." *Journal for Healthcare Quality*, 2013, 35(2), 50-60.

Miles, M., and Huberman, A. *An Expanded Sourcebook: Qualitative Data Analysis.* Thousand Oaks, CA: Sage, 1994.

Mohr, J. J., Mahoney, C. C., Nelson, E. C., and others "Improving Health Care: Part 3. Clinical Benchmarking for Best Patient Care." *Joint Commission Journal on Quality Improvement*, 1996, 22(9), 599-616.

Morse, G. "Health Care Needs a New Kind of Hero: An Interview with Atul Gawande." *Harvard Business Review,* Apr. 2010, 1-2.

Nelson, E. C., Batalden, P. B., Plume, S. K., and Mohr, J. J. "Improving Health Care: Part 2: A Clinical Improvement Worksheet and Users' Manual." *Joint Commission Journal on Quality Improvement,* 1996a, 22(8), 531-547.

Nelson, E. C., Mohr, J. J., Batalden, P. B., and Plume, S. K. "Improving Health Care: Part 1. The Clinical Value Compass." *Joint Commission Journal on Quality Improvement,* 1996b, 22(4), 243-258.

Nelson, E. C., Batalden, P. B., Mohr, J. J., and Plume, S. K. "Building a Quality Future." *Frontiers of Health Service Management,* 1998, 15(1), 3-32.

Nelson, E. C., Batalden, P. B., Huber, T. P., and others. "Success Characteristics of High-Performing Microsystems: Learning From the Best." In E. C. Nelson, P. B. Batalden, and M. M. Godfrey (eds.), *Quality By Design: A Clinical Microsystems Approach.* San Francisco: Jossey-Bass, 2007.

Neubeck, T. "Quality Improvement Within Nonprofit Social Service Providers." School of Health and Welfare, Jönköping University. Dissertation Series No. 68, 2016.

Nordin, A. "Expressions of Shared Interpretation: Intangible Outcomes of Continuous Quality Improvement Efforts in Health- and Elderly Care." School of Health and Welfare, Jönköping University. Dissertation Series No. 084, 2017.

Norman, A. C. "Towards the Creation of Learning Improvement Practices: Studies of Pedagogical Conditions When Change Is Negotiated in Contemporary Healthcare Practices." Linnaeus University. Dissertation Series No. 221, 2015.

Nygårdh, A. "A Quality Improvement Project on Empowerment in Chronic Kidney Care: An Interactive Research Approach." School of Health Sciences, Jönköping University. Dissertation Series No. 44, 2013.

Paltved, C., Morcke, A. M., and Musaeus, P. "Insider Action Research and the Microsystem of a Danish Surgical Ward." *Action Research,* 2016, 14(2), 184-200. doi: 10.1177/1476750315592937

Peters, T. J. *Thriving on Chaos: Handbook for a Management Revolution.* New York: Knopf, 1987.

Peterson, A. "Learning and Understanding for Quality Improvement Under Different Conditions: An Analysis of Quality Registry-Based Collaboratives in Acute and Chronic Care." School of Health and Welfare, Jönköping University. Dissertation Series No. 65, 2015.

Plsek, P. E. "Redesigning Health Care With Insights from the Science of Complex Adaptive Systems." In Institute of Medicine (U.S.) Committee on Quality of Health Care in America, *Crossing the Quality Chasm: A New Health System for the 21st Century.* Washington, DC: National Academy Press, 2001.

Plsek, P. E., and Greenhalgh, T. "Complexity Science – The Challenge of Complexity in Health Care." *BMJ Quality & Safety,* 2001b, 323(7313), 625-628.

Quinn, J. B. *Intelligent enterprise: A Knowledge and Service-Based Paradigm for Industry.* New York: Free Press, 1992.

Rejler, M. "*Quality Improvement in the Care of Patients With Inflammatory Bowel Disease.*" Linköping University Medical Dissertation No. 1324, 2012.

Rutherford, P., Lee, B., and Greiner, A. "Transforming Care at the Bedside." IHI Innovation Series white paper. Boston: Institute for Healthcare Improvement, 2004. (Available at http://www.ihi.org/IHI/Results/WhitePapers/TransformingCareattheBedsideWhitePaper.htm)

Sabadosa, K. A., Godfrey, M. M., and Marshall, B. C. "Trans-Atlantic Collaboration: Applying Lessons Learned from the US CF Foundation Quality Improvement Initiative." *Orphanet Journal of Rare Diseases*, 2018, 13(s1), 5-11. doi: 10.1186/s13023-017-0744-8

Senge, P. M. *The Fifth Discipline: The Art and Practice of the Learning Organization*. New York: Doubleday, 1990.

Stevenson, K., Christina, K., Andersson-Gäre, B., and others. Professionals Learning to Lead Improvement Efforts in Health and Social Care: A Realist Evaluation of an Interprofessional Practice-Based Master's Program. Paper presented at the 17th International Scientific Symposium on Improving Quality and Value in Health Care, Orlando, Florida, Dec. 2011.

Sveriges Riksdag. Patientlag 2014:821 (Patient Law 2014:821)." [https://www.riksdagen.se/sv/dokument-lagar/dokument/svensk-forfattningssamling/patientlag-2014821_sfs-2014-821]. 2014.

Thörne, K., Hult, H., Andersson-Gäre, B., and Abrandt Dahlgren, M. "The Dynamics of Physicians' Learning and Support of Others' Learning." *Professions & Professionalism*, 2014, 4(1), 1-15.

Thörne, K. "Läkare, Lärande Och Interaktion i Hälso- Och Sjukvårdens Praktiker" (Physicians, learning and interaction in healthcare practices). Linköping University Medical Dissertation No. 1615, 2018.

Wheatley, M. J. *Leadership and the New Science: Learning About Organization from an Orderly Universe*. San Francisco: Berrett-Koehler, 1992.

Zimmerman, B., Lindberg, C., and Plsek, P. *Edgeware: Insights from Complexity Science for Health Care Leaders*. Irving, TX: VHA, 1999.

Zimmerman, B., Lindberg, C., and Plsek, P. *Edgeware: Insights from Complexity Science for Health Care Leaders*, 2nd Edition. Irving, TX: VHA, 2008.

Additional Resources

Clinical Microsystem website, http://www.clinicalmicrosystem.org
Cystic Fibrosis Foundation website, https://www.cff.org
Health Foundation (The) website, https://health.org.uk
Improvement Journey (The), https://health.org.uk/publications/reports/the-improvement-journey
Institute for Healthcare Improvement (IHI) website, http://www.ihi.org
Jönköping Academy website, https://center.hj.se/jonkoping-academy/en.html
Sheffield Microsystem Coaching Academy website, https://www.sheffieldmca.org.uk
Vermont Oxford Network of Neonatal Intensive Care Units website, https://public.vtoxford.org

Key Words/Terms

Clinical microsystem: A small group of people (including health professionals and care-receiving patients and their families as well as information and information technology) who work together in a defined setting on a regular basis (or as needed) to create care for discrete subpopulations of patients.

Complex adaptive system: A complex adaptive system includes autonomous but interdependent agents that are capable of adaptation.

Information technology: Tools used to move and share information. This can be as sophisticated as an electronic health record, or as simple as pen and paper.

Interdisciplinary: Involving more than one academic field of study.

Interprofessional: Involving more than one profession (for example, nurses, pharmacists, physicians).

Macrosystem: The larger organization in which mesosystems are embedded, such as a hospital, multispecialty group, or health system.

Mesosystem: Two or more microsystems providing healthcare services for a specified population and context that are linked in some way.

Microsystem: See *Clinical microsystem.*

Model for improvement: A framework developed by Associates in Process Improvement and popularized by the Institute for Healthcare Improvement (IHI) to guide improvement work. It includes three questions: What are we trying to accomplish? How will we know if a change is an improvement? What change can we make that will result in improvement? All of the aforementioned are then addressed through a series of small experiments or plan–do–study–act cycles.

Sensemaking: The process by which people understand or give meaning to experiences.

Sharp end: The place where activity (and problems) can occur; in health care, this often refers to actual interactions with patients and families.

Team coaching model: A framework for developing improvement capabilities of frontline teams through the use of coaching.

Value: Value in health care is often thought of as $\dfrac{Quality + Outcomes}{Costs}$.

APPENDIX 1.1 THE TWENTY SITES EXAMINED IN THE CLINICAL MICROSYSTEM STUDY

Name of Microsystem	Location	Name of Macrosystem
Home Health Care		
Gentiva Rehab Without Walls	Lansing, MI	Gentiva Health Services
Interim Pediatrics	Pittsburgh, PA	Interim HealthCare of Pittsburgh
On Lok Senior Health Rose Team	San Francisco, CA	On Lok Senior Health
Visiting Nurse Service Congregate Care program, Queens Team 11S	New York, NY	Visiting Nursing Service of New York
Inpatient Care		
Henry Ford Neonatal Intensive Care Unit	Detroit, MI	Henry Ford Hospital, Henry Ford Health System
Intermountain Shock/Trauma/Respiratory Intensive Care Unit	Salt Lake City, UT	Latter-Day Saints Hospital, Intermountain Healthcare

(continued)

APPENDIX 1.1 (*Continued*)

Name of Microsystem	Location	Name of Macrosystem
Center for Orthopedic Oncology and Musculoskeletal Research	Washington, DC	Washington Cancer Institute, Washington Hospital Center, MedStar Health
Shouldice Hernia Repair Centre	Thornhill, Ontario CANADA	Souldice Hospital
Nursing Home Care		
Bon Secours Woud Care Team	St. Petersburg, FL	Bon Secours Maria Manor Nursing and Rehabilitation Center
Hospice of North Iowa	Mason City, IA	Mercy Medical Center North Iowa, Mercy Health Network
Iowa Veterans Home, M4C Team	Marshalltown, IA	Iowa Veterans Home, Veterans Commission
Primary Care		
Grace Hill Community Health Center	St. Louis, MO	Grace Hill Neighborhood Health Centers, Inc.
Massachusetts General Hospital Downtown Associatres Primary Care	Boston, MA	Massachusetts General Hospital, Partners Healthcare
Evergreen Woods Office	Bangor, ME	Norumbega Medical, Eastern Maine Healthcare
ThedaCare Kimberly Office Family Medicine	Kimberly, WI	ThedaCare Physicians
Specialty Care		
Dartmouth-Hitchcock Spine Center	Lebanon, NH	Dartmouth-Hitchcock Medical Center
Midelfort Behavioral Health	Eau Claire, WI	Midelfort Clinic at Luther Campus, Mayo Health System
Orthopedic Specialty Practice	Boise, ID	Intermountain Healthcare
Overlook Hospital Emergency Department	Summit, NJ	Overlook Hospital, Atlantic Health System
Sharp Diabetes Self Management Training Center	La Mesa, CA	Grossmont Hospital, Sharp HealthCare

Source: Nelson, E. C. and others, 2007, p. 31-32. Used with permission.

CHAPTER TWO

DEVELOPING HIGH-PERFORMING MICROSYSTEMS

Marjorie M. Godfrey, Tina C. Foster, Steve Harrison, Martin J. Wildman, Julie K. Johnson

AIM

The aim of this chapter is to focus on what it takes, in the short term and the long term, for clinical microsystems – the small, functional frontline units that provide most health care to most people – to attain peak performance guided by the five success characteristics identified in the original microsystem research.

LEARNING OBJECTIVES

By the end of this chapter, the reader will be able to

1. Link the high-performing clinical microsystem's five success categories to its strategy to become a high-performing microsystem.
2. Describe the developmental journey of a clinical microsystem adapting the Dartmouth Microsystem Improvement Curriculum (DMIC) ramp to improve care for a selected population.
3. Define each of the five stages of microsystem development to create a learning health system.

Quality by Design: A Clinical Microsystems Approach, Second Edition. Edited by Marjorie M. Godfrey, Tina C. Foster, Julie K. Johnson, Eugene C. Nelson and Paul B. Batalden.
© 2025 John Wiley & Sons, Inc. Published 2025 by John Wiley & Sons, Inc.

Introduction

This chapter features a case study of the evolution of one particular clinical microsystem, the Cystic Fibrosis Practice in Sheffield, United Kingdom. The five categories of characteristics of high-performing microsystems identified in the original research: leadership, staff, patients, performance, and information and information technology are shown in Figure 2.1 (Nelson and others, 2007a). The case study describes how the Dartmouth Microsystem Improvement Curriculum and these

FIGURE 2.1 SUCCESS CHARACTERISTICS OF HIGH-PERFORMING CLINICAL MICROSYSTEMS.

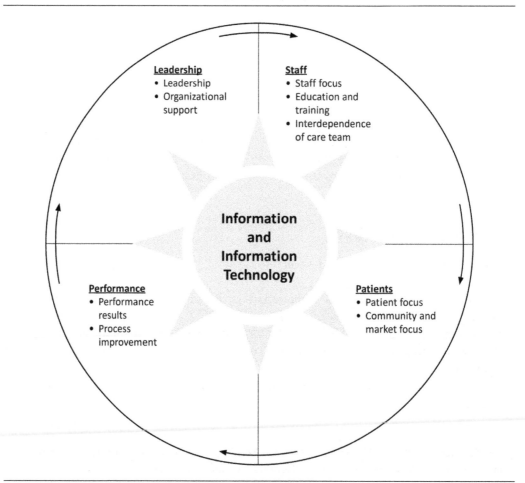

Source: Nelson, E. C. and others, 2007, p. 21. Used with permission.

success characteristics can be used over time to support the development of a continuously improving high-performing microsystem.

The case study introduces a number of additional important principles in the development journey. They include:

- involving all the players.
- focusing on values that matter.
- keeping both discipline and rhythm.
- using measurement and feedback to create a learning system.

It is important to attend to both long-run issues and short-term actions related to attaining high levels of performance that both benefit patients and energize staff.

To become a high-performing clinical microsystem, it is important to have a sense of how actual clinical microsystems can grow, learn, adapt, and improve over extended periods of time. The case study highlights one microsystem's five-year journey toward excellence and offers a framework that reflects a microsystem's developmental journey toward high performance.

Case Study: Maintaining Fidelity in the Face of Complexity – Using Microsystem Improvement to Structure Change in Cystic Fibrosis Care

There is a tension in improvement science between the use of a standardized methodology that can be communicated with fidelity to guide teams and the need to adapt interventions to the complexity of real-world health care. In the cystic fibrosis (CF) case study included here, we demonstrate the strength of the microsystem improvement approach in supporting a wide-ranging program of quality improvement in a complex system. CF is a "Goldilocks" condition in which both individual care units and the national care network are small enough to stimulate the development and iteration of challenging innovations but big enough to adequately test the ability to scale and implement innovations across the whole system. This can also generate learning for other disease areas, which are perhaps more fragmented and more widespread.

Using the Microsystem Improvement Ramp and Team Coaching Model to Support Improvement in CF Care and Services

This case study draws on five years of experience, change, and learning in the CF service at Sheffield Teaching Hospitals Foundation Trust (STH) in the United

FIGURE 2.2 MAP OF AREA AROUND SHEFFIELD UK.

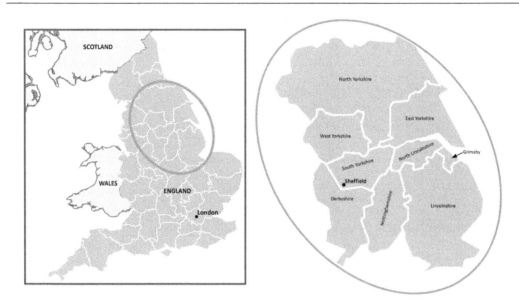

Kingdom. The Sheffield Adult Cystic Fibrosis Center is a regionally and nationally accredited CF Trust unit that opened in 1999. The service treats patients over the age of 16 years who live in Sheffield or the surrounding region, from Lincolnshire to West Yorkshire (Figure 2.2). Patients transition from the Sheffield Children's Hospital Pediatric Cystic Fibrosis Center to the Adult CF Center when they reach 16 years of age. In 2011 there were around 160 adults with CF cared for in the center. Currently 200 patients are treated by the Adult CF Center, with the service growing at the rate of about 10 patients per year. The unit has a 12-bed, state-of-the-art inpatient ward and runs weekly outpatient clinics at the Northern General Hospital.

Cystic fibrosis is an inherited multi-system disease, which typically causes symptoms from birth. The genetic defect affects the bowel causing malabsorption requiring constant attention to nutrition if weight is to be maintained. The lungs are also affected resulting in increased susceptibility to infection necessitating daily physiotherapy and inhaled treatments to keep the lungs healthy (Walshaw, 2019). Adults with CF need to master daily self-care in order to stay well. People with CF are cared for by multidisciplinary teams (MDTs) in just under 30 regional centers in the UK. In 2011, the Sheffield CF unit started to work with a Dartmouth-credentialed team coach from the Sheffield Microsystems Coaching Academy (MCA) to understand how the team could provide the best possible care.

Initial Stimulus and the Pre-Phase – Early 2011

Use of the microsystem approach was in its infancy at Sheffield when the service manager for CF invited a coach from the STH service improvement team to work with the unit in 2011. The manager had seen successful use of the team coaching approach in the Geriatric Falls outpatient service (which she also managed) and hoped a similar level of improvement could be achieved in CF care. The service had pressing issues due to growing patient numbers and the dual need to increase capacity and improve quality.

The team coach spent considerable time reviewing the Team Coaching Model (Figure 2.3) to prepare himself and the team to start working on improvement (Godfrey, 2013). Meetings were held with the clinical leaders to better understand team dynamics, and time was invested in discussing the team coaching approach including the DMIC (see Part Two of this textbook) with the doctors, managers, and senior nurses (Figure 2.4). In addition, support was obtained from the clinical director to enable the work. In this pre-phase period, the coach, leaders, and team agreed on expectations, set a regular weekly meeting time and venue, developed a communication plan, and discussed who would be involved. Patient representation was sought, and the coach spent time visiting the unit to get to know the team before the work started in earnest.

FIGURE 2.3 TEAM COACHING MODEL.

Pre-Phase	Action Phase	Transition Phase
Getting Ready *"Meeting them where they are"*	*Art and Science of Coaching*	*Reflect, Celebrate, and Renew*

◆ **Establish leader relationship**
◆ **Expectations**
  ❖ Clarity of aim
  ❖ Leadership and team discussions about roles and logistics
◆ **Context**
  ❖ Review of past improvement efforts and lessons learned – tools used
  ❖ Preliminary system review – Micro/Meso/Macro
◆ **Site visit**
◆ **Resources (data)**
◆ **Logistics (time)**
	◆ **Relationships**
	  ❖ Helping
	  ❖ Keep on track
	◆ **Communication**
	  ❖ Virtual
	  ❖ Face-to-face
	  ❖ Available and accessible
	  ❖ Timely
	◆ **Encouragement**
	◆ **Clarifying**
	  ❖ Improvement knowledge
	  ❖ Expectations
	◆ **Feedback**
	◆ **Reframing**
	  ❖ Different perspectives
	  ❖ Possibility
	  ❖ Group dynamics – new skills
	◆ **Improvement technical skills**
	  ❖ Teaching
		◆ Reflect on improvement journey
		  ❖ What to keep doing or not do again
		  ❖ Review measured results and gains
		  ❖ Plan how to sustain improvement
		  ❖ Assess team capability and coaching needs, and create coaching transition plan
		◆ Celebrate!
		◆ Renew and re-energize for next improvement focus
		◆ Evaluate coaching
		
		Godfrey, MM (2013 – rev 2019)

Source: Godfrey, M. M., 2013. Used with permission.

FIGURE 2.4 THE IMPROVEMENT RAMP.

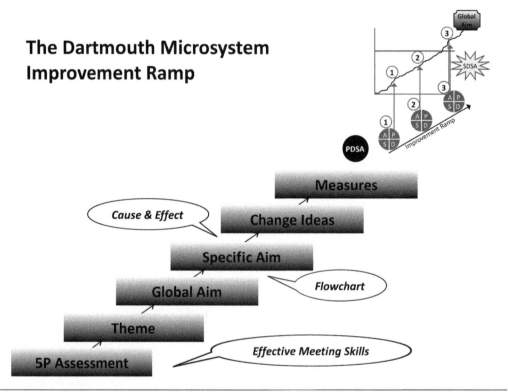

The Dartmouth Microsystem Improvement Ramp

Source: Nelson, E. C. and others, 2007, p. 240. Used with permission.

At the first team meeting in May, the team was further briefed on the approach to assess the microsystem, agreed on ground rules, and had their first go at using effective meeting skills with a timed agenda and clear meeting roles. The team then progressed on to study their system of care delivery using the 5Ps (Nelson and others, 2007a; Nelson and others, 2011).

The 5Ps – Purpose, Patients, Professionals, Processes, Patterns: Seeking Ownership Rather Than Buy-In

The *5Ps* assessment provides a structure for the clinical team to understand the microsystem in which they work. Exploring the 5Ps is similar to the structured history-taking that enables clinicians to rapidly assess patients admitted as emergencies. Decades of experience have taught clinicians the key questions that enable diagnosis. Similarly, the 5Ps are the key variables that guide clinical teams in diagnosing the health of the microsystem. They direct the attention of the members of the microsystem to thinking about purpose, patients, professionals, processes, and patterns.

As the Sheffield CF team used the 5Ps to understand the CF microsystem, they developed a shared understanding of the overall purpose of the CF microsystem. The team agreed that their overall purpose was "to enable people with CF to live as normal a life as possible." The process of discussing the 5Ps unlocked a series of common insights that built a shared understanding, which produced teamwide ownership of the improvement project. Shared ownership built by a team working together in an improvement program builds more motivation and commitment than a program developed by one or two members of a team and then taken to the wider **Multidisciplinary Team** for buy-in. "Ownership builds motivation and commitment" (Lipmanowicz, 2010).

By June 2011 the CF meetings were structured around gathering 5Ps information. This took place over several weeks and was pieced together using a staff and patient survey and a high-level process map created by the team. The team engaged patients to help time activities and waiting times in clinic. Using the "Esther" process developed in Sweden (Nelson and others, 2007b, p. 210–214), the CF team created a representative persona, Brandon, to inform the team's reflection on what they did well and not so well for "Brandon." National benchmarking data was reviewed, as were data from hospital systems specific to the delivery of care for people with CF. The service improvement team helped provide some capacity and demand forecasting to help the team understand what future capacity requirements for appointment slots and staffing might be. However, the real starting point for the change process happened when the team discussed "purpose," which led to what all later agreed had been a moment of epiphany – a sudden realization that typically follows a protracted period immersed in a problem when a new and deeper perspective is gained.

Using the 5Ps to structure inquiry into a microsystem has the potential to lead to breakthroughs or epiphanies in how teams think about care. Systematic exploration of the 5Ps and inclusion of "Brandon" helped the team immerse themselves in the lived experience of their microsystem, prompting connections and insights that would escape more superficial reflection. The insights below show how the 5Ps led to an epiphany in the approach to CF care:

1. Purpose
   • The purpose of our microsystem is to enable people with CF to live as normal a life as possible."
2. Patients
   • Patients find it hard to adhere to prescribed care because they are human beings.
   • Patients self-manage 99.99 percent of the year, but we are not supporting that in a systematic way.

- Discussing adherence can make patients feel guilty and naughty, and patients often are not willing to talk about the complexity of adherence because our clinic processes are slow and patients wait long periods before we see them.

3. Professionals
   - As a healthcare team, we were never taught how to build habits and support behavior change.
   - We also realized that we ourselves also fail to adhere to health advice about weight control and exercise.

4. Processes
   - When patients come to clinic, adherence is invisible because patients can't remember how much treatment they have taken. We need to make the invisible visible.
   - If you can't measure it, you can't manage it.

CF care throughout the world is practiced "under the lamppost" (Wildman and Hoo, 2014) and as a result care can be inappropriate and ineffective. (See Figure 2.5, Sidebar "Patient story: The importance of moving care beyond the lamppost.")

5. Patterns
   - People with CF are often admitted to hospital for highly disruptive, unscheduled rescue therapy.
   - Rescue therapy is often necessary because patients find it hard to take preventive therapy.

FIGURE 2.5 I DROPPED MY QUARTER.

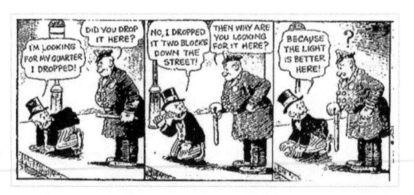

Patient story: The Importance of Moving Care Beyond the Lamppost

Typically, when an adult with CF comes to clinic, we measure the things that are easy to measure and concentrate our attention under the lamppost – "where the light is." Lung function and weight are measured, and if either has fallen, the team attempts to understand why. In most CF clinics, adherence data is not available so teams might send off sputum cultures to look for new infections (such as abscessus or cepacia), diabetes might be suspected, and a glucose tolerance test or blood sugar series ordered. In the UK, guidance suggests that if patients deteriorate despite twice daily inhaled tobramycin, they can be escalated to thrice daily aztreonam. All these strategies take place under the lamppost. A patient story explains why a different approach can be transformative.

An independent 22-year-old woman who we will call Jane attended clinic with her mother. This was unusual; normally we never saw Jane's parents. On entering the clinic room, Jane was slumped in her chair staring at the floor, her mother was perched anxiously on the edge of her chair staring intently at the clinician. Jane's mum hurriedly described the last few weeks during which Jane had started to cough whenever she talked, was out of breath on the stairs, and had started to cough blood. It was clear that both Jane and her mother thought that CF had won and Jane was dying. Had we been under the lamppost we might have ordered a blood sugar series, sent off sputum, and perhaps switched from tobramycin to aztreonam. We would have prolonged the agony as we waited for tests and waited for aztreonam to work a miracle.

In fact, what we did was look at the metrics that matter as seen above (Figure 2.6), which shows Jane's adherence downloaded from a nebulizer with an electronic chip that recorded how much treatment had been taken during the six months leading up to the clinic appointment. Equipped with these metrics we were able to say, "It's OK, you are not dying from CF, it's just that you have untreated CF and the wonderful news is that CF treatment works and we need to work with you to help you take the treatment that will keep you well."

FIGURE 2.6 LAMPPOST FIGURE – SPC CHART OF ADHERENCE DATA.

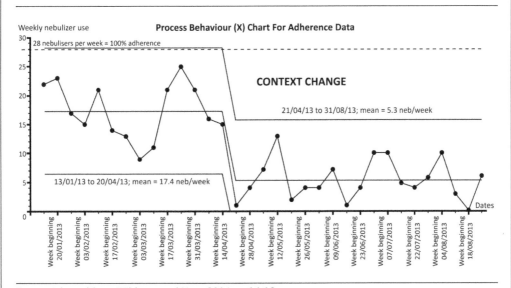

Source: Adapted from Wildman and Hoo, 2014, p. 16-18.

- Data shows that in adults with CF the median amount of preventive inhaled therapy taken is 36 percent (Daniels and others, 2011). If patient characteristics are used to estimate completion of treatment, the rate drops even lower (Hoo and others, 2020).
- CF care involves a dynamic balance between disruptive rescue and strategic prevention; our team can influence this balance.

The 5Ps exercise built consensus and ownership within the CF team as they began to settle on a number of *themes for improvement*, which ultimately are all interconnected. These were

1. Clinic flow – In order to support behavior change in our patients, we needed to redesign our clinic system to eliminate waiting wherever possible. We learned from the 5Ps and "Brandon" that the main issue patients described was long waits in clinic. Providers reported poor flow in clinic resulting in rushed appointments with patients (who were irritated by the time they were seen due to the long wait). Neither the patients nor the providers were in a good place to have a conversation about self-care and behavior change in this environment. Clinic change work was essential to create the conditions for a better consultation.
2. Capacity – The team needed more outpatient capacity to deal with increasing numbers of patients while also allowing time for complex behavior change interventions in clinic.
3. Adherence – This is the metric that matters to "make the invisible visible."

Clinic Redesign – A Journey Up the Improvement Ramp

To support this new vision for the adult CF service, the team decided to work on the clinic flow theme first and move forward using the steps outlined in Part Two of *Quality by Design* (2007). In order to structure this process, the team was coached using the Dartmouth Microsystem Improvement Ramp (Figure 2.7), detailed in the following text.

After reviewing the 5Ps and identifying the first theme of clinic flow, the first task was to draft a global aim statement to more clearly define the process the team wished to improve. The global aim statement agreed upon was:

> *We aim to improve the efficiency and quality of the service of the CF outpatient clinic for staff and patients. The process begins with first contact with the patient and ends with them arriving back to their home after the visit. By working on the process, we expect: the Do Not Attend (DNA) rate to improve, for there to be less waiting for patients, improved efficiency for patients and staff, and to achieve a greater standard of our quality markers. It is important to work on this to improve the clinic experience for patients, meet CF trust standards, and to provide an area of clinical excellence.*

FIGURE 2.7 BEGINNING THE IMPROVEMENT JOURNEY: THE STAR INDICATES THE THEME OF IMPROVEMENT.

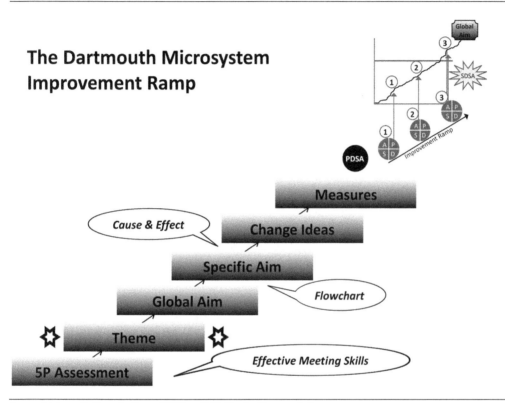

Source: Nelson, E. C. and others, 2007, p. 240. Used with permission.

The team then created a detailed process map of the CF clinic visit. Doing this helped team members increase their understanding of the role of others in the CF clinic and generated many ideas for improvement. At meetings, ideas were captured on a "parking lot" list (Scholtes, Joiner, and Streibel, 2010, p. 3-11) so they could be revisited later in the improvement journey. Figure 2.8 shows the actual process map or flowchart, created with brown paper, markers, and Post-it® notes. This step was messy and protracted but built real knowledge and consensus around the need to change and the way to improve the clinic.

After reviewing the 5Ps and the flowchart, the team chose to reduce patient waiting time as their first specific aim: "We aim to reduce average total patient waiting time within the two CF outpatient clinics by 50 percent from our baseline measure of 40 minutes by the end of October 2011."

FIGURE 2.8 THE CF CLINIC FLOWCHART.

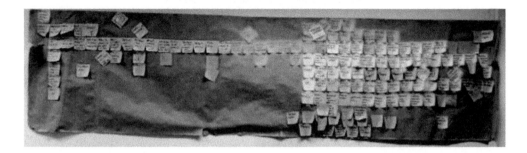

The team realized that meeting this specific aim was unlikely to be achieved through one intervention alone – patients waited in clinic for many reasons and achieving the aim was likely to be complex and iterative. In order to further understand why patients were waiting, the team continued up the improvement ramp and created a cause and effect or fishbone diagram, listing all the reasons why delays occurred, as shown in Figure 2.9.

After reviewing the fishbone diagram, the team discussed many interventions to improve flow and settled on four main change ideas that they would proceed to test using plan–do–study–act (PDSA) cycles.

Four main change ideas emerged:

1. Get everything we need – The fishbone identified several items such as scales, nebulizers, and prescription refills that were not readily at hand in clinic, which impeded flow. Supported by the service management team, the unit ensured everything essential was available in all clinic rooms.
2. Change the clinic schedule – Analysis of the cycle-time data captured in clinic by patients initially during the 5Ps assessment followed up by staff collection of data showed a mismatch between patient arrivals and availability of resources, leading to long patient waits. The team decided to change the clinic schedule template to smooth the arrival rate. Further measurement of how long each step of the process took was completed. From this data (displayed using run charts) and by understanding the variation in each step, a new ideal clinic template was designed (Figure 2.10). Each block shows planned activity per patient from the different members of the MDT across the clinic.
3. Communicate – It became clear that communication among team members about patients and their needs from the clinic was not as good as it might be. The team decided to test the use of an electronic diary system, which could be accessed

FIGURE 2.9 CAUSE AND EFFECT FOR PATIENT WAITING IN CF CLINIC.

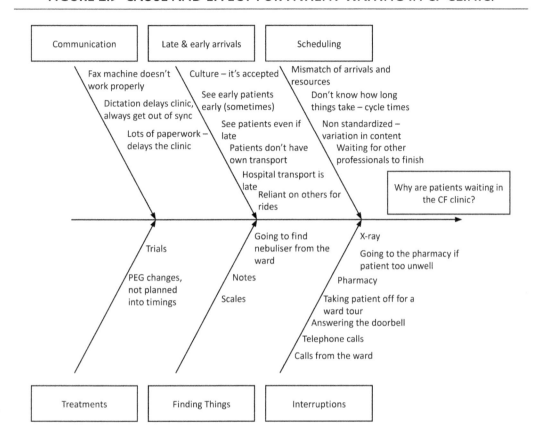

FIGURE 2.10 CF CLINIC REDESIGN PROCESS FLOWCHART.

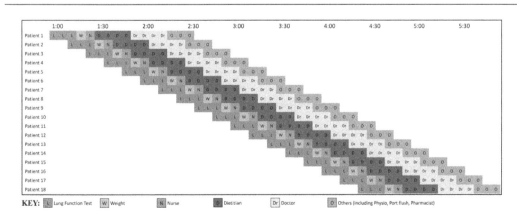

by the whole team. The diary had details of all the patients in clinic and their specific needs, such as the requirement for a port flush, percutaneous endoscopic gastrostomy (PEG) tube change, or social worker input.

4. Manage the process – The CF clinic had always used a whiteboard to manage clinic flow. The team redesigned the use of the whiteboard, adding in patient timings and dedicating a clinic nurse to supervise the flow of the MDT through the clinic schedule.

The team tested all the listed change ideas using PDSA cycles discussing, debriefing, and planning new changes at the weekly, coached improvement meetings. Measures were identified to determine if there were improvements or not. Using the structure of the *value compass* described in Chapter Eight to aid thinking, the team chose the following balancing measures to track over time while testing their change ideas:

- Do Not Attend rate (DNA) or "no show rate" as a proxy measure for patient satisfaction.
- Staffing numbers per clinic as a proxy measure for cost.
- Attendance numbers to ensure less waiting did not impact capacity.

Over time the changes began to take effect, and eventually waiting time dropped from an average of 40 minutes to an average of eight minutes per patient with no impact on clinical contact time or the balancing measures (see Figure 2.11).

Through this process, the team realized that waiting time was a key metric. Following the scheduling redesign, they continued to consistently measure wait time per patient and test new ideas if the data identified problems – a standardize–do–study–act process (SDSA). An example of this occurred when the clinic moved to a new outpatient location and habits established in the physical space of the old clinic were lost, resulting in an increase in waiting time. This increase was immediately noticed as wait times were measured and discussed regularly, and the team proceeded with new PDSA cycles to address the waiting time issue in a new context.

One 5Ps – Many Improvements

Following the initial clinic improvement work, the team went on to improve many aspects of the service, which are summarized in Figure 2.12. Driven by the weekly coached improvement meetings using the DMIC improvement ramp, redesign work was started on all of the themes with multiple aims identified and PDSA cycles undertaken. Subsequent work has seen the team begin improving the inpatient

FIGURE 2.11 SPC CHART OF WAITING TIMES IN THE CF CLINIC.

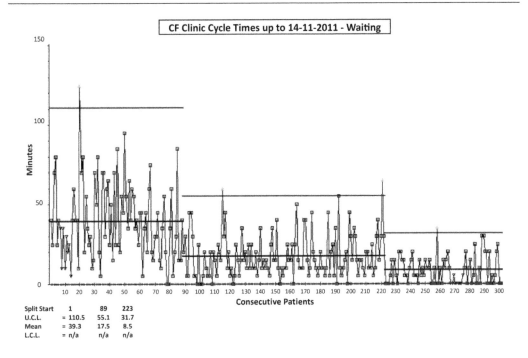

Split Start	1	89	223
U.C.L.	= 110.5	55.1	31.7
Mean	= 39.3	17.5	8.5
L.C.L.	= n/a	n/a	n/a

ward, initiating daily huddles to improve communication, and beginning a research project designed to "stratify" patients by need into different types of clinics to maximize clinic efficiency to support adherence.

The team focus on the theme of adherence has resulted in the Sheffield CF service developing and leading innovative work, which has subsequently been adopted by many UK CF centers. Initial work focused on making the invisible visible by using an electronic process of "chipping" patients' iNeb devices to monitor adherence; the chip recorded the actual use of the nebulizer, allowing patients and clinicians to see actual use data versus prescribed use. The team was trained in motivational interviewing to support conversations with patients in clinic. Recent developments have stretched beyond the CF unit with the team winning a large program grant to build a national team and a data observatory to embed adherence measures and transform CF care across the entire UK (NIHR, 2015; Sheffield Teaching Hospitals, 2015). This work created a digital learning health system, CFHealthHub, which was evaluated in a 19-center, 600-patient randomized controlled trial that demonstrated significant improvements in self-care maintained to 80 weeks. CFHealthHub is now in use in more than 50 percent of Adult CF units in the UK.

FIGURE 2.12 OVERVIEW OF CF IMPROVEMENT ACTIVITIES.

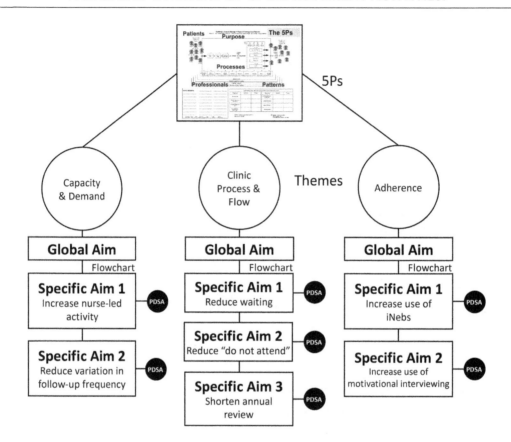

The Sheffield Teaching Hospital CF case study reveals a high-performing clinical unit united around a common purpose: "To enable patients with CF to live as normal a life as possible." The 5Ps process built consensus and ownership for change while the microsystem method and team coaching helped move the team forward in designing a new service around their purpose. The case study embodies the following principles that may be helpful in guiding other microsystems' progress toward the best possible performance.

Begin by uniting the microsystem around a common purpose. The 5Ps exercise was a transformational moment for the CF team in Sheffield. They considered what they did as a clinical unit and united around what mattered to "Brandon": to live as normal a life as possible. All subsequent work was guided by this purpose. "The team ethos has changed with the patient more firmly at the central point. The outpatient processes have been streamlined and have more efficiency, effectiveness, timeliness, etc. Patient adherence has been accepted by all the team as a critical outcome of CF care. We identified that we needed to move our care from rescue to prevention" (CF Physician; Sheffield Teaching Hospitals, 2011).

Involve all team members. Over time the CF leaders and coach found ways to involve all of the microsystem players in the improvement activities. Interprofessional staff, stakeholders from supporting microsystems, patients, managers, and leaders have all become involved in the action of analyzing and improving processes and outcomes, which has strengthened teamwork and improved morale on the unit. "This process has been really inspiring. For the first time I have felt that we've been able to implement changes to help the service run more efficiently for patients and staff" (CF Medical Resident; Sheffield Teaching Hospitals, 2011).

Focus on the metrics that matter. The CF team quickly identified a series of measures that helped sustain a positive and virtuous cycle of improvement. These included process measures of clinic performance (waiting times) and an outcome measure of adherence (nebulizer use). "If you can't measure it, you can't improve it. We needed to make the invisible visible and did this by increasing the number of electronically chipped nebulizers in use. We understood that consultations under the 'lamppost' were inappropriate" (CF Physician; Sheffield Teaching Hospitals, 2011).

Be thoughtful about behavior change. Improvement will always involve change. While we often focus on what it will take to change patients' behavior, it is equally important to think about how health professionals can change their own and their teams' behavior. As the work developed in Sheffield, the team recognized that supporting adults with CF to self-manage their care required an understanding of behavior change. An exploration of the behavior change literature revealed a multiplicity and complexity of behavior change models; the team settled on the Capability, Opportunity, and Motivation Behavior (COM-B) system developed by Susan Michie (2011) at University College London. As the CF team began to customize the COM-B model to capture the particular challenges of behavior change required to support patient self-management in CF, they realized that behavior change on the part of health professionals was also needed to support both optimal patient self-management and to sustain their own improvement (Figure 2.13). The COM-B model provides an easily communicated yet powerful tool that can equip clinical teams to understand behavior change. In the United States justice system, the prosecution is required to demonstrate the motivation, capability, and opportunity of the accused to commit the crime. The COM-B model uses the same domains of motivation, capability, and opportunity to gain an understanding of behavior. When using the COM-B model, it is usual to start with

FIGURE 2.13 ADAPTED COM-B BEHAVIOR CHANGE MODEL.

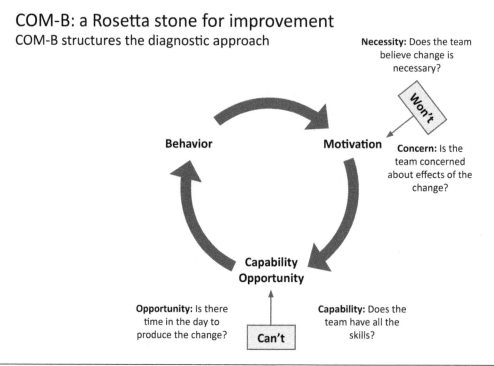

COM-B: a Rosetta stone for improvement
COM-B structures the diagnostic approach

Necessity: Does the team believe change is necessary?

Won't

Behavior   Motivation

Concern: Is the team concerned about effects of the change?

Capability
Opportunity

Opportunity: Is there time in the day to produce the change?

Can't

Capability: Does the team have all the skills?

Source: Adapted from Michie and others, 2011, p. 42.

motivation – does the individual have the will to change? If the motivation to change develops, the individual then faces capability and opportunity issues; does he/she have the skills, ability, time, and space to change? If these issues are overcome, the behavior change may occur but will only be sustained if new habits and routines are formed (Wildman and others, 2021).

Similarly, the improvement team had discovered motivation through their work to understand their microsystem and "Brandon's" experience, and now needed to develop new capabilities and take advantage of opportunities to practice new skills and sustain new habits. The team adopted the simple behavior change model (see Figure 2.13) to understand and diagnose change interventions. This model was not only routinely used by the team to understand how to think about changing behaviors with patients, but also as a way of understanding how to change staff behaviors to achieve improvement. "We identified that we needed to expand our skill set to understand behavior change and habit formation. To do that, we secured a grant to train the team in motivation interviewing, and we developed expertise in COM-B" (CF Physician; Sheffield Teaching Hospitals, 2011).

Keep both discipline and rhythm. Improvement work can be sustained over time and become part of a unit's culture when leaders instill new habits and new patterns that produce an internal discipline and reliable rhythm. Regular, coached, weekly meetings utilizing the DMIC improvement ramp helped instill this discipline and rhythm within the CF team.

Use measurement and feedback. Both discipline and rhythm – essential for fostering learning – are sustained by the use of continuous measurement and feedback. To inform and sustain their improvement work, the CF team paid rigorous attention to the metrics that matter. "We now have a re-energized team no longer daunted by increasing workload but motivated to find ways to work more effectively – and through measurement seeing them work" (CF Specialist Nurse; Sheffield Teaching Hospitals, 2011).

Create a learning system. The members of the CF team are on a learning journey as they redesign their system and attempt to achieve their purpose. By testing changes and reflecting on the results, by becoming more scientific when making improvements, by becoming keen participant observers of their own processes and the related outcomes, and by sharing ideas and methods about what works and what fails, they are creating a learning system that provides conditions under which staff members can learn and discover, test out new ideas, and attempt to innovate. "I have enjoyed this experience immensely and have a passion for making things better for the patients. It has been satisfying for me personally to be able to do this with a system that I thought we were stuck with and that we all hated – staff and patients" (CF Nurse; Sheffield Teaching Hospitals, 2011).

Transformation of Improvement Patterns

The Sheffield CF case study reveals a clinical unit that always had the intention to achieve superior results but lacked an effective method for doing so. This case study embodies the following principles, which may be helpful in guiding other microsystems' progress toward the best possible performance.

Begin with the intention to excel. Improvement is initiated and sustained with the intention to achieve the best possible results. This aim is motivated not so much by the desire to capture the high ground or to bask in the limelight but by the desire to do what is best for the patients and families who have the potential to benefit from care.

Involve all the players. The leaders who are successful will, over time, find a variety of opportunities and ways to involve all the microsystem players – interdisciplinary staff and patients and families – in the action of analyzing and improving processes and outcomes.

Focus on values that matter. The leadership activity that will sustain a virtuous cycle of improvement in performance is one that connects change to core values that matter to patients, families, and staff.

Keep both discipline and rhythm. Improvement work can be sustained over time and become part of a clinical microsystem's culture when leaders inculcate new habits and new patterns that produce an internal discipline and reliable rhythm.

- Discipline. Discipline relates to such things as the use of the scientific method and open, respectful inquiry into authentic causes and full effects.
- Rhythm. Rhythm relates to devoting some time to improving patient care even as large amounts of time are spent on providing patient care. Weekly improvement meetings and daily huddles are examples of devoting time and creating rhythm.

Use measurement and feedback. Both the discipline and the rhythm – the patterns essential for fostering learning systems – are aided and abetted by the use of measurement and feedback to assess the gap between current results and the desired state.

Create a learning system. A statement often attributed to Galileo holds that "you cannot teach anyone anything, you can only help him find it within himself." People learn in many ways – by being confronted with a worthy challenge, by taking action and reflecting on the results, by using the scientific method, by becoming keen participant observers of their own work processes and the related outcomes, by exchanging ideas and methods about what works and what fails, and so on. It is important to create a learning system and thereby the conditions under which staff members can learn and discover, test out new ideas, and identify what works and what fails while realizing their own potential and attempting to innovate.

A Model of Development and a Curriculum to Catalyze Microsystem Growth

In this section, we first provide a general model that portrays a clinical microsystem's developmental journey toward best possible performance. We then introduce a curriculum that can be used to jump-start clinical microsystems to embark on their own paths toward peak performance.

A Microsystem's Developmental Journey

To complement the previous case study, which details one particular microsystem's developmental journey, Figure 2.14 provides a general model for the journey. The model is based on work with and observations of hundreds of clinical microsystems over the past two decades. It calls attention to five stages of growth over time.

Stage 1: Create awareness of the clinical microsystem as an interdependent group of people (microsystem members including patients and families) with the capacity to make change. Often it is the invitation to create a graphic representation of the microsystem's work that initiates that microsystem's enhanced self-awareness. Members of the clinical microsystem often see routines, habits, or processes that do not work very well or that do not make sense when they look at the system's functioning as a whole

FIGURE 2.14 A MODEL FOR A MICROSYSTEMS DEVELOPMENTAL JOURNEY.

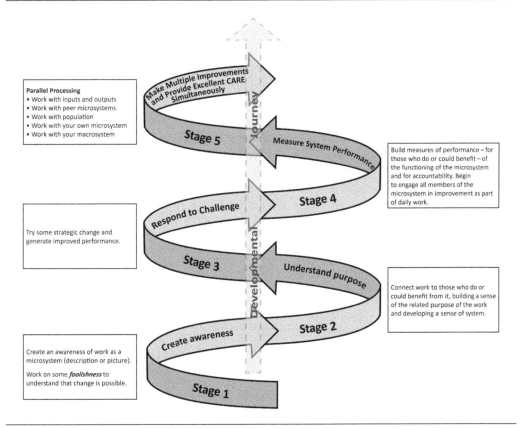

Parallel Processing
• Work with inputs and outputs
• Work with peer microsystems
• Work with population
• Work with your own microsystem
• Work with your macrosystem

Make Multiple Improvements and Provide Excellent CARE Simultaneously

Stage 5

Measure System Performance

Build measures of performance – for those who do or could benefit – of the functioning of the microsystem and for accountability. Begin to engage all members of the microsystem in improvement as part of daily work.

Respond to Challenge

Stage 4

Try some strategic change and generate improved performance.

Stage 3

Understand purpose

Connect work to those who do or could benefit from it, building a sense of the related purpose of the work and developing a sense of system.

Create awareness

Stage 2

Create an awareness of work as a microsystem (description or picture).

Work on some *foolishness* to understand that change is possible.

Stage 1

Source: Adapted from Kolb, A. and Kolb, D., 2018, p. 9.

and may decide to change them. The experience of working on what some describe as the "foolishness of work" – the things no one wants to admit to, much less brag about (such as confusion and rework in patient flow) – can lead to staff members' realization that change is possible. The sense that "we" can take action on "our" microsystem begins a journey of empowerment for the microsystem.

Stage 2: Connect routine daily work to the high purpose of benefiting patients; see the system. Once its members have a sense of agency (the ability to take action on one's own work), a team is often able to come to a deeper realization of its purpose (Leitch, 2019). With this clarification of an aim – to benefit a defined population of patients – it is easier for everyone to see the providers, processes, and patterns as a system (Godfrey and others, 2003; Wasson and others, 2003). This step of relating the needs of a population of patients to the hurly-burly world of everyday work is a challenge that clinical microsystems have often skipped.

Stage 3: Respond successfully to a strategic challenge. When a microsystem that has a sense of itself as a system faces a strategic challenge, such as "eliminate waiting for access to appointments in primary and specialty care" or "cut costs by 15 percent in the CF program," it can successfully change its processes and make things work better. However, for a clinical unit lacking this self-awareness, responding to a challenge such as this is often a matter of "following a recipe" or "looking like we are moving forward and attending to the issue when we are really walking in place." The results usually show up later as a slow decline in the changed performance to the previous unsatisfactory level (following the recipe) or as no measurable improvement after all (walking in place but looking attentive). Clinical microsystems that have well-developed identities as systems are better able to integrate large and small changes into their regular operations – their identity – and as a result they sustain them over time. As noted in the case study, a model for behavior change can be very helpful in this effort.

Stage 4: Measure the performance of the system as a system. The clinical microsystem that has made some changes, developed an explicit sense of itself as a system, and is producing many important outcomes tends to be curious about its results and wants to track its performance. Visual reminders of performance in the form of data walls (large, detailed displays of results) are often present (Nelson and others, 2003). Data walls are designated areas in the clinical microsystem where data over time are displayed for all members of the microsystem to review and take action on. Data walls typically include data over time from:

- Strategic measures that might be collected by the larger organization such as patient and staff satisfaction.

- Mesosystem-level data such as time to catheterization laboratory for a cardiac microsystem and infection rates for a surgical service.
- Clinical microsystem data that reflect current performance data such as cycle time from the time a patient enters the microsystem until they leave in an ambulatory practice, length of stay in an inpatient unit, number of days from last infection, and other improvement-cycle data specific to current improvement activities.

Measurement becomes a friend of forward progress and of the microsystem's enhanced sense of understanding. The microsystem often begins to track important indicators of its process for providing services and its outcomes to gain a better understanding of what is happening and to put itself in a better position to manage and improve care. The leaders of the microsystem begin to engage all the staff in the work of improving and innovating.

Stage 5: Successfully juggle multiple improvements while taking excellent care of patients and continuing to develop an enhanced sense of the system. With self-understanding and the ability to change, track, and reflect on its performance, the clinical microsystem is able to engage its context – the macrosystem in which it works and the other microsystems with which it regularly interacts. It is now in a better position to

- Analyze, modify, and standardize its own operations such as the internal flows (from input to output).
- Reach out and involve all members of the clinical microsystem, including those who are only marginally connected to this newfound identity.
- Focus renewed energy on finding ways to meet the needs of each individual patient one by one and the needs of the population of patients the microsystem serves. The clinical microsystem finds it is now possible to engage many people in many ways in taking actions to provide and improve care, to run multiple tests of change simultaneously, and to create a work environment that recognizes good work and promotes personal and professional growth (Huber and others, 2003). It finds ways to foster a virtuous cycle, or positive, upward evolutionary spiral. A microsystem's developmental journey does not always work this way.

"All models are wrong, some are useful," as Box (1978, p. 202) reminds us. A model such as the microsystem improvement curriculum is depicted in a stagewise, linear fashion. However, the microsystem's developmental journey does not necessarily occur in this sequence; it has interactions, barriers, detours, and feedback loops (see Figure 2.15).

FIGURE 2.15 MIXED UP IMPROVEMENT RAMP.

The reality of the
Dartmouth Microsystem
Improvement Ramp

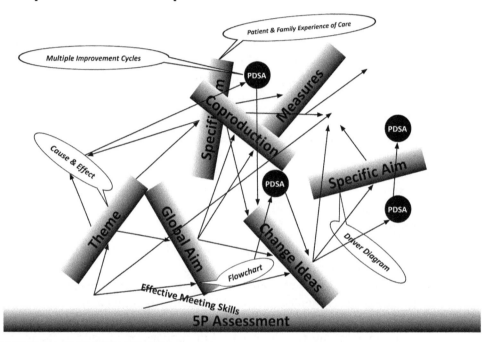

Source: Cary, Jamie L., 2019. Used with permission.

Despite this reality, learning and forward progress are possible and can lead to improved patient and family experience and outcomes, and a new sense of joy in work for professionals, as the case study illustrates so well.

Although we often speak of the microsystem as an entity, many clinical microsystems resemble a loosely coupled group rather than a tightly linked interdependent crew (Scott, 1981; Weick, 2001). Working on the microsystem can foster tighter linkages and appreciation for interdependencies. This developmental model has proven helpful for members and leaders of clinical microsystems who are eager to reflect on their work and on their efforts to attain the highest levels of quality, safety, service, and efficiency. A developmental journey is not an overnight occurrence; leadership that seeks knowledge, takes action, and reviews and reflects can help keep everyone's focus on the journey (Batalden and others, 2003).

A Model Curriculum for the Developmental Journey

Researchers can sometimes identify clinical units and clinical programs that are extraordinary. Most health systems have many exemplary clinical units. However, most health systems also recognize that what they need is not a few "pockets of gold" but a total system that is "solid gold." How does a health system begin the evolution toward a solid-gold health system, one that is composed of many small systems that are excellent in what they do? Recall that the patient's healthcare journey often requires him or her to interact with many small clinical units that come together into a care continuum that addresses the patient's changing health needs (Nelson and others, 2002).

There are many answers to this fundamental and challenging question, "How might we embark successfully on improving the health system by improving the small systems of which it is composed?" One very good answer is offered in Chapter Four of this book. That chapter demonstrates the powerful strategic value of applying microsystem thinking to the problem of organization-wide improvement in large, complex health systems.

Another complementary (and partial) answer to this question of organization-wide transformation is to provide each and every clinical and supporting microsystem with a basic learning program that will enable each individual microsystem to gain the skill and knowledge needed to start and sustain its own self-improvement from the inside out. Part Two of *Quality by Design* (Nelson and others, 2007b) introduced the Dartmouth Microsystem Improvement Curriculum, which was based on more than 10 years of direct experience working with clinical units as they redesign their work or design completely new healthcare programs. (Table 10.1, in Chapter Ten, provides an overview of this curriculum.) This curriculum performs the following functions:

- Helps clinical staff acquire the fundamental knowledge and skills they will need to master if they are to increase their capacity to attain higher levels of performance.
- Uses *action-learning theory* and sound educational principles to provide people with the opportunity to learn, test, and gain some degree of mastery.
- Involves people in the challenging real work of improving, assessing, diagnosing, and treating the small systems in which they work, in ways that will matter.

This curriculum has been applied to diverse clinical units – primary care practices, specialty medical practices, inpatient clinical units, home health teams, and clinical support units, such as pharmacy, radiology, and pathology – in North America and in many settings throughout Europe. It has been offered in various formats – one day per month for six months, one day per week for 10 weeks, and an accelerated workshop running for five consecutive half-days.

Two points about the Dartmouth Microsystem Improvement Curriculum learning model merit special emphasis.

Studio course principles. Donald Schön (1983) uses the architectural studio course as a model for effective learning to emphasize creating the conditions under which people can learn rather than focusing mostly on direct teaching or skills training. We base the microsystem improvement curriculum on Schön's studio-course model and capitalize on the power of these strategies:

- Giving people a meaningful challenge to work on, for example, improve access, reduce errors, and delight patients.
- Offering longitudinal learning, a by-product of working on the challenge.
- Evoking the magic of interactive learning, which involves peer-to-peer exchanges, teacher-to-student dialogues, microsystem-to-microsystem discussions, and microsystem-to-macrosystem conversations.
- Learning from concrete experience and reflecting on the experience.
- Drawing on other life experiences and knowledge bases and applying them to the challenge at hand. Many healthcare professionals do not regularly take the time to reflect on their practice. Once they have protected time to do this, self-awareness grows.

Three-thread tactic. The aim of the Dartmouth Microsystem Improvement Curriculum is to intertwine three vital threads and develop them in learners over time. These three threads are:

1. Finding ways to better meet each patient's special needs.
2. Making the work experience for staff meaningful and joyous through their learning to work in an interdisciplinary manner to design and provide patient-centered care.
3. Increasing each staff person's capability to improve his or her work and to contribute to the betterment of the system as a whole.

Several years ago, Donald Wolfe (1980) called attention to the needed competence within microsystems and macrosystems for work in the "applied behavioral sciences." He noted that *competence* always has a context (the microsystem work life), is rooted in a knowledge base and analytical skills (clinical knowledge and improvement knowledge), is inevitably interdependent with values, and involves the whole person (unity of organizational mission with personal values). The Dartmouth Microsystem Improvement Curriculum and the style of teaching that accompanies it are designed to reflect these themes.

In this second edition of *Quality by Design*, Part Two provides processes and insights into advancing from clinical microsystems to clinical mesosystems. Recognizing most care and services involve multiple microsystems, connecting mesosystems to work through their shared purpose for multiple populations can be enhanced with the new Part Two.

Conclusion

The challenge for all of us, leaders of health systems and people who work in those systems, is to provide high-quality, patient-centered care that is safe, effective, timely, equitable, and efficient (IOM, 2001). Despite almost two decades of efforts to improve safety, we have not met the goals set by the IOM and still have the opportunity to achieve the goals (AHRQ, 2009). We can do this if and only if we can redesign our systems. We need system-based improvement methods to make lasting improvements in the healthcare system.

A successful redesign requires creating the conditions for learning, improvement, and accountability at multiple levels – the large-system level (populated by macro organizations that exist in reimbursement, legal, policy, and regulatory milieus), the mesosystem level (that consists of individual microsystems providing care and services to multiple subpopulations) and the small-system level (characterized by clinical microsystems such as outpatient clinics, inpatient units, and other frontline delivery teams and clinical support groups). We must pay close attention to the large-system issues; if we fail to do so, our progress will be limited. However, we must also pay close attention to the small-system realities if we are to meet the quality challenge. There are many reasons why this is so. As noted earlier in this book, a small system can be described as:

- A basic building block of health care.
- A unit of clinical policy-in-use.
- A place where good value and safe care are made.
- A locus of control for most of the variables that account for patient satisfaction.
- A setting for interdisciplinary professional formation.
- A locus of control of most of the work-life dissatisfiers and many of the genuine motivators for health professionals' pride and joy in work.

For us, the joy of these insights is that they allow us to see the familiar with "new eyes," as Marcel Proust observed about the discovery process (Nelson and others,

2007c). The challenge comes from using our new eyes to see and asking ourselves questions such as:

1. What will it take for the processes of health professional education and development to recognize the cooperative and interdependent work of professionals from different disciplines and prepare these professionals accordingly?
2. What will help health system leaders recognize the opportunities they have to actively foster the development of clinical microsystems on which their macrosystem depends, and what will help those macrosystem leaders hold their microsystems accountable for the quality, value, and safety of patient care?
3. What structures of organization and work will enable clinical microsystems to regularly improve value by facilitating the never-ending removal of waste and cost?
4. What practices and disciplines in clinical microsystems will hold and honor the vitality of the paradox of the health care of the individual and the health of populations (that doing what seems best for the health of the individual and doing what seems best for the health of the population may seem to or may actually conflict)?

We hope that this book, by focusing attention on clinical microsystems – the places where patients and care teams meet – will contribute to lasting improvements in patient care as well as betterment of the working lives of those who provide care.

Mesosystem Considerations

The case study in this chapter describes a clinical microsystem's developmental journey as it developed and then worked to fulfill its purpose of "enabling people with CF to live as normal a life as possible." Their efforts began within the outpatient clinic, but later spilled over into the inpatient unit, demonstrating natural spread through the mesosystem. Creating a "solid gold" health system will be impossible without robust mesosystem involvement and mesosystem-level work on understanding purpose, context, and change. Systems are systems; just as many of the approaches to understanding clinical microsystems can be applied in nonclinical settings, many of the principles of microsystem inquiry readily apply to the mesosystem. Chapter Ten in this volume provides a fuller exploration of the approach to understanding a mesosystem and improving the care it provides. Members of the microsystem are acutely aware of the mesosystem – both the other microsystems they regularly interact with as well as the larger system within which they are embedded. The Dartmouth Microsystem Improvement Curriculum described in this chapter develops the ability of those members to see systems and appreciate the importance of how they relate to and interact with other microsystems in their mesosystem. Just as the microsystem must be aware of other elements of the mesosystem, the mesosystem must be aware of the specific microsystems it comprises: their purposes, contexts, and function. This requires mesosystem leaders to recognize and appreciate improvement efforts at the microsystem level, and to communicate those successes across microsystems and upward to the macrosystem, while simultaneously translating high-level institutional goals into terms that make sense for a microsystem. This is the essential challenge of "leading from the middle," which we will continue to explore throughout this book.

Summary

A microsystem's journey of self-discovery begins with the 5Ps assessment, including a robust discussion of purpose. Moving on to global and specific aims for improvement and working to achieve those aims can produce better patient and family experience and outcomes and enhance joy in work for professionals in the microsystem. The stages of this developmental journey are similar across many different settings; this journey has in turn informed the development of the Dartmouth Microsystem Improvement Curriculum, which offers an experiential learning approach to developing the capabilities of all microsystem members – professionals, patients, and families.

Review Questions

1. Describe three ways in which the 5Ps process helped the Sheffield CF team gain insight into the care processes and outcomes.
2. What is the purpose of balancing measures?
3. Briefly review the five steps of a microsystem's developmental journey.

Discussion Questions

1. The Sheffield team developed a persona to help them in their work, "Brandon." Can you describe a persona that might help you gain insight into the patient experience in a microsystem you are familiar with?

2. The Sheffield team found the COM-B model helpful for their own behavior change. Why might a specific model be helpful for change?

3. The Microsystem Improvement Curriculum is based on "experiential learning" using a "studio course" approach. What do these terms mean to you? Can you think of learning experiences you have had that embodied these principles?

Additional Activities

1. Apply the 5Ps to a small system you are a part of, such as your family, a class, or a nonclinical workplace.

2. Explore how the Esther persona has been used in Sweden to improve care.

References

Agency for Healthcare Research and Quality. *Advancing Patient Safety: A Decade of Evidence Design and Implementation.* Rockville, MD: Agency for Healthcare Research and Quality, Nov. 2009. AHRQ Publication No. 009(10)-0084. [https://www.ahrq.gov/patient-safety/resources/advancing.html]

Batalden, P. B., Nelson, E. C., Mohr, J. J., and others. "Microsystems in Health Care: Part 5. How Leaders Are Leading." *Joint Commission Journal on Quality and Safety,* 2003, 29(6), 297-308.

Box, G. *Statistics for Experimenters: An Introduction to Design, Data Analysis and Model Building.* Hoboken, NJ: Wiley-Interscience, 1978.

Daniels, T., Goodacre, L., Sutton, C., and others. "Accurate Assessment of Adherence: Self-Report and Clinician Report Vs Electronic Monitoring of Nebulizers." *Chest,* 2011, 140, 425-432.

Godfrey, M. M., Nelson, E. C., Wasson, J. H., Mohr, J. J., and Batalden, P. B. "Microsystems in Health Care: Part 3. Planning Patient-Centered Services." *Joint Commission Journal on Quality and Safety,* 2003, 29(4), 159-170.

Godfrey, M. M. "Improvement Capability at the Front Lines of Healthcare Helping Through Leading and Coaching." School of Health Sciences, Jönköping University. Dissertation Series No. 46, 2013.

Hoo, Z. H., Curley, R., Walters, S. J., and Wildman, M. J. Exploring the Implications of Different Approaches to Estimate Centre-Level Adherence Using Objective Adherence Data in an Adult Cystic Fibrosis Centre – A Retrospective Observational Study." *Journal of Cystic Fibrosis,* 2020, 1, 162-167. doi: 10.1016/j.jcf.2019.10.008

Huber, T. P., Godfrey, M. M., Nelson, E. C., and others. "Microsystems in Health Care: Part 8. Developing People and Improving Work Life: What Front-Line Staff Told Us." *Joint Commission Journal on Quality and Safety,* 2003, 29(10), 512-522.

Institute of Medicine (U.S.) Committee on Quality of Health Care in America. *Crossing the Quality Chasm: A New Health System for the 21st Century.* Washington, DC: National Academies Press, 2001.

Leitch, J. "Why Activating Agency Is Essential for Improvement." Boston, MA: Institute for Healthcare Improvement. [http://www.ihi.org/communities/blogs/why-activating-agency-is-essential-for-improvement], Feb. 21, 2019.

Lipmanowicz, H. "Buy-In Versus Ownership." Liberating Structures, 2010. [http://www.liberatingstructures.com/hl-articles/].

Michie, S., van Stralen, M. M., and West, R. "The Behaviour Change Wheel: A New Method for Characterising and Designing Behaviour Change Interventions." *Implementation Science,* 2011, 6(42), 1-11.

National Institute for Health Research. "Development and Evaluation of an Intervention to Support Adherence to Treatment in Adults with Cystic Fibrosis (ACtiF)." NIHR Award ID RP-PG-1212-20015, 2015. [https://fundingawards.nihr.ac.uk/award/RP-PG-1212-20015]

Nelson, E. C., Batalden, P. B., Huber, T. P., and others "Microsystems in Health Care: Part 1. Learning from High-Performing Front-Line Clinical Units.*" Joint Commission Journal on Quality Improvement,* 2002, 28(9), 472-493.

Nelson, E. C., Batalden, P. B., Homa, K., and others. "Microsystems in Health Care: Part 2. Creating a Rich Information Environment." *Joint Commission Journal on Quality and Safety,* 2003, 29(1), 5-15.

Nelson, E. C., Batalden, P. B., Huber, T. P., and others. "Success Characteristics of High-Performing Microsystems: Learning from the Best. In E. C. Nelson, P. B. Batalden, and M. M. Godfrey (eds.), *Quality by Design: A Clinical Microsystems Approach.* San Francisco, CA: Jossey-Bass, 2007a.

Nelson, E. C., Batalden, P. B., and Godfrey, M. M. (eds). "Part Two: Activating the Organization and the Dartmouth Microsystem Improvement Curriculum." In *Quality by Design: A Clinical Microsystems Approach.* San Francisco, CA: Jossey-Bass, 197-383, 2007b.

Nelson, E. C., Batalden, P. B., Edwards, W. H., and others. "Developing High-Performing Microsystems." In E. C. Nelson, P. B. Batalden, and M. M. Godfrey (eds.), *Quality by Design: A Clinical Microsystems Approach.* San Francisco, CA: Jossey-Bass, 2007c.

Nelson, E. C., Batalden, P. B., Godfrey, M. M., and Lazar, J. S. (eds). *Value by Design: Developing Clinical Microsystems to Achieve Organizational Excellence.* San Francisco: Jossey-Bass, 2011.

Scholtes, P. R., Joiner, B. L., and Streibel, B. J. *The TEAM® Handbook.* Edison, NJ: Oriel STAT A MATRIX, 2010.

Schön, D. A. *The Reflective Practitioner: How Professionals Think in Action.* New York: Basic Book, 1983.

Scott, W. R. *Organizations: Rational, Natural and Open Systems.* Upper Saddle River, NJ: Prentice Hall, 1981.

Sheffield Teaching Hospitals. "Microsystem Coaching Evaluation." *SurveyMonkey,* distributed on October 20, 2011.

Sheffield Teaching Hospitals. *Development and Evaluation of an Intervention to Support Adherence to Treatment in Adults with Cystic Fibrosis (ACtiF).* National Institute for Health Research Programme, Grants for Applied Research, Reference No RP-PG-1212-20015, 2015.

Walshaw, M. J. "Cystic Fibrosis: Diagnosis and Management – NICE Guideline 78." *Paediatric Respiratory Reviews,* 2019, 31, 12-14. doi: 10.1016/j-prrv.2019.02.006

Wasson, J. H., Godfrey, M. M., Nelson, E. C., and others. "Microsystems in Health Care: Part 4. Planning Patient-Centered Care." *Joint Commission Journal on Quality and Safety*, 2003, 29(5), 227-237.

Weick, K. E. *Making Sense of the Organization*. Malden, MA: Blackwell, 2001.

Wildman, M. J., O'Cathain, A., Maguire, C., and others. "Self-management Intervention to Reduce Pulmonary Exacerbations by Supporting Treatment Adherence in Adults with Cystic Fibrosis: A Randomised Controlled Trial." *Thorax*, 2022, 77(5), 461–469. doi: 10.1136/thoraxjnl-2021-217594.

Wildman, M. J., and Hoo, Z. H. "Moving Cystic Fibrosis Care from Rescue to Prevention by Embedding Adherence Measurement in Routine Care." *Paediatric Respiratory Review*, 2014, 15(S1), 16-18.

Wolfe, D. M. "Developing Professional Competence in the Applied Behavioral Sciences." In E. Byrne and D. E. Wolfe (eds.), *New Directions in Experiential Learning: Developing Experiential Learning Programs for Professional Education*, No. 8. San Francisco: Jossey-Bass, 1980.

Additional Resources

CFHealthHub website, http://www.cfhealthhub.org
Microsystem website, http://www.clinicalmicrosystem.org/
Sheffield MCA, https://www.sheffieldmca.org.uk/00.89

Key Words/Terms

5Ps: The 5Ps place improvement themes into context and are a great place from which to start your improvement work.

Action-learning theory: Action learning is an approach to problem-solving that involves taking action and reflecting upon the results. This helps improve the problem-solving process as well as simplify the solutions developed by the team.

Balancing measures: Looking at a system from different directions or dimensions and asking if the changes are designed to improve one part of the system and cause new problems in other parts of the system.

Clinical value compass: A clinical value compass has four cardinal points (1) functional status, risk status, and well-being; (2) costs; (3) satisfaction with health care and perceived benefit; and (4) clinical outcomes.

Data wall: Designated areas in the clinical microsystem where data over time specific to the microsystem are displayed for all members of the microsystem to review and take action on. Data walls typically include data over time from organization-strategic measures, service line data, and clinical microsystem data that reflect current performance such as cycle time or length of stay.

Multidisciplinary team (MDT): A team of healthcare professionals who are members of different disciplines (e.g., psychiatrists, social workers, pharmacists, nurses, etc.), each providing specific services to the patient that work together toward a specific set of goals.

Parking lot: A list of tangential topics or issues that arise in a meeting that should be dealt with later.

PDSA (Plan–Do–Study–Act): Schema for continuous quality improvement originally developed by Walter Andrew Shewhart and made popular by W. Edwards Deming, who ascribed inherent variation in processes to chance and intermittent variation to assignable causes. The PDSA cycle is a four-part method for discovering and correcting assignable causes to improve the quality of processes.

SDSA (Standardize–Do–Study–Act): Steps taken following a successful PDSA cycle to achieve the original aim. The purpose is to hold the gains that were made using PDSA cycles and standardize the process in daily work.

Value compass: See *Clinical value compass*.

CHAPTER THREE

LEADING IMPROVEMENT OF HEALTHCARE SERVICE SYSTEMS: MICROSYSTEMS, MESOSYSTEMS, AND MACROSYSTEMS

Paul B. Batalden, Edgar H. Schein, Don Caruso, Marjorie M. Godfrey, Tina C. Foster, Julie K. Johnson

AIM

The aim of this chapter is to review the essentials of leadership including similarities and differences of leading at the micro-, meso-, and macrosystem levels.

LEARNING OBJECTIVES

By the end of this chapter, the reader will be able to:

1. Describe how leaders can nurture their organization's capability to improve through vertical and horizontal integration of micro-, meso-, and macrosystems.
2. Provide an example of leading by taking action at multiple levels in an organization.
3. Understand the role of leaders in aligning micro-, meso-, and macrosystem vision and values in enabling transformative change.
4. Create a short list of priorities for leading the improvement of healthcare services.

Quality by Design: A Clinical Microsystems Approach, Second Edition. Edited by Marjorie M. Godfrey, Tina C. Foster, Julie K. Johnson, Eugene C. Nelson and Paul B. Batalden.
© 2025 John Wiley & Sons, Inc. Published 2025 by John Wiley & Sons, Inc.

Introduction

The work of leadership is extensively explored in much contemporary writing. In this chapter, leadership at multiple levels and the importance of alignment is highlighted with specific attention to the work of providing high-quality, high-value healthcare services.

Leading the improvement of a healthcare service system begins by appreciating and understanding its work as a system with multiple levels: microsystems, mesosystems, and macrosystems. First, it is necessary to understand that services are always *coproduced* between patients, families, and healthcare professionals. This understanding, coupled with the exploration of leadership strategies and processes, can be used to develop leaders and improve overall organizational leadership.

Today, healthcare service system leaders must nurture their organization's capability to continuously improve the quality, safety, and value of the contributions that healthcare services make to better health. They do this by attracting the energies of people and by forging agreement on the actions needed to improve the shared work. Leaders begin by fostering a relationship of trust and respect among themselves and others. As the ancient teacher Abba Felix observed about the relationship between culture and learning, "they permit learning by creating a space in which obedience to truth is practiced" (Palmer, 1983).

The systems they lead need knowledge, skill, and habits that fit and that can help meet the formidable challenges of today and tomorrow. This chapter begins with an overview of the working systems involved in daily healthcare service and what leading each system level involves. The accompanying leadership case study illustrates the work at multiple system levels that is needed to achieve real change (Figure 3.1).

FIGURE 3.1 A VIEW OF THE MULTILAYERED HEALTH SYSTEM.

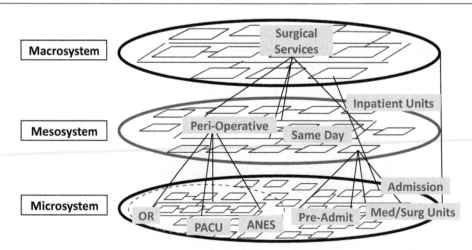

Source: Adapted from Nelson and others, 2011, p. 10. Used with permission.

Multiple System Levels

The first, or top level, referred to as the macrosystem, represents the whole of the organization and is led by senior leaders such as the chief executive officer (CEO), chief operations officer (COO), chief financial officer (CFO), chief medical officer (CMO), chief nursing officer (CNO), and chief information officer (CIO). It is guided by a governing board. The second level, termed the mesosystem, represents major divisions or clusters of work found in a healthcare service organization, such as the department of medicine, the department of nursing, and information services as well as clinical service programs and service lines such as oncology, cardiovascular, and women's health. The mesosystem also is two or more microsystems working together for a population and can include microsystems from multiple departments and programs. The third level, populated by what we call clinical microsystems, represents the frontline places where patients, families, and professionals meet and together create health-care services.

A clinical microsystem can be described as a small group of people with a shared purpose who work together on a regular basis – or as needed – to design, create, and offer healthcare services together with the individuals who receive those services and the information and information technology that is helpful. We see these small systems as the locus of the value-creating work of healthcare service today.

An overview of these systems and their work is presented in the following illustrations and case study.

Case Study: Leadership

The setting is a 1,000-physician, *multispecialty group practice* providing healthcare services in a rural region of the United States. It is the clinical arm of an academic medical center with four affiliate hospitals in two neighboring states and multiple subsidiary group practices, which had historically practiced quite independently. In the early 2000s, this healthcare organization, already in one of the lowest-cost settings in the United States, understood that to be sustainable, it needed to *bend the cost-curve* growth over time even further toward better value.

The macrosystem leadership understood that transformative change would be needed to meet this challenge. The organization now faced living with two different payment systems: one traditional "fee-for-service" and the other, called "value-based care," which paid better for lower-cost, higher-quality healthcare services. Leadership described this as trying to stand in "two canoes." The culture and processes of the system were part of the historical fee-for-service world, but to thrive in a value-based care world, these needed to change. In the inaugural Center for

Medicare and Medicaid Pay-for-Performance Quality Incentive Program in 2005, the organization struggled in its first value-based reimbursement program (Thomas and Caldis, 2007; McWilliams and others, 2015). Despite an organizational philosophy that emphasized the importance of data and outcomes, there was little population-level data. At the level of the macrosystem, leaders perceived the need to continue to accept both forms of payment. The mesosystems lacked the infrastructure to pursue service design in any mode other than traditional fee-for-service. The microsystems were left to invent change one process at a time to try to optimize their service reimbursement. Many observed the inherent conflict in the two methods of payment. Despite this, the organization managed to perform well in pay-for-performance and continued its vision of data-driven quality improvement for populations.

Macrosystem

In 2014, this healthcare system fully embraced *Population Health*, a strategic decision with widespread implications. In the Population Health world, the processes would need to be patient-centric and preventive in nature and had to incorporate *community-based interventions*, despite historic clinical processes that responded to financial incentives to increase volume and number of services in the practices (Kindig, Asada, and Booske, 2008). Systematic information about clinical quality or value-added care was difficult to get. Dismantling the volume-based approach to health care and replacing it with a health environment that included the community, incorporated new technology, and offered visits that did not require physicians was an enormous challenge. The macrosystem would need to ensure financial solvency during the transition and articulate expectations for the development of meso- and microsystems infrastructure to enable transformation-of-care processes.

The macrosystem began by incorporating Population Health into its mission and vision statements, but there were no concomitant transformative changes in service design and improvement. The senior leadership became committed to creating a sustainable health community and not just a healthcare system. Fully understanding that payment models drive process design, the organization committed to engaging in the new *Accountable Care Organization* (ACO) payment models with risk-sharing approaches (Porter, 2008). These payment methods would allow reimbursement for types of healthcare services not historically reimbursable in the traditional fee-for-service environment. Nurse-based visits and technology-supported home interventions, as well as home visits by community health workers, would now be reimbursed. Macrosystem leadership was now able to step out of the "two canoes" that had effectively created mixed messages and hampered the ability to change processes.

FIGURE 3.2 EXAMPLE OF LOCAL AREAS OF AUTONOMY COMPARED TO SERVICE LINES: CARDIOVASCULAR CARE.

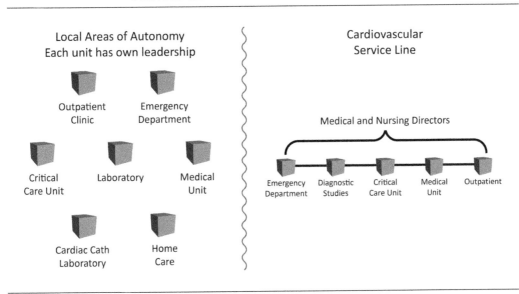

The macrosystem leadership recognized the need to create a methodology to introduce these changes in a systematic fashion across the entire organization. Evidence-based population health approaches needed an infrastructure that would allow evidence-based change at the practice level and disseminate best practices across the *health continuum* (Barr and others, 2003). To accomplish this, "service lines" structured around specialties were developed (see Figure 3.2).

Mesosystem

The service-line structure enabled one leader across a specialty healthcare service line to make decisions for that specialty, which was intended to reduce variation across all practices. This was very different from the previous structure, which effectively created local areas of autonomy at the microsystem level within a specialty practice. Service lines in the organization allowed autonomy at the mesosystem level. This autonomy gave the service line the ability to embrace fee-for-service models of care as needed, as well as alternative models of care that made sense in the ACO's *globally capitated* economic environments. In the service line approach, leadership could create singular service-line-specific approaches, which allowed the macrosystem leadership to maintain its desired goal of reduced variation.

The primary care service-line mesosystem leader, with the new autonomy granted by the macrosystem, understood the need to allow the microsystems to engage locally in service redesign and improvement work, and simultaneously replicate the best practices across the mesosystem. Mesosystem leaders also understood the barriers of compensation connected to a volume-based world that rewarded more service, not better value. At the mesosystem level, the new compensation approach that paid physicians based on the quality outcomes of care, rather than the number of patients seen, improved physician engagement and enabled care teams to redesign workflow and to create a new model of care.

The service-line leader was empowered to align primary care compensation embracing value rather than volume by discontinuing pay based on "relative value units" (RVUs) and creating a "base" salary compensation with bonuses connected to quality outcomes.

This was an essential element in the transformation. The mesosystem also disseminated quality improvement toolkits to individual practices to facilitate workflow analysis and enable tests of change (see Tables 3.1 and 3.2). The individual microsystems

TABLE 3.1 HYPERTENSION IMPROVEMENT MATRIX.

Root Cause	Improvement
Work flow inconsistencies	Universal evidence-supported triage and treatment algorithms for primary care, specialty care, and community
Poor communication between staff	Single blood pressure brochure with care plan prompt used throughout the community for consistent messaging along with regular upkeep of Electronic Medical Record (EMR)
Multiple brands of equipment	Standardized future purchasing
Lack of timely maintenance and calibration of equipment	A process to make sure all blood pressure cuffs are calibrated appropriately
Lack of resources to effectively manage registries	Individual provider registries and monthly data transparency with increased number of registry managers
Cost barrier of blood pressure re-checks and lack of consistent centralized process	Nurse clinic with no-cost blood pressure re-checks and triaging
Patient education	Single blood pressure brochure campus-wide and "Know your Numbers" campaign
Community involvement	Working together with Healthy Monadnock 2020, home healthcare agencies, YMCA, and senior centers to bring awareness, screenings, distribution of "Know Your Numbers" cards, education, and improvement opportunities to our community

Source: Cheshire Medical Center Dartmouth-Hitchcock Keene NH, Hypertension Improvement Team. Used with permission.

TABLE 3.2 BEST PRACTICE IMPROVEMENT TOOLKIT FOR HYPERTENSION.

Document Name	Description
Meeting Agendas	
Kick-off Meeting	This agenda provides the topics and instructions to introduce the project and complete the project charter.
Document Current Process Meeting	This agenda provides the topics and instructions on how to lead a successful meeting to document the current process.
Root Cause Analysis Meeting	This agenda provides the topics and instructions to identify the main barriers to improved hypertension control for your department.
Improvement Brainstorming Meeting	This agenda provides the topics and instructions to lead the project team through the exercise of identifying the improvements from the toolkit that will best help your department.
Ongoing Project Status Meeting	This agenda provides a template to manage and track the improvements.
Patient Education	
Blood Pressure Poster	This poster for exam rooms helps educate patients on normal blood pressure numbers.
BP Tracking Card	This is a card for patients to record their blood pressure readings over time. It also helps to educate about blood pressure numbers.
DH Hypertension Brochure	Patient education brochure.
Selecting a BP Cuff Tips for Home BP Monitoring	This is an information sheet for patients about how to most accurately monitor their home blood pressure.
Dash Diet Handout Dash Diet - In Brief	This is a patient education handout about the DASH diet.
Staff Education	
Blood Pressure Competency Training	This is a training powerpoint from Linda Savinsky, RN, that reviews the correct method for measuring blood pressure.
Documenting Blood Pressure in a Flow Sheet	BP is not recorded into the data warehouse unless it is entered correctly. Use this to review how repeat BP readings should be documented in CIS.
JNC-7 Guidelines	This is an excellent summary of the evidence-based evaluation and treatment guidelines for high blood pressure.

(continued)

TABLE 3.2 (*Continued*)

Document Name	Description
Meeting Agendas	
Plan of Care for Hypertension	This document outlines the elements in a plan of care for hypertension. A plan of care must be documented to receive full credit through CMS and NCQA for appropriate care of a hypertensive patient.
Support Staff Workflow and Script	This document describes the support staffs workflow when they room patients who are found to have elevated blood pressure. It describes how they assist in patient education and use the room posters and handout cards.
Registry Management	
How to Use the Hypertension Registry	A user guide for maximizing the use of the registry tools for proactive patient management.
Hypertension Registry Management Process Flow	Flow chart that details the roles and responsibilities of the registry process.
Patient Contact Protocols	Scripting for contacting patients that require a visit with their provider to check on their hypertension.
Physical Environment	
Blood Pressure Room Setup	The physical layout of the exam room can influence the accuracy of the blood pressure reading. This describes optimal room layout.
Completed HTN Project Presentations	
Hudson Family Practice	This powerpoint illustrates how the Hudson office used an improvement process and best practice tools to make improvements in blood pressure control for their patients.
Manchester IM/FM	This powerpoint shows how Manchester used improvement processes and best practice tools to make dramatic improvements in blood pressure control across their whole division.
Additional Resources	

Source: Dartmouth-Hitchcock Manchester NH, Quality and Outcomes Improvement Committee. Used with permission.

were thus exposed to evidence-based best practice workflows, which were created through a collaborative effort across service lines (see Figures 3.3 and 3.4).

The mesosystem also inquired about needed resources at a service-line level, allowing mesosystem leaders to deploy these resources (such as nurse care coordinators

FIGURE 3.3 FINAL HYPERTENSION WORK FLOW – PRIMARY CARE.

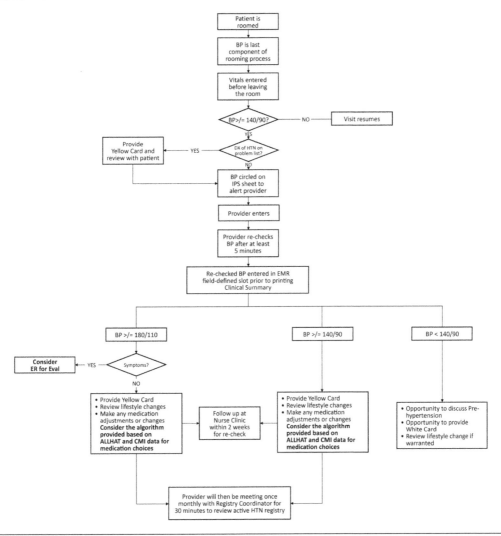

Source: Cheshire Medical Center Dartmouth-Hitchcock Keene NH, Hypertension Improvement Team. Used with permission.

FIGURE 3.4 FINAL HYPERTENSION WORK FLOW – SPECIALTY CARE.

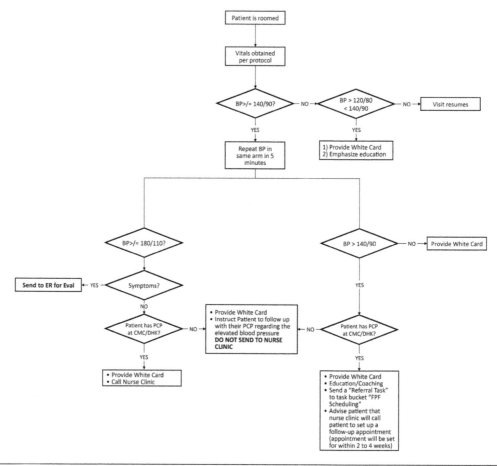

Source: Cheshire Medical Center Dartmouth-Hitchcock Keene NH, Hypertension Improvement Team. Used with permission.

and social workers within the microsystem) across the organization where there was an identified need.

Microsystem

The new primary care service line (mesosystem) comprised multiple microsystems. Local microsystem leader triads (physician, nurse, and administrator) recognized the need to manage change in a way that the physicians in the practice would embrace. They also realized that this would require that physician and staff values

FIGURE 3.5 TEAM-BASED CARE MODEL OF SERVICE LINE RESOURCES.

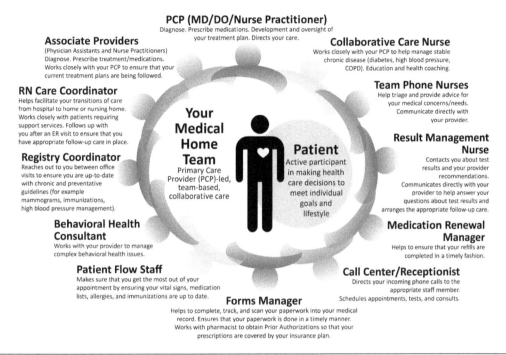

PCP (MD/DO/Nurse Practitioner)
Diagnose. Prescribe medications. Development and oversight of your treatment plan. Directs your care.

Associate Providers
(Physician Assistants and Nurse Practitioners)
Diagnose. Prescribe treatment/medications.
Works closely with your PCP to ensure that your current treatment plans are being followed.

Collaborative Care Nurse
Works closely with your PCP to help manage stable chronic disease (diabetes, high blood pressure, COPD). Education and health coaching.

RN Care Coordinator
Helps facilitate your transitions of care from hospital to home or nursing home. Works closely with patients requiring support services. Follows up with you after an ER visit to ensure that you have appropriate follow-up care in place.

Team Phone Nurses
Help triage and provide advice for your medical concerns/needs. Communicate directly with your provider.

Registry Coordinator
Reaches out to you between office visits to ensure you are up-to-date with chronic and preventative guidelines (for example mammograms, immunizations, high blood pressure management).

Result Management Nurse
Contacts you about test results and your provider recommendations. Communicates directly with your provider to help answer your questions about test results and arranges the appropriate follow-up care.

Your Medical Home Team
Primary Care Provider (PCP)-led, team-based, collaborative care

Patient
Active participant in making health care decisions to meet individual goals and lifestyle

Behavioral Health Consultant
Works with your provider to manage complex behavioral health issues.

Medication Renewal Manager
Helps to ensure that your refills are completed in a timely fashion.

Patient Flow Staff
Makes sure that you get the most out of your appointment by ensuring your vital signs, medication lists, allergies, and immunizations are up to date.

Call Center/Receptionist
Directs your incoming phone calls to the appropriate staff member. Schedules appointments, tests, and consults.

Forms Manager
Helps to complete, track, and scan your paperwork into your medical record. Ensures that your paperwork is done in a timely manner. Works with pharmacist to obtain Prior Authorizations so that your prescriptions are covered by your insurance plan.

Source: Andrew Tremblay, MD and Family Medicine Cheshire Medical Center, Dartmouth-Hitchcock, Keene, NH. Used with permission.

align with those of the service-line leaders (mesosystem) and ultimately with the macrosystem vision. Through collective meeting management, individual clinician values quickly aligned with local leadership's vision – a vertical alignment. A *Team-Based Care model* was jointly developed by the microsystems under the direction of the service-line leader, allowing a "horizontal" alignment across microsystems (see Figures 3.5 and 3.6).

This aligned set of changes (Table 3.3) enabled the transformative events that followed. The microsystems trained in improvement techniques were able to use the toolkits provided to transform their care model using small tests of change with measured results (see Table 3.4 for improvement training methods; see Figure 3.7 for hypertension improvement over time).

As each team was committed to evidence-based approaches driving value and not volume, dissemination of practices and outcomes occurred through daily morning *huddles* at service-line microsystems, leadership-level weekly meetings, and monthly mesosystem meetings. Replication of best practices that had been shown to add value

FIGURE 3.6 TEAM-BASED CARE MODEL: HORIZONTAL ALIGNMENT ACROSS MICROSYSTEMS.

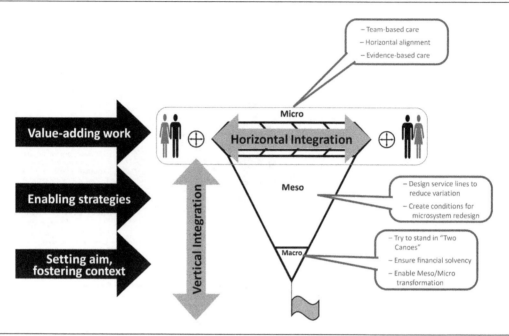

Source: Adapted from Batalden and others, 2005, p. 7. Used with permission.

TABLE 3.3 SUMMARY OF CHANGES.

Macrosystem	Mesosystem	Microsystem
Sustainable Population Health Focus	Service Lines	Team-Based Care
Value-Based Care	Quality Tool Kits	Best Practice Approaches
New Payment Models	New Compensation Models	Base Salary with Quality Bonus

Source: Cheshire Medical Center Dartmouth-Hitchcock Keene NH, Hypertension Improvement Team. Used with permission.

occurred widely as a result of the multi-level communications. Early wins focused on care coordination of the "top five percent," or "sickest of the sick," collaborative care for the stable, chronic disease population, and Screening, Brief Intervention, and Referral to Treatment (SBIRT) interventions for the well population.

Having individual practices focus on the subpopulations that they cared for, rather than focus on individuals, required a new mindset (see Figure 3.8). Clinicians were used to thinking about resource needs one patient at a time. They began to use

TABLE 3.4 IMPROVEMENT TRAINING METHODS.

Quality Improvement Program Training
DAY ONE — AGENDA

Times		Faculty
8:00–8:30 30 min	**WELCOME AND INTRODUCTIONS – ONE**	Linda/Vicki
8:30–8:45 15 min	**SPONSORSHIP – TWO** *Objective: Discuss the role of the sponsor in supporting improvement work.*	Don
8:45–9:15 30 min	**INTRODUCING THE DMAIC MODEL – <u>THREE</u>** *Objective: Explain the purpose of the DMAIC process.*	Vicki
9:15–10:15 60 min	**MANAGING COMPLEX CHANGE – <u>FOUR</u>** *Objective: Define Complex Change Model and understand how workplace culture affects change.*	Linda
10:15–10:30 15 min	**BREAK**	
10:30-11:45 75 min	THE **D**MAIC MODEL – EXPLORING HOW TO <u>DEFINE</u> AN ISSUE – <u>FIVE</u> *Objective: Define the components of an effective Project Charter/ Aim Statement, Functions of a team.*	Vicki
11:45–12:30 45 min	**LUNCH**	
12:30–1:30 60 min	THE D**M**AIC MODEL – FUNDAMENTAL SKILLS OF <u>MEASURE</u> – <u>SIX</u> *Objective: Explain the purpose of measurement to monitor progress.*	Vicki
1:30–2:30 60 min	**MEETING SKILLS - <u>SEVEN</u>** *Objective: Demonstrate how effective meeting skills help teams achieve their purpose.*	Linda
2:30–2:45 15 min	**BREAK**	
2:45–3:45 60 min	THE D**M**AIC MODEL – FUNDAMENTAL SKILLS OF <u>MEASURE</u> – FLOWCHARTING – <u>EIGHT</u> *Objective: Learn to create and use flowcharting in process improvement and redesign.*	Vicki
3:45–4:15 30 min	**WRAP UP, HOMEWORK, EVALUATION** *Objective: Review concepts and learning from the day and assign homework to be completed with site leaders.*	Linda
	Quality Improvement Program Training DAY TWO — AGENDA	
8:00-8:15 15 min	**WELCOME AND OVERVIEW OF DAY**	Linda/Vicki
8:15-9:00 45 min	THE D**M**AIC MODEL – FLOWCHARTING – <u>NINE</u> *Objective: Review and create a process flow chart.*	Linda

(continued)

TABLE 3.4 (*Continued*)

Times		Faculty
9:00–10:00 60 min	THE D**M**AIC MODEL – MORE ON FUNDAMENTAL SKILLS OF <u>MEASURE</u> – <u>TEN</u> *Objective: Demonstrate the value of using various data displays to present and analyze data.*	Vicki
10:00–10:15 15 min	**BREAK**	
10:15–11:30 75 min	**MANAGING COMPLEX CHANGE – <u>ELEVEN</u>** *Objective: Demonstrate how vision and leadership are essential components of improvement work.*	Linda
11:30–12:15 45 min	**LUNCH**	
12:15–1:30 75 min	THE DM**A**IC MODEL – FUNDAMENTAL SKILLS OF <u>ANALYZE</u> – <u>TWELVE</u> *Objective: Learn how to conduct a root cause analysis using fishbone and 5 Why techniques.*	Vicki
1:30–2:30 60 min	THE DMA**I**C MODEL – FUNDAMENTAL SKILLS OF <u>IMPROVE</u> – <u>THIRTEEN</u> *Objective: Learn how to utilize brainstorming, affinity sorts, prioritizing matrix, and multi-voting techniques to generate improvement ideas.*	Linda
2:30–2:45 15 min	**BREAK**	
2:45–3:15 30 min	THE DMA**I**C MODEL – FUNDAMENTAL SKILLS OF <u>IMPROVE</u> – **5**S – <u>FOURTEEN</u> *Objective: Learn how to utilize 5S techniques to create efficiency and reduce waste.*	Vicki
3:15–3:45 30 min	THE DMAI**C** MODEL – FUNDAMENTAL SKILLS OF <u>CONTROL</u> – <u>FIFTEEN</u> *Objective: Learn the key factors for closing and monitoring an improvement project.*	Vicki
3:45–4:15 30 min	**WRAP UP, EVALUATION**	Linda/Vicki

DMAIC = Define, Measure, Analyze, Improve, and Control

Source: Cheshire Medical Center Dartmouth-Hitchcock Keene NH, QIP Program Vicki Patric MS, LSSBB; Linda Patchett RN; Don Caruso MD, MPH. Used with permission

this new framework of considering subpopulations and their care needs, such as preventive, acute, chronic, and palliative care. In the new model of care, specific resources could be dedicated to subpopulations based on their specific needs. *Care coordination* for the top five percent was attractive to clinicians. At the same time,

FIGURE 3.7 HYPERTENSION IMPROVEMENT OVER TIME.

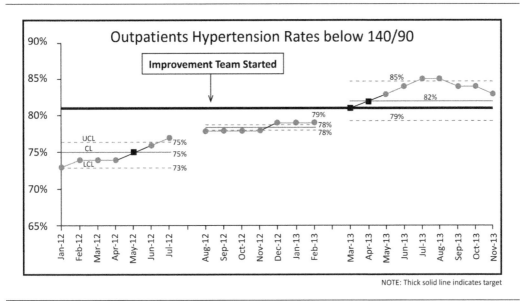

NOTE: Thick solid line indicates target

Source: Cheshire Medical Center Dartmouth-Hitchcock, Keene, NH. Used with permission.

FIGURE 3.8 MICROSYSTEM PREVENTATIVE, ACUTE, CHRONIC, AND PALLIATIVE SUBPOPULATIONS.

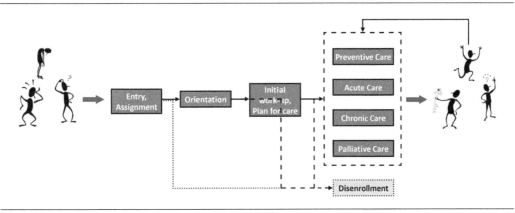

Source: Nelson and others, 2011, p. 52. Used with permission.

professional roles were "repurposed" based on population need and skills. Expensive resources were used where the population need was the greatest. These resources were not new but repurposed professionals based on population need and skills. Because these tests of change were measured and seen to be highly successful, they were rapidly replicated and disseminated.

Lessons Learned

We learned from the case study that when the macrosystem leaders created a clear vision and enabled it with structure, resources, and leadership, the mesosystems were able to ensure the successful improvement efforts of the microsystems. The vision, strategy, and tactics were all in alignment from macrosystem to mesosystem to microsystem, allowing the organizational practices and clinician values to align.

In this model, the macrosystem, sometimes called the blunt end of service delivery because it is the part of the healthcare system that does not come in direct contact with patients, contrasts with the microsystem, the sharp end of service delivery, because the microsystem is the point where the service is created and where the patient directly contacts the professional resources of the system. The view shown in Figure 3.1 reflects a system of service that is exceedingly complex, which makes clear the need for a fresh approach that will reflect the intricacies of today's healthcare service system while still focusing primary attention on the front lines of healthcare service where patients, families, and groups of professionals meet. It also illustrates the importance of aligning the different levels of the system so that waste is minimized and services are optimized (Batalden and others, 2005).

Figure 3.9 provides another way to frame the challenges faced by healthcare leaders today. It retains the macro-, meso-, and microsystem format shown in Figure 3.1 but turns the image upside down. This diagram is based on J. Brian Quinn's observations on the requirements needed to become a world-class leader in the service sector (Quinn, 1992). The inverted pyramid offers a contrast to the more typical representation of a healthcare service organization by putting the patients and frontline staff at the top of the system and suggesting that the rest of the organization really exists to support the myriad of important interactions that take place at the front line of healthcare service.

Clinical microsystems are the naturally occurring building blocks that form the front line of all healthcare service systems. These small systems form around the patient and family to provide care for shorter or longer periods of time as health needs evolve. For example, if a person has an acute myocardial infarction (AMI) and survives, he or she will typically receive care in a series of clinical microsystems. Paramedics stabilize, transport, and begin treatment; the emergency department diagnoses and treats; the catheterization lab assesses, diagnoses, and treats as indicated; the cardiac care unit assesses and treats; the inpatient telemetry unit assesses, treats, and discharges; cardiac rehabilitation services assist with the full recovery; and the outpatient cardiology clinical practice, with or without the assistance of home healthcare services in the community, follows the patient over time to minimize risk of a new cardiac event. Together these microsystems act separately and together as a mesosystem at the front line of healthcare service for that individual

FIGURE 3.9 THE HEALTHCARE SYSTEM AS AN INVERTED PYRAMID.

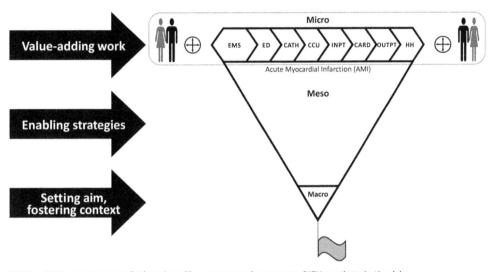

NOTE: EMS = emergency medical services; ED = emergency department ; CATH = catheterization lab;
CCU = cardiac care unit; INPT = inpatient telemetry unit; CARD = cardiac rehab; OUTPT = outpatient cardiac;
HH = home health

Source: Adapted from Batalden and others, 2005, p. 7. Used with permission.

patient. Figure 3.9 shows the collection of AMI microsystems at the top of the inverted pyramid that come together to function as a mesosystem.

The quality and value of service for any single patient, or for a cohort of patients such as people who have had an AMI, fully depend on the quality of the operations of the healthcare service system. The quality of the healthcare system (Q HS) is the sum of the quality of service provided within each contributing microsystem (Q m1, Q m2, Q m3, and so forth) plus the quality of the *handoffs* and integration that occur in the organizational "white spaces" between microsystems (for example, handoffs of the patient, information and data about the patient, and services needed for the patient).

Clinical microsystems form the front line of the healthcare system – they represent the place where quality is made and costs are incurred. The special knowledge, skills, and resources of the clinical staff are used in the clinical microsystem to meet the special needs of an individual patient. It is the place where innovation opportunities are most often found. It is the place where, with discretion, things that are flexible can be customized and where, with discipline, things that are standardized can be made routine.

The inverted pyramid goes from the microsystem level to the mesosystem and the macrosystem level, respectively. The mesosystem includes the areas that contribute to the integrated healthcare service for the patient with a specific need requiring diverse knowledge and skills found in the following:

- clinical departments (for example, medicine, nursing, surgery)
- clinical support departments (for example, radiology, pathology, anesthesiology, pharmacy, medical information, healthcare service management)
- aggregated mid-level structures (such as specific centers for oncology, cardiovascular health, women's health).

The macrosystem, at the bottom of the inverted pyramid, is populated by senior leaders (for example, those in the "C" suite of offices, the CEO, CFO, CMO, CNO, and CIO). Figure 3.5 also contains a flag representing a governing board that guides (and oversees) senior leaders to help shape the context of work in core areas such as vision, mission, values, guiding principles, strategy, and finance. Working down through the inverted pyramid can be compared to working through a *root cause analysis* that moves progressively away from the sharp end and toward the blunt end of the system as staff ask the "why" question repeatedly.

We turn now to a consideration of the work of leading each level of system. The essential work of leadership is gaining knowledge, taking action, and reflecting, which occurs at all leadership levels of an organization. The following insights on these three leadership actions are presented specifically for the clinical microsystem. We suggest that leaders at every level of the organization consider all three actions.

Leading Clinical Micro-, Meso-, and Macrosystems

The original research exploring high-performing healthcare microsystems that Nelson, Batalden, and colleagues conducted focused on the observations and impressions of healthcare professionals and staff working in high-performing microsystems (Nelson and others, 2007). It was believed that their reflections and observations about the work of their leaders would offer a direct view of the content of the work that leaders do in actual work settings. We acknowledge that patients may have been able to offer additional observations and perspectives about "leader work" in these settings, but we did not interview them systematically for their impressions.

Building Knowledge

Leaders build knowledge of the basic structural characteristics of the microsystem: its organization and language; its physical arrangements and the technology to promote flow of services; its intended – and its practiced – policy about healthcare services and work; the constraints that impede daily good work; and the current skills and knowledge base of those who work in it. They foster inquiry into the processes of work, the sources of unwanted variation in those processes, and the methods associated with better practice performance, including ways of measuring and monitoring processes (covered in Chapter 8). They create a local context for open inquiry, learning, and creativity by their attention to the relationships, patterns, habits, and traditions, which helps everyone focus on the patients' aims and capabilities (Revans, 1964; Schein, 2013). Leaders help people notice what might need to be changed and support the work of testing and making change.

When we asked health professional workers in these high-performing microsystems to describe the work of their leaders, they told us about the diverse set of behaviors, actions, and approaches that their leaders use to "build knowledge" (shown in Table 3.5).

TABLE 3.5 BEHAVIORS, ACTIONS, AND APPROACHES THAT LEADERS USE TO "BUILD KNOWLEDGE".

- Observe the actual context of work.
- Have a predictable presence.
- Be interested in follow-up.
- Lead learning as needed.
- Focus on what, not who.
- Encourage proactive thinking.
- Foster a common language for the common work.
- Determine the need for new services based on community availability.
- Use data to characterize problems and foster change.
- Create widespread information about operational performance.
- Seek information from every helpful source.
- Encourage use of imagination and ideas by listening and implementing them.
- Share their theories, assumptions.
- Make it easy to do the right thing.
- Recognize desired behaviors.
- Instill confidence.
- Have a passion for the future.
- Move information everywhere.
- Show rather than tell.
- Directly experience the work of others in order to better understand the system.
- Build knowledge of how issues are dealt with.
- Encourage conversations about the future.
- Create predictable space for communication in the midst of busyness.
- Find ways to learn informally, even from personal and family issues.
- Foster inquiry – by everyone.

Leaders in these clinical microsystems were curious, focused, and transparent. They invited the participation of all in the microsystem. They were building knowledge for themselves and for the whole microsystem. Their knowledge was "for action" (Argyris and Schön, 1996).

Taking Action

The second major characteristic of these leaders was "taking action." Their action-taking involved will, ideas, and execution as Nolan and others have observed (Nolan, 2007; Berwick, 2014). Those who worked with these leaders observed many different behaviors for making things happen, executing plans, and making good on intentions. The actions involved ranged from the way people are hired and developed to the way work gets done and the way the work is held accountable.

The attributes, concrete steps, and behaviors that workers in high-performing microsystems associated with the actions their leaders took are listed in Table 3.6.

As a review of Table 3.6 reveals, leading means taking action on the structure to create and modify formal reporting relationships, clearly identifying go-to people for the multitude of different microsystem processes, and changing the physical arrangements for work when they stand in the way of an optimal workflow. It means championing the integration of information technology into the healthcare service processes. It means managing the flow of talent and hiring people who share the purpose and values of the clinical microsystem, bringing the right people together at the right time. It means noticing what needs to be done and having the courage to initiate action while also inviting others to join in the detailed specification of work processes.

Leading by taking action means having specific processes for making things happen. It involves having explicit, authentic respect for all the people who are necessary for the work of creating service in the clinical microsystem. It means involving the patients and families as full members in the co-creation and coproduction of the healthcare services (see Chapter 6) that the microsystem creates and offers. It means being vigilant about ways that the current processes might fail, are failing, or might be a hazard. It usually involves active engagement of the leader in the daily workings of the microsystem and in the actions to be taken. It means using process knowledge to cross-train members of the microsystem to increase the reliability and resilience of the system's capabilities.

Leading involves taking action on the patterns of work to promote the cooperative functioning of all microsystem members and to recognize their interdependence. It means caring for one another. It means celebrating in the midst of the work. It involves fostering the daily practices necessary for trust and respect among the

TABLE 3.6 ATTRIBUTES, CONCRETE STEPS, AND BEHAVIORS ASSOCIATED WITH LEADERS IN HIGH-PERFORMING CLINICAL MICROSYSTEMS.

- Taking timely actions.
- Acting together to encourage ideas and suggestions.
- Hiring for shared values.
- Sharing information in a format that connects to taking action.
- Fostering process literacy as an adjunct to clarity of work definition.
- Taking action on issues of concern.
- Dealing openly and directly with conflicting points of view.
- Accepting coworkers as colleagues, and promoting their individual development.
- Supporting others.
- Minimizing the gap between what you say and what you do.
- Following through, connecting your voice and your actions.
- Taking the actions you say you are going to take – predictably.
- Recognizing the others who depend on you.
- Maintaining the respect of others by the actions you take.
- Enabling others to act.
- Providing the technology needed to do a good job.
- Recognizing the potential of people, and taking steps to enable it.
- Acting in a way that reflects your own values.
- Making daily work and those values congruent.
- Building process knowledge, including the underlying rationale for the process.
- Treating people so they feel respected.
- Working to earn respect and trust.
- Being reliably available and accessible.
- Fostering an environment of respect and love for patients.
- Telling the truth about what isn't working well.
- Offering room for others to solve the problem.
- Helping people work better by helping them work differently.
- Recognizing the part of the work that is factual and objective.
- Caring for one another.
- Demonstrating interest in others.
- Celebrating whatever you can.
- Recognizing interdependence.
- Leading by example.
- Asking others to do only what you would do yourself.
- Being clear about what needs to be done, inviting people to contribute to how it might be done.
- Recognizing the need to be in the middle of the action.
- Being aware of the others needed for leadership of the work.

Source: Adapted from Berwick, D. M., 2014, p. 57-58.

diverse patients and staff. It means paying attention to the ways that differences and conflicts are addressed.

Leaders build knowledge and take action, but the leaders in these high-performing settings are also active in reviewing and reflecting on their own work.

Reviewing and Reflecting

Reviewing and reflecting in leading usually involves creating some structure for *reflection.* This structure often begins with having a vision of what the clinical microsystem is trying to become. This vision provides insight into how the system's patterns, processes, and structure will enable the desired work to get done, what success will look like, and what the next steps will be after success is accomplished. It means creating time space – and geographical space – in which people can gather to have meaningful conversations about their work. Part of the structure of review and reflection is the leaders' awareness of the temporal limits on members' participation in the work of the microsystem and their anticipation of the time when the current leaders' turns will be over (Geus, 1997; Batalden, 2010).

Leading by reviewing and reflecting means having a process for honestly asking, "Is the work necessary?" and "If so, is it getting done?" and "Is there a good match between the needs of the patients (and other beneficiaries) and our work?" and "Do the outputs we measure reflect the patients' aims as well as the use of good science?" It means that people are regularly invited to assess the degree to which their own professional growth and development are addressed. Exploring and noticing the predicted and unforeseen effects of change are also parts of leaders' reflection on the work of the microsystem (Table 3.7).

Colleagues recognized that another aspect of leading is demonstrated in the ways that their leaders reflect on the patterns in practice and the assumptions driving them. This involves analyzing the ways in which the care and work processes connect to the structures of the microsystem. It calls for exploring the relationships of changes envisioned (or already made) in the microsystem's patterns, structures, and processes. It invites attention to the critical leadership task of framing and reframing the work (Bolman and Deal, 1992).

Leading the Clinical Mesosystem

Mesosystems comprise microsystems that must work together to achieve a common purpose – usually two or more clinical and/or supporting microsystems. Usually they are clusters of associated microsystems necessary to meet the needs of a population of patient-beneficiaries. The transfer of information and the flow of patient-beneficiary and healthcare service from one microsystem to another are key

TABLE 3.7 HOW LEADERS REVIEW AND REFLECT.

- Created definitions of success that serve the present and the future.
- Grounded interpretations of the past and present in data and had conversations that connected to the actual realities that we were facing.
- Fostered an understanding of the imperative of leaving the past behind.
- Created regular time for communication and conversation about the work.
- Invited the outside connections of the microsystem to honor the time spent in review and reflection.
- Let the reflective process serve the needs of the people involved.
- Centered the review on the population served.
- Recognized the microsystem as a place experienced by others.
- Were mindful of the signature (the way the microsystem is known, recognized by others) of the microsystem.
- Explored the relation between joy and success.
- Were explicit about the contributions that people could make to the work that went on beyond them as individuals.
- Reviewed the positioning of leaders and followers.
- Revisited the mission and the relation of the mission to what each person does.
- Encouraged reflection on the connection between individual's identity and the work itself.
- Appreciated the aesthetics of interdependent work.
- Focused on the enhancement of people as professionals—in both formal and informal ways.
- Were mindful of the professional and disciplinary focus that can compete with attention to the patient.
- Explored the ways technology can help (and hinder) the work.
- Regularly scanned for the reality of the environment, and explored its implications for leadership of the work.
- Helped visualize, understand and remember those served by the microsystem in the daily conversations about the work.
- Were clear about what next will look like.
- Recognized change in our midst, certifying it as the help it was.
- Continually reviewed the vision informing the direction of the work.
- Explored the threats that eroded a focus on the vision.
- Had conversations about the competing commitments that crowd the vision.
- Created a safe, open place where truthful conversations about the facts of performance could occur.

to the effective functioning of a clinical mesosystem. The transition from one microsystem to another requires some attention to the designated outputs of the first microsystem and the required inputs of the next. Patients and professionals who are able to co-create those transitions transparently from microsystem to microsystem have the possibility of better fidelity of information and service flow.

TABLE 3.8 NEEDS IDENTIFIED BY MESOSYSTEM LEADERS.

- Vision of a desired microsystem/mesosystem future.
- Connection of desired future to the current reality.
- Clarification of implications of change(s).
- Idea/option generation.
- Ability to design and conduct pilot tests of change.
- Balance between local innovation, creativity and the needs of the commons.
- Appropriate standardization of the work and work flow.
- Methods of responding to signals that "all is not well."
- Resource allocation strategies that address the functioning of the clinical microsystem and the whole mesosystem, macrosystem.
- Approaches to advocacy for the microsystem with the macrosystem.
- Development of useful measures of clinical microsystem performance.
- Identification of microsystem staffing, leadership and staff professional development needs.
- Integration of professional educational function with daily patient care realities.
- Methods for receiving and processing complaints.
- Execution of plans.
- Convene microsystems and macrosystems.

Mesosystem leaders are in a privileged position to help develop microsystem leaders. They can also help identify the information support that will facilitate the coordinated work of the multiple microsystems. From the perspective of the mesosystem, it is possible to identify and reduce waste in the aggregate work. Mesosystem leaders are also able to see the hazards and risks of the coordinated work of the several microsystems involved.

Mesosystems frequently occupy the organizational space between the "front offices" and the "front lines" of healthcare systems. They become the crucible where the macrosystem's vision meets the daily reality of patient/beneficiary's need. They enable the changes needed for the future and some measure of stability based on a clear understanding of "what works" in the current reality.

As we interviewed mesosystem leaders, they identified the following needs shown in Table 3.8.

When queried, "What knowledge, skill has proven helpful in your work as a clinical mesosystem leader?" they provided a long list of "how to" items (see Table 3.9).

What emerges from these reflections on leading mesosystems is the value of insight into the two worlds of the microsystem and the macrosystem, and what is necessary to foster alignment amongst all three levels of work.

TABLE 3.9 HELPFUL KNOWLEDGE AND SKILLS FOR CLINICAL MESOSYSTEM LEADERS.

- How to develop knowledge of healthcare as a system, process.
- How to understand patient need, illness burden.
- How to measure, display, and analyze variation in the daily processes of healthcare.
- How to lead, follow.
- How to attract cooperation across health professional disciplinary traditions.
- How to plan, work in a socially accountable way.
- How to design, test change.
- How to link "evidence" to the processes and systems of the local context.
- How to follow the patient's journey—especially between and into the "other" department(s).
- How to "see" the ways that the process of interaction could "automatically" throw off data.
- How to use data to understand unreliability and/or poor quality of care.
- How to work together to test changes in the process(es) of interaction.
- How to establish ownership of the processes of leverage in the "space between" microsystems.
- How to establish processes for review of shared care.
- How to focus on "flow" of care, information, and patient need.

Leading the Clinical Macrosystem

Clinical macrosystems are aggregates of mesosystems and microsystems that come together to achieve a shared aim. They "face in" to the smaller systems and "face out" to the community and the populations served by the healthcare systems. From interviews with several clinical macrosystem leaders, six commonly recognized needs emerged (Table 3.10).

As these leaders described their work against these perceived needs, they took pains to contextualize their own efforts to create a "language commons" that allowed

TABLE 3.10 SIX COMMONLY RECOGNIZED NEEDS.

- Bring meaning to the work. . .show why it makes a difference.
- Create the context of the whole.
- Define possibilities and limitations.
- Create supportive infrastructures for health information and human resources.
- Stay connected to the clinical microsystem and create the conditions for growing capability from the inside out.
- Drive out fear of changing.

people to work together (Hardin, 1968; Senge and others, 1994; Senge, 2006). The work done against each of the identified needs requires adaptation to the local setting, but a brief set of suggestions emerged for each need.

Bring meaning. . .show why work in this macrosystem makes a difference in the lives of those served. This included creating system aims that were grounded in the real burdens of illness that patients and beneficiaries experienced. Efforts were grounded in the reality that healthcare professionals were often more loyal to patients and their needs than to the healthcare service organization. Macrosystem leaders described stories that connected patients, communities, and the daily work of healthcare professionals. They knew that deeply held values often grounded their successful efforts to foster professional development, professional formation, and professional growth. These leaders knew that every individual could be invited to a personal engagement in safeguarding and improving healthcare service. While macrosystem leaders were often personally held directly accountable for addressing external organizational challenges, they realized that these same challenges were no more than secondary motivators for most of those who worked inside their macrosystem.

Create a context of the whole by establishing a clear vision and strategy that can be understood by all. When this understanding was in every organizational unit, macrosystem leaders could begin to attract the engagement of each person – at the level and place of his/her own work. All had to understand how both doing and improving their own work could become a contribution to the continual improvement of patient outcomes. A never-ending curiosity about change within, between, and across microsystems and mesosystems really helped these leaders achieve the results they sought.

Define the possibilities and limitations that live in the connections between work in the system and life in the "real world" that workers in the macrosystem confront every day. Clinical macrosystem leaders realized that choices were made by each person about what needs to be done as part of the work of the macrosystem and what work needs to be done by others. Regulatory and reimbursement mechanisms are daily reminders of the social accountability that microsystems, mesosystems, and macrosystems face. These leaders realized that each level of system makes a contribution to the aims and well-being of the whole macrosystem. Leaders at all levels need recognition of their efforts to connect the multiple levels.

Create a supportive human resources infrastructure that recognizes and rewards individuals and groups and fosters alignment of efforts to create, maintain, and improve quality, efficiency, and flexibility. Paul O'Neill succinctly suggested that macrosystem leaders need to create a work context where every worker is able to "strongly agree" to each of the statements in Table 3.11 about their work life (O'Neill, 2001).

TABLE 3.11 POSITIVE WORK-LIFE CONTEXT STATEMENTS.

- "I'm treated with dignity and respect everyday by everyone I encounter. . . and it doesn't have anything to do with hierarchy."
- "I'm given the opportunity and tools that I need to make a contribution and this gives meaning to my life."
- "Someone noticed that I did it."

Source: Adapted from O'Neill, P. H., 2001. p. xiii.

TABLE 3.12 SUPPORTIVE INFORMATION INFRASTRUCTURE QUESTIONS.

- What are microsystems trying to do?
- How is information helping or making harder the action needed at the point of healthcare service?
- How can information technology take work out of the clinical microsystem?

Create a supportive information infrastructure that is readily accessible and easy to use. This includes real-time, "feed forward" and "feedback" data. It involves using *balanced metrics* of performance (Table 3.12).

Stay connected to the clinical microsystem and create conditions for growing capability "from the inside out." Wise clinical macrosystem leaders never forget that the value of their enterprise is created in the microsystems of healthcare service where professionals and patients are working together. Physically "showing up" in those settings gives clinical macrosystem leaders the opportunity to demonstrate their own curiosity, their ability to encourage the curiosity and creativity of others, and their personal recognition of the fundamental importance of continual learning. They recognize that not all clinical microsystems and mesosystems are equally capable of self-development. They know that as macrosystem leaders they can help create an environment that encourages learning, action, and reflection on the work.

Drive out fear of changing by challenging microsystem and mesosystem leaders to learn how to change and sustain helpful improvements. Encouraging rapid tests of change at all levels of the macrosystem is made "natural" when the curiosity of the macrosystem leader drives the inquiry. The requirements of a "hospitable space for change" will vary from setting to setting. The clinical macrosystem leader can be transparent about efforts to foster such a setting and can seek regular feedback about the current state of the "hospitable space." Insightful clinical macrosystem leaders are aware of the dangers of "trapped" thinking and know the benefit of creating a learning environment where assumptions and conclusions are continually challenged. It is

TABLE 3.13 FACTORS THAT INFLUENCE OUR THINKING.

- Time, space, causality
- Information organization
- Identity
- Memory
- Classification/labels
- Big decisions of right/wrong, life/death

Source: Adapted from Douglas, M., 1986.

TABLE 3.14 TIME ESTIMATES TO DO THE WORK.

- Manage self – one's own integrity, character, ethics, knowledge, wisdom, temperament, words, and acts. (50%)
- Manage those with authority over you – bosses, supervisors, directors, regulators, and others. (20%)
- Manage one's peers – those with no authority over you and over whom you have no authority: associates, competitors, suppliers, customers. (20%)
- Manage those over whom you have authority. (5%)

Source: Adapted from Hock, D., 2005, p. 48-49.

important to recognize that fear of change is a major source of waste in a hierarchical organization – and it is next to impossible to remove fear "from the bottom up."

In some ways the words about leadership and institutions never end, in part because institutions and our systems of work influence our thinking (Douglas, 1986; see Table 3.13).

Dee Hock, the innovative banker-developer of the Visa® card suggested that leaders can only recognize and modify conditions that prevent superlative performance; perceive and articulate a sense of community, a vision of the future, a body of principle to which people are passionately committed; then encourage and enable them to discover and bring forth in everyone the extraordinary capabilities that lie trapped, struggling to get out. To do this work, Hock rank ordered, with time estimates, the tasks that leaders need to address (Hock, 2005; see Table 3.14).

Some Current Priorities for Leading the Improvement of Health and Health Care

Good leaders know the benefit of a "short list" to help stay focused on the important "what-to-work-on" priorities in times when the contexts of work seem buffeted in a world that seems to be volatile, uncertain, complex, and ambiguous (Bennett and Lemoin, 2014). They know they serve two realities: the current situation and the future that they are trying to create. They also know that no one else can construct their list, which must address the local situation they face and the challenges that fit their "turn" as a leader (Batalden, 2010). In an effort to help initiate such a list for leaders of improved service at all levels of healthcare service systems, we wish to offer a "short list" of themes to consider.

Focus on Basics

There are three inextricably linked aims at the heart of systems of healthcare services that are capable of ongoing, generative, sustainable improvement: reducing the burden of illness for individuals and for them as a population; improving system quality, safety, and value performance; and developing and maintaining a lifetime of professional competence, pride, and joy in the daily work that includes making these gains (Batalden, 2012).

To achieve these linked aims, assessment of outcomes must include an understanding of what system changes and professional competence contributed to them. The development of professional competence must include an understanding of the relation of that competence to the achievement of desired outcomes in the patient and population, as well as the intended gains in system quality, safety, and value performance. We must recognize that efforts to coproduce services that offer better quality, safety, and value require attention to measurement of outcomes that reflect the use of good science and the attainment of patients' goals (Batalden and others, 2016).

We have resisted linking these basic aims because we have pretended that competence, joy, and pride in health professional work can be separated from achieving system change and better coproduced outcomes for individuals and their communities. When competence, joy, and pride are not linked to system change, we deprive settings and leaders of the energies necessary for generating and sustaining the changes needed. Yet, linking them is not easy when clear responses to urgent mandates for "less cost" tempt quick but incomplete responses by leaders.

Relentlessly Reduce Waste and Add Value

We have yet to develop a sense of embarrassment about waste in health care. We would do well to recall the shame and embarrassment associated with the Japanese word *muda*, which means "action without value" (Ohno, 1988).

Some waste in health care is easy to see – needlessly repeated services, procedures and tests, delays experienced but not required, and added transport because things that needed to be close together were not historically recognized as such.

Some waste is harder to see – the information gaps and the behaviors that arise from habit rather than science.

Still even harder to see is the waste embedded in the business models we have grown to love but have the effect of constraining our thinking and design. Waste also lives in some of our cherished myths, such as the persistent notion that health care today is largely a matter of soloist work independent of other people and professionals, information, and technology. Rather the independent work must work well together as functioning systems to achieve a reduction in the burden of illness in the lives of those served (Batalden, Ogrinc, and Batalden, 2006).

Seek and Use Good Science

Diverse methods are required for doing "good science" in health care. The words "evidence" and "science" are not interchangeable. For example, a randomized controlled trial works best for assessing the effectiveness of a drug or new therapy, and a carefully detailed case report may work best to help explain or discover a new approach (Vandenbroucke, 2008).

The coproduction of healthcare service will require new knowledge-building methods that honor the unique combinations of science and patient goals that are often no less "personalized" than the match of therapy to a specific genotype (Kravitz and Duan, 2014).

We can be clear about which methods work best for what situation and model the integration of science into the daily work of coproduced service. We have no choice but to honor the diverse ways of knowing. Our old habits of "doing biomedical science" and "achieving social change" must be seen as a synergistic invitation to leaders to bring very different traditions together and to foster learning from the experience of designing and making real and needed change.

Enable Continual Inquiry into the "Unchanged Present" and Offer the Social Support that Fosters It

Living systems continually change in response to the circumstances around them and within them. Change is resisted as a manifestation of the competing commitments and assumptions working together to hold the unchanged present in place (Lewin and Lewin, 1948; Kegan and Lahey, 2009). Inquiry into the unchanged present involves understanding both the driving and the restraining competing forces.

Change mastery requires habits that seek the understanding of actual daily performance-in-context and its contrast with theoretic limits of what is possible. Fostering the never-ending desire to improve requires social support that appreciates the creativity, the discipline, the courage, and the satisfaction that comes with changing one's own work (O'Neill, 2001; Lucas and Nacer, 2015).

Recognize and Foster Community

There is a mode shift underway in today's workplaces. The coproduction of healthcare services requires new ways of professionals and patients working together. The new way will include new levels of cooperation among professionals from different disciplines and organizations. The competitive drives might change from a focus on "us versus them" to a focus on a collaborative competition versus the unmet social need for health. This collaborative competition can build camaraderie and appreciation for diverse gifts, ideas, and talents.

If our aim is large, we know we cannot make it alone, and cooperation with others is obligatory, not merely a preference. We need to overcome the deep habits that have fostered unnecessary competition among people and the implicit covenants of neglect about unmet needs. The needs and the tasks are much larger than one's life-career space. We must enjoy and encourage each other in the community of practice.

The design lessons from the alignment of providers and the beneficiaries of care in the early HIV-AIDS experience offer a striking example of what this might look like (Gamson, 1989). If we are going to work better together, we have to be prepared to make promises to one another and to be prepared to seek forgiveness for those promises not kept (Arendt, 1998). The words popularly attributed to Albert Einstein are a helpful reminder: "We cannot hope to solve problems with the same level of thinking that created them."

Model the Work of Leader as "Reflective Learner"

Donald Schön (1983) helped us see that there are natural limits to the technical knowledge of any professional. He suggested that the gap between that limit and the need of a specific person or specific application of the professional's knowledge involves empirical exploration of possibilities and reflection on those attempts to span the gap.

Edgar H. Schein, an icon in the organizational development field and professor emeritus at the Massachusetts Institute for Technology (MIT) Sloan School of Management, has helped us recognize the regenerative power of helpful inquiry in the reflective process (Schein, 2013).

Note from the editors: We have had the privilege to learn and work with Professor Edgar H. Schein for the past decade and asked him to share his perspectives and insights about leading at different levels and in different cultures of the organization. We offer his unique reflections here.

Co-creating Health Through Relationships that Align Micro-, Meso-, and Macrosystems

My goal, in these brief comments, is to supplement the excellent analysis on what needs to be changed in order to create co-creating, high-performing health systems. I am viewing this from the perspective of a marginal outside observer who tries to understand and help. I have had a variety of contacts with health systems, especially the work of Gary Kaplan at Virginia Mason Hospital in Seattle and with Amicus, the consultants who work with the *physician "compact."* My main concern has been with safety issues in the nuclear power industry, which has great implications for patient safety and the quality of patient experience.

What I think I have learned about organizations as systems is based largely on Kurt Lewin's famous dictum: You don't really understand an organization until you try to change it (Lewin and Lewin, 1948). I was fortunate during my professorial years at MIT's Sloan School of Management to have had a chance to work with a variety of organizational leaders on various programs of change and improvement. I learned how to be a helper from mentors such as Douglas McGregor (1960) and Richard Beckhard (1969; 1987). So, what have I learned and how does it apply to the coproduction of health?

Point 1. Leaders at the micro-, meso-, and macrosystem levels have to have faith in people, what McGregor labeled a set of optimistic assumptions about human desires to work and to contribute to organizational goals (McGregor, 1960). He called this Theory Y and contrasted it with the more cynical Theory X, the assumption that people do not really want to work or contribute hence have to be motivated, incentivized, rewarded and punished, and, most important of all, monitored and controlled. I do not believe it is possible to achieve quality, safety, and value with Theory X leadership at any level. The implication is that macro leaders have to hold Theory Y assumptions for the meso- and microsystem levels to achieve the desired goals. A further implication is that Boards who appoint and support macro leaders have to learn to assess this fundamental attitude and ensure that the people at the very top have this optimistic view of human nature. The detailed list of what effective leaders do in this paper are basically a reflection of a Theory Y attitude.

Point 2. Macro leaders have to hold their immediate direct reports accountable for creating a climate of inquiry, openness, and trust (Schein, 2009, 2013, 2016). In order to do that, they must exhibit those behaviors themselves and regularly inquire of their direct reports how they are creating such an environment for their direct reports and how they are holding them accountable. An accountability system based on Theory Y focuses on the senior person being clear about the mission and targets to be achieved, discussing this with direct reports until true consensus is achieved, and regularly sitting down with each direct report to ask how it is going and what help is needed. The senior person does not "measure" in the quantitative or monitoring sense, but regularly (weekly or monthly) has an open dialogue with each direct report and/or with the whole group if they are interdependent. Accountability is created through the leaders' curiosity and regular dialogues with the direct reports.

Point 3. How things work is all about the quality of the relationship across hierarchical and functional boundaries. We design structures and processes but fail to design relationships. In most cultures, the "default" relationship position is what I would call Level 1, or transactional relationships, which incidentally includes professional relationships such as doctor-patient and doctor-nurse. However, there is nothing in Level 1 relationships that guarantees openness and trust. To elicit openness and trust we must move to what I have called a Level 2 more personal relationship (Schein and Schein, 2018, 2019). We do not have to be intimate across these boundaries, we do not even have to be friends, but we must acknowledge the other person as a whole person not just someone who plays a "role" like patient or nurse. It is easy to glibly specify that in an effective system there will be trust and openness, but there is very little said in our various literatures about how to achieve that magical condition of trust and openness. In my recent books on helping, I have noted that what our macro culture designates as an appropriate relationship across such boundaries should be respectful and "professionally distant" (Schein, 2013, 2016). But that is a Level 1 transactional relationship, which, in proposing professional distance, actually undermines openness and trust. Instead, managers should have an appropriately personalized relationship with their direct reports (Level 2) and I have tried to illustrate how one achieves such a relationship through appropriate humble inquiry and being more personal oneself. To get there of course requires Theory Y attitudes and shared learning.

Point 4. The goals of co-created healthcare services are very clear, as are the conditions that have to be present to achieve them. What is much less clear is what kind of a joint learning process will have to occur to get there (Edmondson, 2012). There is an amazing lack of clear theorizing about what it takes for groups and systems to learn new ways of doing things. We have formal learning theories that derive from organizational sociologists and social psychologists (Schön, 1983; Edmondson, 2012), we have business change theorists such as Kotter (1996), we have all the methods and theories that derive from the production improvement models of the Toyota Production System and "Lean" (Plsek, 2014), and we have the change theories that grew out of the Tavistock Institute and Lewin's group dynamics theories (Lewin and Lewin, 1948; Beckhard and Harris, 1987; Trist and Murray, 1990; Bunker and Alban, 1997) but amazingly little cross referencing or aligning of these models. We learn that micro-, meso-, and macrosystem can coordinate their activities and produce dramatic improvements but we do not yet have a model of the learning process that gets us there. We need to document how the leaders at each level learned the right attitudes and skills, and how they passed those on in the system.

Point 5. The essence of that learning process will be how to forge new Level 2 "personized" relationships. It will be less about individual competencies and more about how to learn together in dialogic modes based on a spirit of inquiry (Bushe and Marshak, 2015). It will be about getting the right people into the room together and then stimulating a new kind of conversation based on personal stories of goals, worries, and achievements. Each of the systems at each level will have developed its own culture based on occupational background and shared organizational experience. To make co-creation work will require mutual understanding of each other's cultures and, based on such understanding, forging a new "macro culture" that will preserve what is best in each local subculture but align its activities with the work of other subcultures (Schein, 2010).

Point 6. Examine carefully what the conditions are that facilitate motivation to learn something new. What data do we see that tells us that things are not working properly and need to be improved? The motivation to improve comes inevitably from some sense of dissatisfaction, we are disconfirmed in some way, and that can come in two forms. One, things we expected to work no longer work, and, two, the things that work still fall short of our ideals, of where we want to be (Schein, 2009). I believe that disconfirmation is an essential first step to learning because it produces uncomfortable feelings of anxiety, failure, and disappointment. When our new efforts initially fail, we have to remind ourselves that the old effort was failing as well, so we must try again. Failure is a source of learning and, therefore, must be accepted and analyzed. In that regard, near misses and close calls are equally important stimuli to learning. However, it takes a Theory Y leader and manager to create a climate of psychological safety for direct reports so that they can report near misses, close calls, and actual failures and be rewarded for reporting them so that everyone can learn.

In conclusion, I think the goals that the micro-, meso-, and macrosystem alignments espouse are clearly critical for the future of co-created health. What the successful efforts teach us is that it is possible. However, I believe it is only regularly possible with a certain kind of leadership at every level that honors and values more personal relationships and creates the conditions that allow people to trust each other and be open with each other.

Conclusion

Leading at the micro-, meso-, and macrosystem of an organization is the same, and yet it is different. The leaders' work at each of the levels includes gaining knowledge, taking action, and reviewing and reflecting. Leaders at the macro and mesosystem levels may have more ability to create vertical alignment of the organization's vision, mission, and values. Leaders at the micro- and mesosystem levels have deeper knowledge of the coproduced care necessary to meet the needs of populations through horizontal alignment of microsystems into service lines that can move organizations toward value-based care.

Summary

In this chapter, we have reviewed the work of leading at multiple organizational levels to achieve value-based care. Structural redesign, current leadership priorities, and understanding of what leading looks like in a multilevel organization can result in new leadership for today and the future. Professor Edgar H. Schein rounds out the chapter reflecting on the importance of leaders creating conditions for relationships, joint learning, and productive group dynamics.

Review Questions

1. Define microsystem, mesosystem, and macrosystem.
2. What three activities comprise the work of the leader?
3. Describe how the work of micro-, meso-, and macrosystem leaders differs.
4. Review the six priorities of leading healthcare improvements. Provide an example of each.
5. What is the difference between a Level 1 and Level 2 relationship?
6. Define "personized" in defining relationships.

Discussion Questions

1. Consider Figures 3.1 and 3.2 – what makes the most sense to you? Discuss your choice building off your own experiences in health care and/or leadership.
2. Review the six priorities for leading healthcare improvement. How do you see these reflected in the case study? Do you have examples from your own experience?
3. Dr. Schein discussed our failure to "design relationships." What does that mean?

Additional Activities

1. Draw a picture of your organization's alignment of micro-, meso-, and macrosystem levels.
2. Create an action plan to intentionally design relationships in your work setting.
3. Interview leaders at each level of the organization (micro-, meso-, and macrosystem) about their strategies to lead actions at each level of the organization.
4. The leadership case study discusses having feet in two different canoes. What metaphor would you use to describe leadership in your organization?

References

Arendt, H. *The Human Condition.* Chicago, IL: University of Chicago Press, 1998.

Argyris, C., and Schön, D. A. *Organizational Learning II: Theory, Method and Practice.* Reading, MA: Addison-Wesley, 1996.

Barr, V. J., Robinson, S., Marin-Link, B., and others. "The Expanded Chronic Care Model: An Integration of Concepts and Strategies from Population Health Promotion and the Chronic Care Model." *Healthcare Quarterly,* 2003, 7(1), 73-82.

Batalden, P. B., Nelson, E. C., Gardent, P. B., and Godfrey, M. M. "Leading the Macrosystem and Mesosystem for Microsystem Peak Performance." In S. Berman (ed.), *From Front Office to Front Line: Essential Issues for Health Care Leaders.* Oakbrook Terrace, IL: Joint Commission Resources, 2005, 1-40.

Batalden, P. B., Ogrinc, G., and Batalden, M. K. "From One to Many." *Journal of Interprofessional Care,* 2006, 20(5), 549-551.

Batalden, P. B. "Make the Most of Your Turn. In P. Batalden (ed.), *Lessons Learned in Changing Healthcare . . . And How We Learned Them.* Toronto, ON: Longwoods Publishing Corporation, 2010.

Batalden, P. B. "The Evolutionary Beginnings of the Model." In P. Batalden and T. Foster (eds.), *Sustainably Improving Health Care: Creatively Linking Care Outcomes, System Performance and Professional Development.* Boca Raton, FL: CRC Press, 2012.

Batalden, M. K., Batalden, P., Margolis, P., and others. "Coproduction of Healthcare Service." *BMJ Quality & Safety*, 2016, 25, 509-517. doi:10.1136/bmjqs-2015-004315

Beckhard, R. *Organization Development: Strategies and Models.* Reading, MA: Addison-Wesley, 1969.

Beckhard, R., and Harris, R. T. *Organizational Transitions: Managing Complex Change.* Reading, MA: Addison-Wesley, 1987.

Bennett, N., and Lemoin, C. J. "What a Difference a Word Makes: Understanding Threats to Performance in a VUCA World." *Business Horizons*, 2014, 57, 311-317.

Berwick, D. M. *Promising Care: How We Can Rescue Health Care by Improving It.* San Francisco, CA: Jossey-Bass, 2014.

Bolman, L. G., and Deal, T. E. "Reframing Leadership: The Effects of Leaders' Images of Leadership." In K. E. Clark, M. B. Clark, and D. Campbell (eds.), *Impact of Leadership.* Greensboro, NC: Center for Creative Leadership, 1992.

Bunker, B. B., and Alban, B. T. *Large Group Intervention: Engaging the Whole System for Rapid Change.* San Francisco, CA: Jossey-Bass, 1997.

Bushe, G. R., and Marshak, R. J. (eds). *Dialogic Organization Development: The Theory and Practice of Transformational Change.* San Francisco, CA: Berrett-Koehler, 2015.

Douglas, M. *How Institutions Think.* Syracuse, NY: Syracuse University Press, 1986.

Edmondson, A. C. *Teaming: How Organizations Learn, Innovate, and Compete in the Knowledge Economy.* San Francisco, CA: Jossey-Bass, 2012.

Gamson, J. "Silence, Death and the Invisible Enemy: AIDS Activism and Social Movement 'Newness.'" *Social Problems*, 1989, 36(4), 351-367.

Geus, A. "The living Company." *Harvard Business Review*, 1997, 97, 51-59.

Glass, K. P., and Anderson, J. R. "Relative Value Units: From A to Z (Part I of IV). *The Journal of Medical Practice Management*, 2002, 17(55), 225-228.

Hardin, G. "The tragedy of the commons." *Science*, 1968, 162(3859), 1243-1248. doi: 10.1126/science.162.3859.1243

Hock, D. *One from Many: VISA and the Rise of Chaordic Organization.* San Francisco, CA: Berrett-Koehler, 2005.

Kegan, R., and Lahey, L. *Immunity to Change.* Boston, MA: Harvard Business Press, 2009.

Kindig, D. A., Asada, Y., and Booske, B. "A Population Health Framework for Setting National and State Health Goals." *JAMA* 2008, 299(17), 2081-2083. doi:10.1001/jama.299.17.2081

Kotter, J. P. *Leading Change.* Boston, MA: Harvard Business School Press, 1996.

Kravitz, R. L., and Duan N. (eds), and the DEcIDE Methods Center N-of-1 Guidance Panel (Duan, N., and others). *Design and Implementation of N-of-1 Trials: A User's Guide. AHRQ Publication No. 13(14)-EHC122-EF.* Rockville, MD: Agency for Healthcare Research and Quality, 2014. [www.effectivehealthcare.ahrq.gov/N-1-Trials.cfm]

Lewin, K., and Lewin, G. W. *Resolving Social Conflicts: Selected Papers on Group Dynamics, 1935-1946.* New York, NY: HarperCollins, 1948.

Lucas, B., and Nacer, H. *The Habits of an Improver: Thinking About Learning for Improvement in Health Care.* London: The Health Foundation, 2015.

McGregor, D. M. *The Human Side of Enterprise.* New York, NY: McGraw-Hill, 1960.

McWilliams, J. M., Chernew, M. E., Landon, B. E., and Schwartz, A. L. "Performance Differences in Year 1 of Pioneer Accountable Care Organizations." *New England Journal of Medicine*, 2015, 372(20), 1927-1936. doi: 10.1056/NEJMsa1414929

Nelson, E. C., Batalden, P. B., and Godfrey, M. M. "Success Characteristics of High Performing Microsystems." In E. C. Nelson, P. B. Batalden, and M. M. Godfrey (eds.), *Quality by Design: A Clinical Microsystems Approach.* San Francisco, CA: Jossey-Bass, 2007.

Nolan, T.W. *Execution of Strategic Improvement Initiatives to Produce System-Level Results.* IHI Innovation Series White Paper. Cambridge, MA: Institute for Healthcare Improvement, 2007. (Available on www.ihi.org)

Ohno, T. *Toyota Production System: Beyond Large-Scale Production.* Cambridge, MA: Productivity Press, 1988.

O'Neill, P. "Foreword." In T. Cox (ed.), *Creating the Multicultural Organization.* San Francisco, CA: Jossey-Bass, 2001.

Palmer, P. J. *To Know As We Are Known: A Spirituality of Education.* New York, NY: Harper & Row, 1983.

Plsek, P. *Accelerating Health Care Transformation with Lean and Innovation.* Boca Raton, FL: CRC Press, 2014.

Porter, M. E. "Value-Based Health Care Delivery." *Annals of Surgery,* 2008, 248(4), 503-509.

Quinn, J. B. *Intelligent Enterprise: A Knowledge and Service Based Paradigm For Industry.* New York, NY: Free Press, 1992.

Revans, R. W. *Standards for Morale: Cause and Effect in Hospitals.* London: Oxford University Press, 1964.

Schein, E. H. *Helping: How to Offer, Give, and Receive Help.* San Francisco, CA: Berrett-Koehler, 2009.

Schein, E. H. *Organizational Culture and Leadership,* 4th edition. San Francisco, CA: Jossey-Bass, 2010.

Schein, E. H. *Humble Inquiry: The Gentle Art of Asking Instead of Telling.* San Francisco, CA: Berrett-Koehler, 2013.

Schein, E. H. *Humble Consulting: How to Provide Real Help Faster.* San Francisco, CA: Berrett-Koehler, 2016.

Schein, E. H., and Schein, P. *Humble Leadership: The Power of Relationships, Openness, and Trust.* Oakland, CA: Berrett-Koehler Publishers, Inc., 2018.

Schein, E. H., and Schein, P. *The Corporate Culture Survival Guide,* 3rd edition. Hoboken, NJ: John Wiley & Sons, Inc., 2019.

Schottenfeld, L., Petersen, D., Peikes, D., and others. *Creating Patient-Centered Team-Based Primary Care.* AHRQ Pub. No. 16-0002-EF. Rockville, MD: Agency for Healthcare Research and Quality, 2016.

Schön, D. A. *The Reflective Practitioner: How Professionals Think in Action.* New York, NY: Basic Books, 1983.

Senge, P. M., Kleiner, A., Roberts, C., and others. *The Fifth Discipline Fieldbook: Strategies and Tools for Building a Learning Organization.* New York, NY: Currency Doubleday, 1994.

Senge, P. *The Fifth Discipline: The Art and Practice of the Learning Organization.* New York, NY: Currency Doubleday, 2006.

Silversin, J., and Kornacki, M. J. "Creating a Physician Compact That Drives Group Success." *Medical Group Management Journal,* 2000, 47(3), 54-58, 60, 62.

Thomas, F. G., and Caldis, T. "Emerging Issues of Pay-For-Performance in Health Care." *Health Care Financing Review,* 2007, 29(1), 1-4.

Trist, E., and Murray, H. (eds). *The Social Engagement of Social Science: A Tavistock Anthology,* Vol. 1. Philadelphia, PA: University of Pennsylvania Press, 1990.

Vandenbroucke, J. P. "Observational Research, Randomized Trials, and Two Views of Medical Science." *Public Library of Science Medicine,* 2008, 5(3), e67, 339-343.

Additional Resources

Catalyst/Transforming Healthcare/Healthcare Leadership, https://createvalue.org/

Dartmouth Institute Microsystem Academy (The), http://www.clinicalmicrosystem.org/

Emerging Nurse Leader – a leadership development blog, https://www.emergingrnleader.com/

Habits of an improver (The), http://www.health.org.uk/sites/health/files/ TheHabitsOfAnImprover.pdf

Harvard Business Review – Leading the way, https://www.harvardbusiness.org/leadership-learning-insights/blog/

Human Synergistics, https://www.humansynergistics.com/home

Institute for Healthcare Improvement (IHI), http://www.ihi.org/

Organizational Culture and Leadership Institute, http://www.scheinocli.org/

Key Words/Terms

Accountable care organization: Groups of doctors, hospitals, and other healthcare providers, who come together voluntarily to give coordinated high-quality care to the Medicare patients they serve.

Balanced metrics: A well-rounded set of measures that reflect important dimensions of quality and performance.

Bend the cost curve: To drive down medical costs.

Care coordination: The deliberate organization of patient care activities between two or more participants involved in a patient's care to facilitate the appropriate delivery of health-care services.

Community-based interventions: Refer to multicomponent interventions that generally combine individual and environmental change strategies across multiple settings aiming to prevent dysfunction and to promote well-being among population groups in a defined local community.

Coproduction: Describes health care as a service, which is co-created by healthcare professionals in relationship with one another and with people seeking help to restore or maintain health for themselves and their families.

Fee for service: A payment model where services are unbundled and paid for separately. In health-care, it gives an incentive for providers to provide more treatments because payment is based on the quantity of care, rather than the quality of care.

"Feed forward": The modification or control of a process using its anticipated results or effects.

"Feedback": The modification or control of a process or system by its results or effects.

Globally capitated (Global capitation): A payment model specifically for integrated healthcare delivery. By accepting a defined fixed payment to provide contracted services, providers assume the financial risk for their patients, usually including both insurance risk and technical risk.

Handoffs: To pass from one to another.

Health continuum: Describes the delivery of health care over a period of time and refers to an integrated system of health care that follows a patient through time or through a range of services. The goal of a health continuum is to offer more comprehensive patient care.

Huddles: To gather together to strategize, motivate, or celebrate, usually for a short duration.

Multispecialty group practice. The presence of two or more providers offering various types of medical specialty care within one practice.

Physician "compact": Popularized by Dr. Jack Silversin, founder of Amicus Consulting, a physician compact is where the healthcare organization and their physicians choose to engage with each other to understand their respective perspectives of the changing healthcare landscape, and to negotiate a new set of mutual expectations (Silversin and Kornacki, 2000).

Population health: An interdisciplinary, customizable approach that allows health departments to connect practice to policy for change to happen locally. This approach uses non-traditional partnerships among different sectors in the community – public health, industry, academia, health care, local governments, etc. to achieve positive health outcomes.

Reflection: Careful thought or consideration.

Relative value units (RVUs): Originally developed as a physician payment mechanism, RVUs have expanded into a valuable practice management tool that allows common denominator analyses and per-unit comparisons for both clinical productivity and expense data. Use of RVUs in practice management falls into three broad categories: productivity, cost, and benchmarking (Glass and Anderson, 2002).

Root cause analysis: A systematic process for identifying "root causes" of problems or events and an approach for responding to them. Root cause analysis is based on the idea that effective management requires finding ways to prevent problems that develop.

Team-based care model: A delivery model where patient care needs are addressed as coordinated efforts among multiple healthcare providers and across settings of care (Schottenfeld and others, 2016).

Value-based care. A payment model that rewards healthcare providers for providing quality care to patients. Under this approach, providers seek to provide better care for their patients and better health for populations at lower cost.

White space. In organizations it is where unmet and unarticulated needs are uncovered to create innovation opportunities. It is where products and services don't exist based on the present understanding of values, definition of business or even existing competencies.

CHAPTER FOUR

DEVELOPING PROFESSIONALS AND IMPROVING WORK LIFE

Marjorie M. Godfrey, Tina C. Foster, Gay L. Landstrom, Joan Clifford, Julie K. Johnson

AIM

In this chapter, we focus on two new case studies to provide a real-world context for the guiding principles, useful insights, and practical methods that can help microsystem leaders develop their workforce and cultivate a positive working environment.

The aim of this chapter is to illustrate these innovative leadership strategies and principles including *team coaching* to create the conditions where staff at the front line of care can be the best they can be.

LEARNING OBJECTIVES

By the end of this chapter, the reader will be able to:

1. Identify current stressors in the workplace and their impact on quality of work and staff morale.
2. Compare key principles and models of leading that engage frontline staff to own improvement and change.
3. Discuss the impact of organizational investment in leadership development to create high-performing microsystems.
4. Describe the benefit of team coaching skills for a microsystem leader.
5. List the results that can be achieved in a microsystem as a result of leading differently.

Quality by Design: A Clinical Microsystems Approach, Second Edition. Edited by Marjorie M. Godfrey, Tina C. Foster, Julie K. Johnson, Eugene C. Nelson and Paul B. Batalden.
© 2025 John Wiley & Sons, Inc. Published 2025 by John Wiley & Sons, Inc.

Introduction

The previous chapters have focused on the *success characteristics of high-performing clinical microsystems*, with illustrations from research, cystic fibrosis care, and organizational leadership. Another key success characteristic is an intentionally designed workplace that promotes a culture in which everyone matters. Leaders who enable all staff to make the most out of their talent, training, and skills (Godfrey and others, 2003) can raise levels of performance not previously reached.

The genesis of this chapter is in our detailed qualitative study of 20 high-performing clinical microsystems. During the research we listened to the people who staffed those outstanding clinical microsystems and learned key tips and ideas to achieving work environments that yield outstanding outcomes (Nelson and others, 2002). We have added updated insights from two nursing leaders who describe their focus on creating environments where leaders at the frontline and staff can be the best they can be.

Despite the recognition of the importance of staff, staff development, and workplace culture, the clinical workplace is experiencing high rates of burnout, dissatisfaction, low staff morale, and high turnover rates in the United States. In 2015, 37 percent of newly licensed registered nurses were thinking of leaving the profession, 54 percent of physicians were burned out, and 60 percent of surveyed physicians were considering leaving their jobs (Shanafelt and others, 2015).

A 2019 survey of physicians in the United States and Europe reported on average 10 percent of physicians were feeling burned out and depressed (Popa, 2019). Nursing strikes have become more common. Nurses are seeking improved work conditions (many with implications for patient safety) such as time for breaks, elimination of mandatory overtime, and better patient ratios (Lardieri, 2019).

Based on 30 years of workplace tracking in the United States and across the globe, Clifton and Harter (2019) report that to address declining economics and productivity, organizations need to address their biggest failure to maximize human potential. Learning how to address and lead the new "will" of today's workforce can result in improved economics and productivity and a happier workforce. They further remind us that Gallup's 80 years of research identifies that 70 percent of the variance in team engagement is directly related to the frontline leader or manager.

The first case study describes a strategically planned intervention in a rural academic medical center led by the system chief nursing officer (SCNO) with the aim of transforming the mental model of leaders from one of hierarchy to one of distributed leadership attentive to maximizing the potential of staff.

The second case study is a *Doctor of Nursing Practice (DNP)* formal project that aimed to improve quality improvement education and skill development through frontline leadership. Interviews from these managers reveal the importance of new leadership knowledge, skills, and attitudes to create an inspiring work environment for all. New leadership approaches that optimize the work of each and every staff member and promote a culture where everyone matters allow the microsystem and mesosystems to attain levels of performance not previously experienced.

Case Study One: Dartmouth-Hitchcock Frontline Clinical Manager Development

A crucial, early task for a new clinical executive entering a healthcare organization is the detailed assessment of the capabilities of frontline managers. This was no different when a new SCNO arrived at Dartmouth-Hitchcock, a regionally distributed academic health system located in New Hampshire and Vermont. She held *focus groups* and individual meetings and analyzed a recent educational needs assessment report conducted for the organization's nurse managers and other clinical leaders. The SCNO's assessment led to a number of conclusions:

1. The healthcare system had invested little in the skills and development of the clinical managers, many of whom had held their leadership role for less than two years.
2. The leaders held a mental model of leadership that was predominantly hierarchical. *Shared governance* had stalled. *Distributed decision-making models of leadership* were not part of their overall mental model of leadership. The managers felt overwhelmed by their responsibilities, especially since they believed they had to shoulder their responsibilities alone.
3. The traditional hierarchical approach to leadership was reinforced and modeled by the leaders to whom these managers reported.

The challenge for the new SCNO was threefold:

- First, new expectations needed to be established throughout the organization, and a perceived urgency for change ignited (Kotter, 2002; see Sidebar 4.1).
- Second, a significant number of the frontline clinical managers needed intensive skill development focused on engaging staff in the work of the clinical microsystem.
- Third, the organizational culture needed to change in order to foster and support a new style of leadership.

Kotter's Eight-Step Process for Leading Change

John P. Kotter is an internationally known best-selling author and a widely regarded authority on change and leadership from Harvard. In the book *Leading Change*, Kotter (1995, 1996) identified eight success factors in leading change based on research on 100 organizations going through change.

1. Create a sense of urgency

Kotter suggests that for change to be successful, 75 percent of a company's management needs to "buy into" the change. In other words, you have to work really hard on this first step and spend significant time and energy building urgency before moving on to the next steps. Without motivation people won't help and nothing is accomplished.

2. Build a guiding coalition

You can find effective change leaders throughout your organization – they do not necessarily follow the traditional company hierarchy. To lead change, you need to bring together a coalition, or team, of influential people whose power comes from a variety of sources, including job title, status, expertise, and political importance. Help them develop a shared assessment of their organization's problems and opportunities, and create a level of trust and communication. Arranging an off-site, two- or three-day retreat is frequently used to accomplish this task.

3. Form a strategic vision and initiatives

A clear vision can help everyone understand why you're asking them to do something and helps clarify the direction in which an organization needs to move. Develop a short summary (one or two sentences) that captures what you "see" as the future of your organization. Practice a vision speech and give it frequently. It's also important to "walk the talk." What you do is far more important – and believable – than what you say. Role model the kind of behavior that you want from others.

4. Enlist a volunteer army

Successful change includes identifying those who are interested in change. Those who are identified are often *early adopters of change* and willing to try out new ideas (Rogers, 1995).

5. Enable action by removing barriers

Put in place the structure for change, and continually check for barriers to it. Removing obstacles can empower the people you need to execute your vision, and it can help the change move forward. Recognize and reward people for making change happen.

6. Generate short-term wins

Create short-term targets – not just one long-term goal. You want each smaller target to be achievable, with little room for failure. Real transformation takes time, and a renewal effort risks losing momentum if there are no short-term goals to meet and celebrate. Most people won't go on the long march unless they see compelling evidence within 12 to 24 months that the journey is producing expected results.

7. Sustain acceleration

Learning and rolling out change successfully requires starting slow and then ramping up with multiple changes. Each success provides an opportunity to build on what went right and identify what you can improve. Most successful transformations have a trajectory of increasing change over time – years, not weeks or months. The SCNO in the case study started with one small group of early, ready-to-learn and open-to-change managers. The roll out to additional managers was in process to build a deeply and emotionally committed team, which according to Kotter and Cohen (2002) would result in sustainable change the longer the early adopters and later change agents were engaged.

8. Institute change

Until new behaviors are rooted in social norms and shared values, they are subject to degradation as soon as the pressure for change is removed. It is important that your organization's leaders continue to support change. This includes existing staff and new leaders who are brought in. If you lose the support of these people, you might end up back where you started. Tell success stories about the change process and repeat other success stories that you hear every chance you can. Kotter's book, *The Heart of Change* (2002), provides additional insights into storytelling and engaging staff in change. Include the change ideals and values when hiring and training new staff. Publicly recognize key members of your original change coalition, and make sure the rest of the staff – new and old – remember their contributions. Create plans to replace key leaders of change as they move on. This will help ensure that their legacy is not lost or forgotten.

The SCNO obtained funding and organizational support for an educational intervention for clinical managers led by The Dartmouth Institute Microsystem Academy (www.clinicalmicrosystem.org). She communicated the importance of fostering empowerment of staff and the need for education and skill development to leadership at all levels of the organization, linking the proposed intervention with key organizational strategic objectives. Her executive message communicated that *only this new style of leadership would be rewarded in the future.* The rewards included the potential for new responsibilities and promotion within the organization. While the SCNO wanted the entire frontline leadership team to experience this training, she sought volunteers for the first cohort. This was an intentional choice to find those who were most motivated to learn a new style of leadership, increasing the likelihood of a successful outcome.

The SCNO believed that learning a new approach to leadership required *experiential learning*, which in turn required opportunities to apply the new skills in real-world, daily leadership challenges with support and reinforcement from the SCNO and the cohort. The world-renowned eCoach-the-Coach (eCTC) program of The Dartmouth Institute Microsystem Academy aligned with this approach (see Sidebar 4.2).

This five-month virtual and in-person experiential learning program provided the opportunity for the Dartmouth-Hitchcock clinical manager cohort to learn how to engage staff in quality improvement and practice new approaches to staff empowerment and engagement in decision-making. As an added bonus, participation in the international eCTC program exposed the Dartmouth-Hitchcock cohort to classmates who came from organizations across the United States and Europe. The clinical managers gained new skills and beliefs about leadership, and also came to recognize that the challenges of their daily work were shared by healthcare leaders all over the globe. This broadening of perspective seemed to unleash their creativity to address challenges in a new way and reduce their previous feelings of isolation and helplessness.

eCoach-the-Coach Program

The eCTC Program is an intensive, dynamic, and highly interactive five-part series (four online sessions and one 3-day onsite session) that offers a unique curriculum that blends the art and science of team coaching with foundational improvement and measurement knowledge and skills along with communication habits necessary to successfully coach frontline teams in their improvement efforts.

Central to the Team Coaching Program is "The Team Coaching Model" developed by the first author, with three phases of team coaching: pre-phase, action phase, and transition phase grounded in multiple disciplines, theories, and original research focused on cultivating improvement and group dynamic capabilities at the frontline of health care (Godfrey and others, 2014a).

The discipline of team coaching builds on Edgar H. Schein's (2009, 2013) work in "helping" groups and using humble inquiry rather than "telling" groups what to do. "Coaches in training" learn and practice that helping and humble inquiry can create supportive relationships with interdisciplinary improvement teams to result in exploring new possibilities, innovation, and improved overall team dynamics.

Ultimately, the overall aim of the Team Coaching Program is to improve the value, safety, and quality of healthcare outcomes through the development of team coaching knowledge, skills, and abilities to coach frontline interdisciplinary clinical and supporting microsystems with knowledge, processes, and tools including the Dartmouth Microsystem Improvement Curriculum. (eCTC has been renamed "The Team Coaching Program" and can be found at www.clinicalmicrosystem.org.)

The five-month program included a three-day, face-to-face meeting coached by expert faculty that allowed the entire class to practice new language, approaches, and skills in person. The experience was enhanced by living, eating, and working together at a beautiful retreat setting. Participants experienced a remarkable level of bonding that yielded long-term commitment to supporting one another through the many months of improvement implementation after the end of the program.

One of the most challenging elements of this program was preparing the organization to receive leaders who had learned to lead in a very different way. The new style of leading in an empowering manner could easily have been extinguished had the organization not been prepared to support and receive the altered approaches of the leaders. It would have been ideal to begin these changes from the highest levels of leadership, organizationally cascading down through vice-presidents and directors before reaching the frontline managers. However, the SCNO appreciated the urgent need for frontline staff to experience leadership that would be more engaging and satisfying; waiting for cascading change could not be tolerated. Turnover across the clinical enterprise was already well above national averages – as high as 28 percent per year in some clinical areas.

The directors for each of the clinical managers received a concentrated educational program to provide an overview and specifics of the development program and the rationale behind it. The SCNO communicated her clear expectations that the directors would support the new empowering leadership style of their managers enrolled in the program.

The SCNO knew that a single cohort of 14 clinical managers would not be enough to change the culture across the organization. Plans were developed and funding secured to continue sending two cohorts of clinical managers through the program each year, until all had completed the program. Unfortunately, a change in executive leadership stalled the implementation of the plan after the third cohort. An early reflection of the benefits of the program was that participants in the first and second cohorts requested additional education and opportunities for skill development, and also volunteered to serve as mentors for participants in later cohorts. Building and compounding the skills, experiences, and expertise of these leaders would accelerate reaching a *tipping point* (Gladwell, 2000).

The change experienced within the leaders was evaluated by focus groups, surveys, examination of the products of their knowledge application projects and knowledge assessments (Godfrey and others, 2016). Results demonstrated that these leaders not only acquired new knowledge and skills, but also acquired enhanced confidence in their ability to lead. (Figures 4.1 and 4.2). Prior to the implementation of the eCTC program, turnover of nurse managers each year was in excess of 20 percent. During the 12 months following the program, turnover of the managers participating in and completing the program in cohorts one and two ($n=19$) was less than six percent, with one of the managers choosing to transfer within the organization to a different leadership position. No program graduates left the organization.

For Dartmouth-Hitchcock, the intervention of an experiential learning program for frontline managers on how to lead improvement and create an empowering environment yielded confident, skilled, and satisfied frontline leaders, with retention serving as a surrogate measure for satisfaction. Further study is needed to understand the numbers required to reach the tipping point for organizational change in leadership style, and to measure the impact of these new leaders on staff satisfaction and the increased productivity resulting from an improved environment of care.

Case Study Two: Exploring a Reflective Team Coaching Model as a Leadership Strategy to Cultivate Frontline Quality and Safety Improvement Capability

This case study is based on a Doctor of Nursing Practice (DNP) project where the candidate addressed quality and safety at the front line of care by increasing each manager's improvement knowledge, skills, and ability to coach frontline staff to

FIGURE 4.1 PARTICIPANT CONFIDENCE WITH CONFLICT MANAGEMENT AND RELATIONSHIPS.

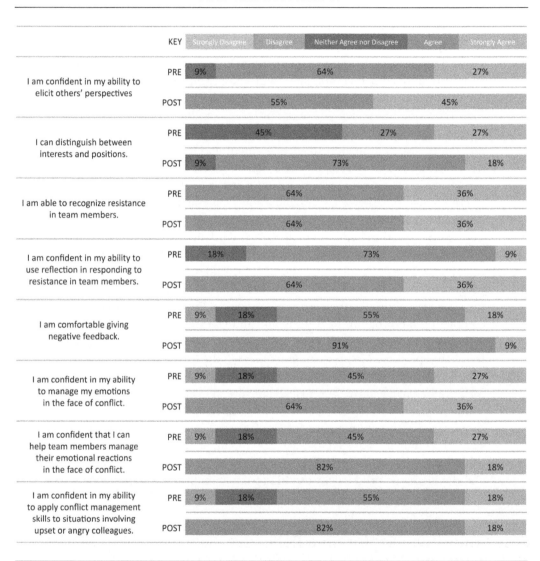

provide care and improve care. Ensuring quality and safety is crucial because we continue to cause harm in medical care in our healthcare systems (IOM, 2007). Optimizing systems to reduce preventable harm is a national priority (AHRQ, 2015). The Institute of Medicine (IOM) reported medical errors cause up to 98,000

FIGURE 4.2 COACHES-IN-TRAINING CONFIDENCE IN COACHING SKILLS.

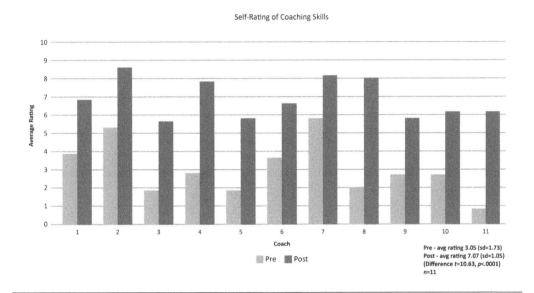

Self-Rating of Coaching Skills

Pre - avg rating 3.05 (sd=1.73)
Post - avg rating 7.07 (sd=1.05)
(Difference *t*=10.63, *p*<.0001)
n=11

deaths and more than one million injuries each year in the United States at an estimated cost of $50 billion per year (IOM, 2000). The Department of Health and Human Services established a goal to reduce *Hospital Acquired Conditions (HACs)* by 20 percent from 2014 to 2019. The baseline of 99 HACs per 1,000 discharges was established to monitor the reduction. This baseline would equate to 79 HACs per 1,000 discharges by 2019. Preliminary data estimated the HAC's in 2017 was 86 HACs per 1,000 discharges. There was a 13 percent reduction in hospital acquired conditions from 2014 to preliminary data for 2017. Hospital patients experienced 1.3 million fewer HACs over the three-year period, approximately 910,000 fewer HACs than if the 2014 rate had persisted. These reductions equated to approximately $7.7 billion in costs saved and 20,500 HAC-related inpatient deaths averted (AHRQ, 2019). Caring for the health and well-being of people is important work – we have to do a better job of doing so safely and reliably.

One of the recommendations of the IOM report was to expand opportunities for nurses to lead and diffuse collaborative improvement efforts (IOM, 2010). It is unclear if the knowledge, skills, and supportive structures to support this recommendation currently exist in acute care settings.

Nurse managers are leaders of their microsystems and must ensure that the unit meets quality and safety objectives. Uniquely positioned to affect the outcomes of their work units, managers need to be able to blend technical, managerial, communication, and relationship skills to promote quality and safety outcomes. However, research suggests that they often do not have adequate leadership skills to do so (Riles and others, 2010; Djukic and others, 2015). Managers need support, education, and skills for their role in leading and cultivating frontline improvement.

The nurse manager has to connect ideas, priorities, and organizational strategy to daily operations. There is a gap between the executive leaders and the clinical microsystems led by nurse managers. The nurse manager knows the patient's journey and can understand how staff providing care to patients and families can connect organizational priorities and clinical microsystems. It is important for managers to own responsibility for every patient's journey (Parand and others, 2014). Further, the nurse manager needs skills to lead the assessment of the unit to identify strengths and improvement opportunities for staff seeking to create an optimal patient journey and find joy in their work.

This gap in organizational alignment from the top to the bottom of the organization (Foster and others, 2007) is a "middle management problem" (Godfrey, 2014b). Focusing on and linking organizational priorities and each microsystem's work is an expectation of the "manager in the middle." However, identifying what really matters and using a team approach to solve problems does not happen naturally. Staff and leaders need to be developed with new knowledge and skills.

Nurse managers need a variety of tools to be successful in managing and leading their microsystems. Reflective team coaching is an effective leadership strategy to develop their own and their staff's knowledge and skills in the science of improvement and in the art of coaching improvement and creating supportive cultures. The skills associated with the art of coaching improvement are useful in many situations involving group dynamics and interprofessional collaboration to provide care and improve care. Incorporating reflective team coaching into nurse manager leadership development plans can assist in creating the conditions to cultivate frontline quality and safety improvement capability and joy in work.

The DNP Project

The Doctor of Nursing Practice project used a *mixed method quality improvement design* with a survey (*quantitative*) and focus group (*qualitative*) evaluative approach. The global aim was to evaluate the impact of the Team Coaching Model's intervention on nurse managers' leadership development through enhanced knowledge and skill in quality improvement and outcomes of care. Specific aims of this project were:

1. To evaluate the change in knowledge, abilities, and skills over time.
2. To describe themes of leadership development from nurse leaders who completed the program, submitted final reflective coaching development plans, and participated in a focus group.

Participants in this development program included five acute care nurse managers in a multidivisional, academic medical center in the Veterans Health Administration (VHA) in West Roxbury, Massachusetts. The nurse managers participated in the eCoach-the-Coach (eCTC) program developed by The Dartmouth Institute Microsystem Academy to develop team coaching skills to improve the workplace and educate staff on improvement (see Sidebar 4.2). Nurse managers coached an improvement team from a unit other than their own to increase the likelihood of success and minimize prior history. Two of the managers coached a team with only nursing staff members; three coached interprofessional teams.

Results

A modified Quality Improvement Assessment (QIA) instrument was used to evaluate the effect of the team coaching model intervention on nurse managers' knowledge and skill in quality improvement (Godfrey, Foster, and Nilsson, 2018). As part of the eCTC program (see Sidebar 4.2), nurse managers completed the online QIA instrument before beginning the program, at the end of the program, and six months after completion of the program. Table 4.1 illustrates the summary of the findings and changes over time.

The end of the eCTC program included participant reflections about the experiential learning experience and included:

- a self-evaluation scale of team coaching skills including a 10-point scale of perceived overall coaching confidence and skill (see Table 4.2).
- a self-development action plan to continue to develop as a team coach.
- a summary narrative of the team coaching experience over the five-month period.

The written work (eCTC Coach Development Plan and Team Coaching Experience) of the nurse managers was analyzed using an iterative approach to identify themes about managers' experiences and lessons learned in the program. The iterative approach (Patton, 2015) is key to gaining insight and developing meaning about an experience. Through a systematic, repetitive, and recursive process of reviewing and reflecting on the pre- and post-Quality Improvement Assessment tool and the narrative from the written eCTC documents these themes emerged.

Learning to listen or "sit on one's hands" and not jump in to fix things. The theme of learning to listen ultimately transcended the coaching role to become something used in daily practice.

> *"I've learned that you have to stop yourself from interrupting when you think you know what the other person is saying – wait until he/she is finished speaking and then repeat back what you think you heard to learn if it's the same message that the other person was trying to convey."*

TABLE 4.1 CHANGES OVER TIME.

Pre	Post	6 months		Time1 – Time2	Time2 – Time3
4.67	3.67	4.33	How important do you consider continuous quality improvement in your professional work?	⇓	⇑
3.00	3.67	3.67	How confident are you that you can make a change to improve health care in your clinic?	⇑	–
3.00	4.00	4.33	Use effective meeting skills (timed agendas/assign meeting roles)	⇑	⇑
2.33	4.00	4.33	Use brainstorming and multi-voting in meetings	⇑	⇑
1.67	3.67	4.00	Assess the 5Ps	⇑	⇑
2.67	4.00	4.33	Use data to determine improvement theme	⇑	⇑
2.00	4.00	4.33	Create process maps (flow charts)	⇑	⇑
2.33	4.00	4.33	Develop specific aim statements	⇑	⇑
2.00	3.33	4.33	Create fishbones (cause and effect diagrams)	⇑	⇑
2.33	4.00	4.33	Identify evidence-based practice for change ideas	⇑	⇑
2.00	3.67	4.00	Adapt Smart Change Ideas to make improvements	⇑	⇑
2.33	3.67	4.33	Develop PDSA cycles (Plan-Do-Study-Act)	⇑	⇑
1.67	3.67	4.33	Develop SDSA cycles (Standardize-Do-Study-Act)	⇑	⇑
1.67	3.33	4.33	Create plays for playbooks (standard operating procedures)	⇑	⇑
2.33	3.33	4.33	Use LEAN improvement knowledge and tools	⇑	⇑
2.0	3.33	4.33	5S (Sort, Set, Shine, Standardize, Sustain)	⇑	⇑
1.67	3.33	4.00	Value stream mapping	⇑	⇑
1.33	3.67	4.00	Create workflow diagrams/ spaghetti diagrams	⇑	⇑
1.33	3.33	4.00	Create and use driver diagrams, including outcome measures	⇑	⇑
1.33	3.33	4.00	Mesosystem improvement including feed forward and feedback data	⇑	⇑
1.67	3.67	4.00	Manage up in the healthcare organization	⇑	⇑
2.00	4.00	4.33	Use observation skills	⇑	⇑

TABLE 4.1 (*Continued*)

Pre	Post	6 months		Time1 – Time2	Time2 – Time3
1.33	3.00	3.33	Conduct force field analysis	⇑	⇑
1.33	3.33	4.00	Explore the ladder of inference	⇑	⇑
1.67	3.67	4.00	Define measures (conceptual and operational definitions)	⇑	⇑
2.00	4.00	4.33	Use Microsoft Excel (basic/ fundamental skills)	⇑	⇑
1.67	4.00	3.67	Collect data using tick and tally sheets	⇑	⇓
1.67	3.67	4.33	Develop a data collection plan	⇑	⇑
1.67	3.67	4.00	Differentiate process, outcome and balanced measures	⇑	⇑
1.33	3.00	3.67	Create clinical value compass	⇑	⇑
1.33	4.00	3.67	Create and interpret run charts	⇑	⇓
1.33	3.00	3.00	Create and interpret statistical process control charts (p Charts, XmR charts)	⇑	–
1.33	3.00	3.67	Create and interpret data walls and dashboards to track improvement over time	⇑	⇑
1.33	3.33	3.33	Determine when to transition to "audit" of measures	⇑	–
0.83	0.77	0.8	I am confident in my ability to elicit others' perspectives	⇓	⇑
0.75	0.87	0.73	I am able to distinguish between interests and positions	⇑	⇓
0.83	0.87	0.87	I am able to recognize resistance in team members	⇑	–
0.67	0.87	0.8	I am confident in my ability to use reflection in responding to resistance in team members	⇑	⇓
0.83	0.87	0.8	I am comfortable giving negative feedback	⇑	⇓
0.75	0.87	0.67	I am confident in my ability to manage my emotions in the face of conflict	⇑	⇓
0.67	0.87	0.8	I am confident that I can help team members manage their emotional reactions in the face of conflict	⇑	⇓
0.07	0.87	0.8	I am confident in my ability to apply conflict management skills to situations involving upset or angry colleagues	⇑	⇓

TABLE 4.2 SELF-EVALUATION WITH COACHING INTERDISCIPLINARY PROFESSIONAL.

Participant	Before	After
A	4	8
B	2	4
C	1	5
D	2	3
E	2	7
Median	2	5

"The best part of this coaching experience was learning to listen and not make assumptions. Have faith in others."

Time and scheduling challenges. A challenge frequently reported was finding the time to coach and focus on improvement.

"Patient acuity along with high census were definite factors in maintaining regular [improvement] meetings."

"Our pace was most impacted by the fact that our group is comprised of healthcare workers that could not always leave the bedside when scheduled to [join meetings]."

"Coaching is not easy. The coaching process (and leadership) is not linear."

"Coaching is an art – difficult to teach the concept of coaching as in there is no Step 1, Step 2, Step 3 (which we often like in nursing), although having set steps in process improvement (ramp) helps keep things structured."

Effective meeting skills are essential. Participants reported they would continue to use the meeting skills that resulted in more organized, staff-engaged, and productive meetings they learned and practiced during the program.

"The biggest thing I learned was effective meeting skills. I know that might seem small but it has made a huge impact in my professional career already. I had never seen a meeting run so well and the practice and skills we got [at eCTC] were so beneficial."

Using learned coaching skills in daily practice and within the system. Nurse managers planned to use their new skills of inquiry, listening, reflecting, reframing, and offering help in their daily practice.

"I will use my experience to facilitate improvement work and improve communication with my own staff as well as future process improvement teams."

"I will help empower my staff to run their own meeting to make improvement on the unit."

Eight months following the completion of the eCTC program, four out of five nurse managers participated in a focus group. Although managers found the program helpful and continued to use some of the skills they learned in their day-to-day practice, they did not feel they had many opportunities to use their coaching skills. All four focus group participants reinforced the benefits of listening skills and "sitting on their hands." Consistent with the identified themes from the iterative analysis, nurse managers did report using effective meeting skills, active listening, and supporting the team to do the work rather than doing it themselves continued eight months after completing the program. Focus group participants felt they had empowered and encouraged frontline staff to lead improvement efforts and that the staff responded positively as noted in the participant quotes.

> *"The morale in my unit's a lot better. There is a lot more engagement. [Staff] need to bring ideas, instead of [nurse managers] just telling [staff] what to do. And it has improved."*

> *"I see so much ownership. . .they actually care about the results and care about how [improvement is] working on the unit, because they're the ones that are leading it."*

> *"[The staff] are the ones doing the leg work and deciding how to implement [improvement] with the input from the rest of the staff. So, they're really owning more of the results and how it's working."*

Barriers frequently mentioned included challenges with time due to variability in workflow on the unit.

Tips from the Case Studies

The two case studies exemplify both general principles and good practices to develop leaders at the front line who can help staff be the best they can be, achieve performance goals, and create a joyful workplace. These tips are relevant to any clinical micro- or mesosystem.

Invest in the leaders of frontline teams. Experiential learning with small cohorts to create a community of learners can provide support and reinforce new knowledge and skills in practice. A culture that provides a safe place to practice, and even fail, will support leaders' experiential learning, while also involving staff with those lessons. A few ways to support learning new knowledge and skills are listed:

- Include exposure to leaders outside one's own organization or microsystem to gain perspectives and see different approaches.
- Provide a place and space to learn where the leaders can unplug to learn, practice, and reflect.

- Hold monthly all-staff meetings to foster good communications, relationships, esprit de corps, and continuous improvement, which will highlight the importance of the work and leadership's commitment to it.
- Communicate and expect a "shared governance" model of leadership (Porter-O'Grady, 1991).

The era of "command and control" leadership is gone. Implementing a shared governance model requires attention to implementing the model and ongoing nurturing. The SCNO in case study one joined the organization with the understanding a shared governance model was in place, when in fact the model was not fully operational. Developing knowledge, skills, and attitudes to engage all staff members and leaders in the identification of strengths and improvement opportunities in their daily work was critical to re-energizing the shared governance model of leadership.

Invite staff into discussions about microsystem performance to create engagement and a sense of ownership, pride in doing the work, and real investment in the results of the work. The leaders' willingness and ability to "sit on their hands" and allow the ideas and solutions to bubble up from the front line is something that nurse managers found gratifying and empowering for frontline staff as they took ownership of their work.

Align leadership at all levels of the organization to support, promote, and invest in the development of new leadership knowledge and skills. The SCNO in case study one clearly sets the expectation of new leadership behaviors from the top of the organization to the front line. The SCNO expected the supervisors to support the new leadership actions and mental model at the front line.

The mission, vision, values, and guiding principles of the organization must be clear to everyone at all levels of the organization, to then specify how specific roles contribute to the mission and vision. This clarity at various organizational levels supports the frontline staff to see how their day-to-day efforts support larger organizational priorities. It is often the work of mesosystem and microsystem leaders to make the "translation" of the organization mission and vision into terms and activities that are specific, actionable, and relevant to the clinical microsystem. A clear vision of excellence (doing the right things right) that staff members can use to navigate the correct path forward in their own work must be created. The alignment of goals that cascade from organizational leadership to the front line allows each member of the microsystem to see how their work reflects the organization's core values and contributes to its mission. When combined with authentic and meaningful interactions at the microsystem level, staff will experience the deep sense of meaning that emerges when head, hands, and heart are united.

Frontline leaders are the connectors in an organization. Batalden (2014) described how the nurse manager needs the skills to help others make connections between the patient-focused work of the organization and that of the clinical microsystem. The improvement and coaching skills used in the Team Coaching Model are helpful in making this connection. Becoming more comfortable in the art and science of improvement and infusing the skills learned through the team coaching program into daily leadership processes will help the nurse manager develop the same abilities in frontline staff. Creating an environment where staff can develop and fully realize their potential is the nurse manager's job.

Link new leadership skills with incentives and promotions. The first case study clearly pointed out how the SCNO articulated and set new expectations that frontline leadership develop new skills and behaviors that would be directly linked to future promotions and opportunities.

Create a positive, even joyful, working climate. Develop a social environment for working that exemplifies respect, interdependency, service, learning, growth, and joy in the work. Through research Google realized work can be designed to actually make people happier, healthier, and more productive (https://rework.withgoogle.com/). Google named the research re:Work and offers a website to help share and push forward the practice and research of data-driven HR. All staff should value each staff member's contribution to meet patients' needs. A social working climate will generate patterns of respect – staff for other staff, staff for patients, staff for families – that enable all staff to handle turbulent times and situations effectively and empathically. In the third edition of *The New Economics*, Deming (2018) describes the relationship between performance and the system, highlighting the role of the manager as a helper – helping everyone do a better job. Schein (2013) reminds us of the importance of humble inquiry and genuine curiosity about the day-to-day work experience. Professor Schein points out that if you want to change behavior, it is often necessary to change the situation. A change in climate can have a marked effect on behavior. Schein and Schein describe four possible levels of relationships (shown in Table 4.3) in the workplace and encourage people to strive for level two relationships by learning more about each other and moving beyond transactional relationships to nurture high-performing workplaces. In *Humble Leadership*, Schein and Schein (2018) further explain that the level two relationship reinforces the interdependence of individuals and requires us to learn more about the whole person, not just a role and function, while building trust.

Multiple researchers (Nembhard and Edmondson, 2006; Carmeli and Gittell, 2009; Edmondson, 2012) have examined the importance of psychological safety for high-performing teams. Building level two relationships increases the psychological safety of staff in the workplace. Team members are more likely to ask questions and speak up without fear; leaders are more apt to listen to and consider input from all voices. In *The Fearless Organization: Creating Psychological Safety in the*

TABLE 4.3 FOUR LEVELS OF RELATIONSHIPS.

Level Minus 1
Total impersonal domination and coercion

Level 1
Transactional role and rule-based supervision, service, and most forms of "professional" helping relationships. Relies on rules, roles, and the maintenance of appropriate professional distance

Level 2
Personal cooperative, trusting relationships as in friendships and effective teams – relationships and group processes

Level 3
Emotionally intimate total mutual commitment

Source: Adapted from Schein and Schein, 2018.

Workplace for Learning, Innovation, and Growth, Amy Edmondson (2019), an internationally known professor of leadership, teaming, and organizational learning from Harvard, reports how psychological safety in the workplace elevates team performance, innovation, learning, and personal success in teams.

Two Jobs. Make sure everyone knows that he or she has two jobs. Staff members have to (1) do their work; and (2) improve their work (Tucker, Edmondson, and Spear, 2001). Providing high-quality care efficiently requires every person to do his or her work well all the time. Finishing today's work that was started yesterday will not improve the system. Therefore, it is important to create a community that has the ability to do today's work today and the ability to improve everyday work. The two case studies inform us about the knowledge, skills, and attitudes needed to coach frontline teams.

Helpful Resources and Methods

How does a clinical microsystem develop into a highly productive and satisfying work environment? How does one engage the head, the hands, and the heart of those involved in the delivery of exceptional health care? We recommend gaining knowledge of the clinical microsystem workplace and its individual staff and then planning action to improve the state of the workplace and its staff. Part Two of this book presents methods and tools for generating this knowledge.

FIGURE 4.3 CLINICAL MICROSYSTEM STAFF SHORT SURVEY.

Clinical Microsystem Staff Survey (Choose only one response for Items 1, 2, 3, and 4.)

1. **How stressful would you say it is to work in this practice?**

   ☐ Very stressful ☐ Somewhat stressful ☐ A little stressful ☐ Not stressful

2. **How would you rate other people's morale and their attitudes about working here?**

   ☐ Excellent ☐ Very Good ☐ Good ☐ Fair ☐ Poor

3. **I would recommend this practice as a great place to work.**

   ☐ Strongly agree ☐ Agree ☐ Disagree ☐ Strongly disagree

4. **How easy is it to ask anyone a question about the way we care for patients?**

   ☐ Very easy ☐ Easy ☐ Difficult ☐ Very difficult

5. **What would make this practice better for patients?**

   _____

   _____

6. **What would make this practice better for those who work here?**

   _____

   _____

Source: Nelson, E. C. and others, 2007, p. 120. Used with permission.

Gaining Knowledge. It is important to understand the workplace's current state and staff capability before initiating efforts to improve. Organizations frequently conduct staff satisfaction or employee engagement surveys that can elucidate what it "feels like" to work in a particular clinical microsystem. For example, a revealing item in one tool, the Clinical Microsystem Staff Short Survey (Figure 4.3), asks staff, "How easy is it to ask anyone a question about the way we care for patients?" (Godfrey, Nelson, and Batalden, 2002). The question taps an important aspect of relationships in the microsystem; answers to it reveal whether the hierarchy within which physicians, associate providers, nurses, and secretaries interact inhibits or promotes inquiry among staff. Creating a joyful work environment starts with a basic understanding of staff perceptions of the organization. Every staff member should complete the survey, anonymously if desired, either electronically or on paper with a box provided where staff can drop off completed surveys. For a longer version of this survey, see Appendix 4.1.

The Relational Coordination Survey is a validated assessment tool used to assess communication and relationships with interprofessional teams in a microsystem or across a mesosystem (Gittell, 2003, 2009, 2016; Carmeli and Gittell, 2009; Havens and others, 2010; Havens, Gittell, and Vasey, 2018; https://heller.brandeis.edu/relational-coordination/). Relational coordination assesses the quality of relationships and

APPENDIX 4.1 STAFF SATISFACTION SURVEY.

1. I am treated with respect every day by everyone that works in the practice.

   ☐ Strongly Agree   ☐ Agree   ☐ Disagree   ☐ Strongly Disagree

2. I am given everything I need—tools, equipment, and encouragement—to make my work meaningful to my life.

   ☐ Strongly Agree   ☐ Agree   ☐ Disagree   ☐ Strongly Disagree

3. When I do good work, someone in this practice notices that I did it.

   ☐ Strongly Agree   ☐ Agree   ☐ Disagree   ☐ Strongly Disagree

4. How stressful would you say it is to work in this practice?

   ☐ Very Stressful   ☐ Somewhat Stressful   ☐ A Little Stressful ☐ Not Stressful

5. How easy is it to ask anyone a question about the care we provide?

   ☐ Very Easy   ☐ Easy   ☐ Difficult   ☐ Very Difficult

6. How would you rate other people's morale and their attitudes about working here?

   ☐ Excellent   ☐ Very Good   ☐ Good   ☐ Fair   ☐ Poor

7. This practice is a better place to work than it was 12 months ago.

   ☐ Strongly Agree   ☐ Agree   ☐ Disagree   ☐ Strongly Disagree

8. I would strongly recommend this practice as a great place to work.

   ☐ Strongly Agree   ☐ Agree   ☐ Disagree   ☐ Strongly Disagree

9. What would make this practice better for patients and their families?

   _____

   _____

   _____

   _____

10. What would make this practice better for those who work here?

   _____

   _____

   _____

   _____

communication involved in the coordination of work through assessing seven dimensions of communication and relationships that are critical when work is complex, uncertain, and time constrained.

Communication

- Frequent
- Timely
- Accurate
- Problem-solving

Relationships

- Shared goals
- Shared knowledge
- Mutual respect

Relational coordination has been found to be significantly related to increased job satisfaction, increased work engagement, and reduced burnout (Havens, Gittell, and Vasey, 2018). Once the survey is completed and results shared with the members of the micro/mesosystem, a discussion pursues to gain insights into the assessments and opportunities for improvement and reinforcement.

Another survey, the Personal Skills Assessment, can be used to help identify specific knowledge and skills an individual may need to perform better in a particular clinical microsystem (Godfrey, Nelson, and Batalden, 2002). For an example of this assessment, see Appendix 4.2. Table 4.4 displays some examples of the personal skills a microsystem might assess. This survey helps microsystems identify people who excel at certain skills and to whom others might turn for assistance. Managers can use survey results to facilitate discussions with individuals as they build their personal development plans.

Taking Action. Buckingham and Coffman (1999) summarized extensive research on the things managers do to create outstanding workplaces, ones that achieve high levels of customer satisfaction, job satisfaction, productivity, and profitability. They contend that great managers create the conditions needed to generate superior performance. They suggest that managers need to focus on these basic tasks:

1. Select for talent.
2. Define the right outcomes.
3. Focus on the strengths of individuals rather than the weaknesses.
4. Find the right fit for individuals based on their talent.

A staff member of a large, multispecialty health system recently said, "I used to love to come to work; I now come to pay my bills." This is a sad commentary; it

APPENDIX 4.2   STAFF PERSONAL SKILLS ASSESSMENT.

Name _____   **Practice Name** _____

Role _____   **Date** _____

Clinical Competencies Please use your list of clinical competencies and evaluate which competencies you are learning.	Want to Learn	Never Use	Use Occasionally	Use Frequently
	☐	☐	☐	☐
	☐	☐	☐	☐
	☐	☐	☐	☐
	☐	☐	☐	☐
	☐	☐	☐	☐
	☐	☐	☐	☐
	☐	☐	☐	☐
	☐	☐	☐	☐
	☐	☐	☐	☐
	☐	☐	☐	☐
	☐	☐	☐	☐
	☐	☐	☐	☐
	☐	☐	☐	☐
	☐	☐	☐	☐
	☐	☐	☐	☐
	☐	☐	☐	☐

Clinical Information Systems (CIS*) What features and functions do you use?	Want to Learn	Never Use	Use Occasionally	Use Frequently
Provider/On-Call Schedule	☐	☐	☐	☐
Patient Demographics	☐	☐	☐	☐
Lab Results	☐	☐	☐	☐
Pathology	☐	☐	☐	☐
Patient and Family Goals and Action Plan	☐	☐	☐	☐
Review Reports/Notes	☐	☐	☐	☐
Documentation	☐	☐	☐	☐
Direct Entry	☐	☐	☐	☐
Note Templates	☐	☐	☐	☐
Medication Lists	☐	☐	☐	☐
Insurance Status	☐	☐	☐	☐
Durable Power of Attorney	☐	☐	☐	☐
Advance Directives	☐	☐	☐	☐
Radiology	☐	☐	☐	☐
OR Schedules	☐	☐	☐	☐

*NOTE: CIS refers to hospital, or clinic-based information systems used for such functions as checking patients in, electronic medical records, and accessing lab and x-ray information. Customize your list of CIS features to determine skills needed by various staff members to optimize their roles.

APPENDIX 4.2 (*Continued*)

Name _____ Practice Name _____

Technical Skills *Please rate the following on how often you use them.*	Want to Learn	Never Use	Use Occasionally	Use Frequently
Clinical Information Systems (CIS)	☐	☐	☐	☐
E-mail	☐	☐	☐	☐
Digital Dictation Link	☐	☐	☐	☐
Word Processing (Word)	☐	☐	☐	☐
Spreadsheet (Excel)	☐	☐	☐	☐
Presentation (PowerPoint)	☐	☐	☐	☐
Database (Access or FileMaker Pro)	☐	☐	☐	☐
Patient Database/Statistics	☐	☐	☐	☐
Internet/Intranet	☐	☐	☐	☐
Registries	☐	☐	☐	☐
Printer Access	☐	☐	☐	☐
Fax	☐	☐	☐	☐
Copier	☐	☐	☐	☐
Voice Mail	☐	☐	☐	☐
Pagers	☐	☐	☐	☐
FaceTime, Skype, Zoom and other video options	☐	☐	☐	☐

Meeting and Interpersonal Skills *What skills do you currently use?*	Want to Learn	Never Use	Use Occasionally	Use Frequently
Effective Meeting Skills	☐	☐	☐	☐
Timed Agenda	☐	☐	☐	☐
Role Assignment During Meetings	☐	☐	☐	☐
Brainstorm/Multi-voting	☐	☐	☐	☐
Decision Making	☐	☐	☐	☐
Delegation	☐	☐	☐	☐
Problem Solving	☐	☐	☐	☐
Open and Effective Communication	☐	☐	☐	☐
Feedback – Provide and Receive	☐	☐	☐	☐
Managing Conflict/Negotiation	☐	☐	☐	☐
Emotional/Spiritual Support	☐	☐	☐	☐

(continued)

APPENDIX 4.2 (*Continued*)

Improvement Skills and Knowledge *What improvement tools do you currently use?*	Want to Learn	Never Use	Use Occasionally	Use Frequently
Surveys – Patient and Staff	☐	☐	☐	☐
Aim Statements	☐	☐	☐	☐
Flowcharts/Process Mapping	☐	☐	☐	☐
Fishbones	☐	☐	☐	☐
Measurement and Monitoring (Ticks and Tallys)	☐	☐	☐	☐
Plan-Do-Study-Act (PDSA) Improvement Model	☐	☐	☐	☐
Standardize-Do-Study-Act (SDSA) Improvement Model	☐	☐	☐	☐
Trend Charts (Run Charts)	☐	☐	☐	☐
Control Charts	☐	☐	☐	☐
Statistical Process Control (SPC)	☐	☐	☐	☐

TABLE 4.4 EXAMPLES OF SKILLS ADDRESSED IN A PERSONAL SKILLS ASSESSMENT.

Personal Skills	Example
Technical skills	Capabilities with e-mail, dictation, handheld computer, fax, copier, phone system, and voice mail
Clinical information system skills	Capabilities with scheduling, test results, problem lists, direct entry, and template use
Meeting and interpersonal skills	Capabilities in meeting management, for example using agendas with a clear aim and timed agenda items, understanding roles that lead to productive meetings, using brainstorming and multi-voting
Improvement skills and knowledge	Ability to use plan-do-study-act (PDSA) process-mapping skills worksheets, fishbone (cause and effect) diagrams, and trend and control charts

suggests a rupture between one's personal values and one's work. There are many books and programs that can be used to involve staff and brighten the workplace (Kotter and Rathgeber, 2017; Campbell, 2020).

Observations of high-performing clinical microsystems led to these suggestions for local leaders:

1. Know every individual in the clinical microsystem and spend time to develop each person's potential. Strive to achieve Schein's level two relationships.

2. Set expectations and develop staff to "be the best they can be" on the basis of education, training, talent, and licensure.
3. Identify and design roles to meet patient and family needs (information to support this task comes from a study of the microsystem's 5Ps – purpose, patients, professionals, processes, and patterns, as described in Chapter two, Part two of this book and Chapter one of *Value by Design*, 2011).
4. Hold regular all-staff meetings inviting everyone's participation. Use timed agendas with clear aims and create a meeting environment that promotes learning and improving together.
5. Actively develop supervisors and managers. Frequently the best and brightest physicians, nurses, and staff are promoted to leadership positions without leadership education. Consider studying "great" managers (Buckingham and Coffman, 1999; Clifton and Harter, 2019; Sherman, 2019).

Clifton and Harter (2019) have further advanced and updated the original work of Buckingham and Coffman (1999) to identify five themes managers should include in their leadership and development of frontline teams (see Table 4.5).

They further reference their research over 80 years to remind us that 70 percent of the variance in team engagement is determined solely by the manager. Additional research data reveals employees leave managers and not the organization. The manager of the workplace can "make or break" a successful workplace where staff can be the best they can be.

6. Try to develop coleaders in microsystems. Virtually all the best microsystems that we have studied enjoyed shared leadership, such as a physician leader who partnered with a nursing leader and/or an administrative leader. These coleaders worked together to set expectations and hold staff accountable.
7. Consider team coaches to support the manager and the team. In the rapidly changing healthcare environment, many leaders are pulled in multiple directions to achieve strategic organizational goals, translate strategy to action at the microsystem level, manage financial performance, and still develop staff at the front line of care (Godfrey, 2013). Team coaches in partnership with leaders can help the frontline staff learn and apply improvement knowledge and skills, which can support leadership goals, organizational mission, and vision and achieve the highest quality, value, and outcomes in care delivery.

TABLE 4.5 FIVE THEMES MANAGERS SHOULD INCLUDE IN THEIR LEADERSHIP AND DEVELOPMENT.

Strategy

Move from "old" will to "new" will

"Old" Will	**"New" Will**
Paycheck	Purpose
Job satisfaction	Pursue development
Bosses	Coaches
Annual reviews	Ongoing conversations
Focus on weakness	Maximize strengths
It's not my job	It's my life

Culture

Identify purpose and brand
Audit all programs and communications
Reposition managers as coaches

Employment Brand

Attract
Hire
Onboard
Engage
Perform
Develop
Depart

Boss to Coach

Establish expectations
Continually coach
Create accountability

Future of Work

Planning how to manage:

A diverse workplace
Remote employees
Artificial intelligence
Gig workers (independent contractors on demand)
The blurring of work and life

Source: Adapted from Clifton and Harter, 2019.

Conclusion

Some healthcare settings enjoy high morale, high quality, and high productivity, but all too often this is not the case. Many clinical microsystems suffer from high staff turnover, high absenteeism, and poor morale. The two case studies, one studying the development of frontline clinical managers and the other studying frontline quality and safety improvement, offer good examples of ways to successfully activate staff and create a positive and dynamic workplace where everyone can be the best they can be. Gaining insight into the current state of the staff and their work life is essential to developing a more engaging workplace that is characterized by high-performing, creative, and fully activated staff.

Mesosystem Considerations

A mesosystem cannot be optimized without tending to the microsystems that comprise it. Microsystems should become curious about their 5Ps and develop competence in deciding on priorities for change and making improvements. Just as different microsystem members come to see their interdependence with other members, analysis of the mesosystem will reveal the important interdependencies between microsystems. Just as we recommend that staff know and value each other's work, each microsystem in a mesosystem should know and value those they are connected to. Similarly, the mesosystem leadership should be able to articulate and role model word and action to illustrate the importance of those relationships and how each microsystem contributes to something that is ultimately greater than "the sum of its parts." As discussed in greater detail in Chapter 10 and the mesosystem workbook, a mesosystem can approach its own analysis in a systematic way. As shown in this chapter, leadership at a mesosystem level can promote educational and coaching experiences at the microsystem level that enhance mesosystem performance. Ideally, experiences and lessons learned can also be shared "up the chain" to macrosystem leadership, which is sometimes distant from the microsystem level. Mesosystem leaders are important connectors across the organization.

Review Questions

1. How might Kotter's eight stages of change provide a template to develop a plan?
2. What five actions can a leader take to enhance the workplace?

3. Thinking about the Schein and Schein four levels of relationships in the workplace, what level of relationship do you experience in your current workplace? What might be done to move to a level two relationship?

Discussion Questions

1. What similarities and differences in the nurse managers' development programs and context can you identify when you compare and contrast the two case studies?
2. Can you describe any scenarios where the cascading leadership message and the frontline leader's actions were inconsistent?
3. Discuss examples in the workplace where psychological safety was low and high. What contributed to the differences in psychological safety?
4. Can you describe the Schein and Schein four levels of relationship in your own workplace?

Additional Activities

1. Distribute the Quality Improvement Assessment Tool to an improvement team you are working with to gain baseline knowledge of improvement capabilities before introducing them to improvement knowledge and skills interventions. Remeasure after the interventions to document any changes and to determine next knowledge and skills activities.
2. Consider developing team coaches to support improvement activities in the micro- or mesosystem of care.
3. Explore www.clinicalmicrosystem.org website and the Google re:Work website (https://rework.withgoogle.com/) for additional guidance and resources.
4. Consider creating a plan for sustainable improvement when executive leadership changes focus. How would you continue the development of managers at all levels of the organization and how would you sustain gains?

References

Agency for Healthcare Research and Quality. *2014 National Healthcare Quality and Disparities Report.* Rockville, MD: Agency for Healthcare Research and Quality, AHRQ Pub. No. 15-0007. [https://archive.ahrq.gov/research/findings/nhqrdr/nhqdr14/]. Apr. 2015.

Agency for Healthcare Research and Quality. *AHRQ National Scorecard on Hospital-Acquired Conditions: Updated Baseline Rates and Preliminary Results 2014-2017.* Rockville, MD: Agency for Healthcare Research and Quality. [https://www.ahrq.gov/sites/default/files/wysiwyg/professionals/quality-patient-safety/pfp/hacreport-2019.pdf]. Jan. 2019.

Ancona, D., and Backman, E. "From Pyramids to Networks: The Changing Leadership Landscape." *MIT Whitepaper.* [http://problemledleadership.mit.edu/wp-content/uploads/MIT_Whitepaper-From_Pyramids_to_Networks.pdf]. Oct. 2017.

Batalden, P. B. Personal conversation with Joan Clifford, *Oct.* 23, 2014.

Buckingham, M., and Coffman, C. *First, Break All the Rules: What the World's Greatest Managers Do Differently.* New York, NY: Simon and Schuster, 1999.

Campbell, B. A. *Where the Hell Is My Bacon? How An Innocent Pork Product Conquered Employee Engagement and Change Management At a Large Midwestern Corporation.* Ocala, FL: Atlantic Publishing Group, 2020.

Carmeli, A., and Gittell, J. H. "High-Quality Relationships, Psychological Safety, and Learning from Failures in Work Organizations." *Journal of Organizational Behaviour,* 2009, 30, 709–729. doi: 10.1002/job.565

Clifton, J., and Harter, J. *It's the Manager: Gallup Finds the Quality of Managers and Team Leaders Is the Single Biggest Factor in Your Organization's Long-term Success.* Washington DC: Gallup Press, 2019.

Creswell, J. W., and Creswell, J. D. *Research Design: Qualitative, Quantitative, and Mixed Methods Approaches,* 5th edition. Thousand Oaks, CA: Sage Publications, 2018.

Deming, W. E. *The New Economics for Industry, Government, Education,* 3rd edition. Cambridge, MA: The MIT Press, 2018.

Djukic, M., Kovner, C., Brewer, C., and others. "Educational Gaps and Solutions for Early-Career Nurse Managers' Education and Participation In Quality Improvement." *Journal of Nursing Administration,* 2015, 45(4), 206-211.

Edmondson, A. C. *Teaming: How Organizations Learn, Innovate, and Compete in the Knowledge Economy.* San Francisco, CA: Jossey-Bass, 2012.

Edmondson, A. C. *The Fearless Organization: Creating Psychological Safety in the Workplace for Learning, Innovation, and Growth.* Hoboken, NJ: John Wiley & Sons, Inc., 2019.

Foster, T., Johnson, J., Nelson, E., and Batalden, P. "Using a Malcolm Baldrige Framework to Understand High-Performing Clinical Microsystems." *Quality and Safety in Health Care,* 2007, 16(5), 334-341.

Gittell, J. H. *The Southwest Airlines Way: Using the Power of Relationships to Achieve High Performance.* New York, NY: McGraw-Hill, 2003.

Gittell, J. H. *High Performance Health Care: Using the Power of Relationships to Achieve Quality, Efficiency and Resilience.* New York, NY: McGraw-Hill, 2009.

Gittell, J. H. *Transforming Relationships for High Performance: The Power of Relational Coordination.* Stanford, CA: Stanford University Press, 2016.

Gladwell, M. *The Tipping Point: How Little Things Can Make a Big Difference.* New York, NY: Little, Brown and Company, 2000.

Godfrey, M. M., Nelson, E. C., and Batalden, P. B. *Assessing Your Practice Workbook* (rev. edn.). Hanover, NH: Dartmouth College, 2002.

Godfrey, M. M., Nelson, E. C., Wasson, J. H., and others. "Microsystems in Health Care: Part 3. Planning Patient-Centered Services." *Joint Commission Journal on Quality and Safety,* 2003, 29(4), 159-170.

Godfrey, M. M. "Improvement Capability at the Front Lines of Health Care: Helping Through Leading and Coaching." Unpublished doctoral dissertation, School of Health Sciences, Jonkoping University, Dissertation Series No. 46, 2013.

Godfrey, M. M., Andersson-Gare, B., Nelson, E. C., and others. "Coaching Interprofessional Health Care Improvement Teams: The Coachee, the Coach, and the Leader Perspectives." *Journal of Nursing Management*, 2014, 22, 452-464.

Godfrey, M. M. Personal conversation with Joan Clifford, November 4, 2014.

Godfrey, M. M., King, A. C., Foster-Johnson, L., and Landstrom, G. L. *Developing Managers to Lead Health Care Transformation at the Front Line of Care Poster*. The Dartmouth Institute Microsystem Academy Retreat, Hanover, NH, 2016.

Godfrey, M. M., Foster, V. L., and Nilsson, M. "Validation of the Quality Improvement Assessment (Qia) Tool." IHI ID 22 Abstract. *BMJ Open Quality*, 2018, 7(s1), a30-a33.

Hackman, J. R., and Wageman, R. "A Theory of Team Coaching." *Academy of Management Review*, 2005, 30(2, Apr), 269-287.

Havens, D. S., Vasey, J., Gittell, J. H., and Lin, W. T. "Relational Coordination Among Nurses and Other Providers: Impact on the Quality of Patient Care." *Journal of Nursing Management*, 2010, 18, 926-937

Havens, D. S., Gittell, J. H., and Vasey, J. "Impact of Relational Coordination on Nurse Job Satisfaction, Work Engagement and Burnout: Achieving the Quadruple Aim." *The Journal of Nursing Administration*, 2018, 48(3, Mar), 132-140. doi: 10.1097/NNA.000000000000587

Institute of Medicine (US). *To Err Is Human: Building a Safer Health System*. Washington, DC: National Academies Press, 2000.

Institute of Medicine (US). *Preventing Medication Errors*. Washington, DC: National Academies Press, 2007.

Institute of Medicine (US). "Committee on the Robert Wood Johnson Foundation Initiative on the Future of Nursing." *The Future of Nursing: Leading Change, Advancing Health*. Washington, DC: National Academies Press, 2010.

Kolb, D. A. *Experiential Learning: Experience as the Source of Learning and Development*. Englewood Cliffs, NJ: Prentice-Hall, 1984.

Kotter, J. P. "Leading Change: Why Transformation Efforts Fail." *Harvard Business Review*, March-April 1995.

Kotter, J. P. *Leading Change*. Boston, MA: Harvard Business School Press, 1996.

Kotter, J. P., and Cohen, D. S. *The Heart of Change*. Boston, MA: Harvard Business School Press, 2002.

Kotter, J., and Rathgeber, H. *Our Iceberg Is Melting: Changing and Succeeding Under Any Conditions*. New York, NY: Penguin Random House, 2017.

Lardieri, A. "Thousands of Nurses Strike for More Staffing, Better Patient Ratios." *US News and World Report*. [https://www.usnews.com/news/health-news/articles/2019-09-20/thousands-of-nurses-strike-for-more-staffing-better-patient-ratios]. Sept. 20, 2019.

Lavrakas, P. *Encyclopedia of Survey Research Methods*. Thousand Oaks, CA: Sage Publications, 2008. doi: 10.4135/9781412963947.n192 [https://methods.sagepub.com/reference/encyclopedia-of-survey-research-methods/n192.xml]

Nelson, E. C., Batalden, P. B., Huber, T. P., and others. "Microsystems in Health Care: Part 1. Learning from High-Performing Front-Line Clinical Units." *Joint Commission Journal on Quality Improvement*, 2002, 28(9), 472-493.

Nembhard, I. M., and Edmondson, A. C. "Making it Safe: The Effects of Leader Inclusiveness and Professional Status on Psychological Safety and Improvement Efforts in Health Care Teams." *Journal of Organizational Behaviour*, 2006, 27, 941-966. doi: 10.1002/job.413

O'May, F., and Buchan, J. "Shared Governance: A Literature Review." *International Journal of Nursing Studies*, 1999, 36, 281-300.

Parand, A., Dopson, S., Renz, A., and Vincent, C. "The Role of Hospital Managers in Quality and Patient Safety: A Systematic Review." *BMJ Open*, 2014, 4(9), 1-15. doi: 10.1136/bmjopen-2014-005055

Patton, M. Q. *Qualitative Research & Evaluation Methods: Integrating Theory and Practice.* Thousand Oaks, CA: Sage Publications, 2015.

Popa, R. "Physician Burnout in the US & Europe: 19 Statistics." *Becker's ASC Review*. [https://www.beckersasc.com/leadership/physician-burnout-in-the-us-europe-19-statistics.html?em=margiegodfrey@gmail.com&oly_enc_id=1761D0018134E0V]. Feb. 15, 2019.

Porter-O'Grady, T. "Shared Governance for Nursing. Part I: Creating the New Organization." *AORN Journal*, 1991, 53(2), 458-459, 461-462, 464-466.

Riles, W., Dis, S., Miller, K., and McCullough, M. "A Model for Developing High-Reliability Teams." *Journal of Nursing Management*, 2010, 18, 556-563.

Rogers, E. *Diffusion of Innovations*, 4th edition. New York, NY: Free Press, 1995.

Schein, E. H. *Helping: How to Offer, Give, and Receive Help.* San Francisco, CA: Berrett-Koehler Publishers, 2009.

Schein, E. H. *Humble Inquiry: The Gentle Art of Asking Instead of Telling.* San Francisco, CA: Berrett-Koehler Publishers, 2013.

Schein, E. H., and Schein, P. A. *Humble Leadership: The Power of Relationships, Openness, and Trust.* Oakland, CA: Berrett-Koehler Publishers, 2018.

Shanafelt, T. D., Hasan, O., Dyrbye L. N., and others. "Changes in Burnout and Satisfaction with Work-Life Balance in Physicians and the General US Working Population Between 2011 and 2014." *Mayo Clinic Proceedings*, 2015, 90(12, Dec), 1600-1613. doi: 10.1016/j.mayocp.2015.08.023

Sherman, R. O. *The Nurse Leader Coach: Become the Boss No One Wants to Leave.* Rose O. Sherman (self-publication), 2019.

Tucker, A., Edmondson, A., and Spear, S. "Why Your Organization Isn't Learning All It Should." *HBS Working Knowledge*. Retrieved Nov. 8, 2005 from [http://hbswk.hbs.edu/archive/2397.html]. Jul. 30, 2001.

Walk-the-talk. In *YourDictionary*, n.d. [https://www.yourdictionary.com/walk-the-talk]

Additional Resources

Brandeis Relational Coordination Research Collaborative, https://heller.brandeis.edu/relational-coordination/

Clinical Microsystem Website, http://clinicalmicrosystem.org/

Emerging Leadership Blog, Rose Sherman, https://www.emergingrnleader.com/

Google re:Work, https://rework.withgoogle.com/

Key Words/Terms

Distributed decision-making models of leadership: Involves leadership practices that are more collaborative, open, and decentralized – designed to mesh more effectively with new forms of work
and new technologies. It is a kind of leadership that blends top-down, and bottom-up
decision-making. And while it is difficult to leave behind models of the pyramid with the
omniscient, omnipotent leader at the top, organizations are beginning to view leadership not
as an individual characteristic, but as a system involving networks of leaders – some formal
and others informal – operating at all levels of an organization and often across organizational boundaries. The result is that organizations can more effectively mobilize the collective
intelligence, motivation, and creative talent of their employees, partners, and customers
(Ancona and Backman, 2017).

Doctor of nursing practice (DNP): The DNP is designed to produce leaders in nursing. DNPs possess
the highest level of nursing expertise to influence healthcare outcomes through organizational leadership, health policy implementation, and direct patient care and work either in a
clinical setting or leadership role upon obtaining the required credentials.

Early adopters of change: These individuals have the highest degree of opinion leadership among
the adopter categories (early adopter, early majority, late majority, and laggards). Early adopters are respected by peers and are the embodiment of successful, discrete use of new ideas.
The early adopter decreases uncertainty about a new idea by adopting it, and then conveying
a subjective evaluation of the innovation to near-peers through interpersonal networks
(Rogers, 1995).

Experiential learning: Experiential learning involves learning from experience. The theory was
proposed by psychologist David Kolb who was influenced by the work of other theorists
including John Dewey, Kurt Lewin, and Jean Piaget (Kolb, 1984).

Focus group: A qualitative research method in which a trained moderator conducts a collective
interview of typically six to eight participants from similar backgrounds, similar demographic
characteristics, or both. Focus groups create open lines of communication across individuals
and rely on the dynamic interaction between participants to yield data that would be impossible to gather via other approaches, such as one-on-one interviewing. When done well, focus
groups offer powerful insights into people's feelings and thoughts and thus a more detailed,
nuanced, and richer understanding of their perspectives on ideas, products, and policies
(Lavrakas, 2008).

Hospital acquired conditions (HACs): A medical condition or complication that a patient develops
during a hospital stay, which was not present at admission.

Mixed methods research: An approach to inquiry that combines or integrates both qualitative and
quantitative forms of research. It involves philosophical assumptions, the use of qualitative
and quantitative approaches, and the mixing or integrating of both approaches in a study
(Creswell and Creswell, 2018).

Qualitative research: A means for exploring and understanding the meaning individuals or groups
ascribe to a social or human problem. The process of research involves emerging questions
and procedures collecting data in the participants' setting, analyzing the data inductively,
building from particulars to general themes, and making interpretations of the meaning of
the data (Creswell and Creswell, 2018).

Quantitative research: A means for testing objective theories by examining the relationship among
variables. These variables can be measured, typically on instruments, so that numbered data
can be analyzed using statistical procedures (Creswell and Creswell, 2018).

Shared governance: A decentralized approach that gives nurses greater authority and control over their practice and work environment, engenders a sense of responsibility and accountability, and allows active participation in the decision-making process, particularly in administrative areas from which they were excluded previously. The primary aim is to support the relationship between the service provider (nurse) and patient (client). It is not a one-time implementation process, with a concrete, fixed set of rules, but rather an ongoing and fluid process, which requires continual assessment and revaluation to be flexible and adaptive to the environment (O'May and Buchan, 1999).

Success characteristics of high-performing clinical microsystems: Robert Wood Johnson-supported research conducted at Dartmouth identified nine success characteristics related to high performance in healthcare systems: leadership, culture, macro-organizational support of microsystems, patient focus, staff focus, inter-dependence of care team, information and information technology, process improvement, and performance patterns. These success factors were interrelated and together contributed to the microsystem's ability to provide superior, cost-effective care and at the same time create a positive and attractive working environment.

Team coaching: Direct interaction with a team intended to help members make coordinated and task-appropriate use of their collective resources in accomplishing the team's work (Hackman and Wageman, 2005).

Tipping point: The tipping point is that magic moment when an idea, trend, or social behavior crosses a threshold, tips, and spreads like wildfire.

"Walk the talk": To do what one said one could do, or would do, not just making empty promises (YourDictionary, n.d.).

CHAPTER FIVE

TRANSFORMING A PRIMARY CARE CLINIC TO AN NCQA-CERTIFIED PATIENT-CENTERED MEDICAL HOME

Marjorie M. Godfrey, Tina C. Foster, Randy Messier, Julie K. Johnson

AIM

The aim of this chapter is to describe the importance of understanding local context and current performance including the 5Ps of purpose, patients, professionals, processes, and patterns) when designing and improving clinical microsystems.

LEARNING OBJECTIVES

By the end of this chapter the reader will be able to:

1. Articulate why context matters in improvement.
2. Name and explain each of the "5Ps" of a clinical microsystem.
3. Connect contextual and performance knowledge with the plan for design or improvement.
4. Compare and contrast "checking the boxes" to meet standards versus engaging the inter-professional team in a developmental improvement journey.

Quality by Design: A Clinical Microsystems Approach, Second Edition. Edited by Marjorie M. Godfrey, Tina C. Foster, Julie K. Johnson, Eugene C. Nelson and Paul B. Batalden.
© 2025 John Wiley & Sons, Inc. Published 2025 by John Wiley & Sons, Inc.

Introduction

This chapter provides an in-depth exploration of the "5Ps" that can describe any microsystem and form a practical basis for understanding the context of improvement work. An understanding of context is essential for system improvement, as it informs a rich understanding of how and why the system works, as well as who is a part of it. The case study presented details how a microsystem-specific understanding of context led to a successful mesosystem transformation.

Strategic focus on clinical microsystems – the small, functional, frontline units that provide most health care to most people – is essential to co-designing high-value, high-quality healthcare services. An understanding of *context* is crucial for this process. Without knowing the needs, desires, and abilities of the patients and families served by the microsystem, without knowing the skills and resources of those who work in the microsystem, without delineating and accessing key processes, without understanding the patterns of outcomes and the culture of the microsystem, the design effort will most likely fail or result in unsustainable change (Øvretveit, 2011; Kaplan and others, 2012; Dixon-Woods, 2014; Kringos and others, 2015).

The starting place for designing or redesigning clinical microsystems is evaluation of the 5Ps: the *purpose* of the microsystem, the *patients* who are served by the microsystem, the *professionals* who work together in the microsystem, the *processes* the microsystem uses to provide services, and the *patterns* that characterize the microsystem's functioning. It is important to note that while we call out "patients" and "professionals" as two distinct "Ps," we view patients and families as members of the microsystem along with clinicians and other staff. While the past two decades have seen widespread use of various tools and approaches to improvement, many efforts to improve care do not result in sustained improvement (Dixon-Woods and Martin, 2016). There are many contributing factors that help explain this phenomenon. This chapter highlights the importance of exploring and understanding the context and current performance as a starting place, rather than beginning with a problem to be solved.

It is relatively uncommon to inquire about the context of where and how clinical health care is provided before starting improvement. Participating in the process of exploring and gathering information about the context provides insights that can be leveraged to engage in more relevant and sustainable improvements. The 5Ps presented in this chapter provide a systematic, accessible, and actionable way to engage members of the microsystem in such learning.

The "improvement formula" described by Batalden and Davidoff (2007) describes the domains of knowledge needed to move evidence into practice, reflecting the complexities of change in healthcare delivery. (See Sidebar "The improvement formula.")

The Improvement Formula (Batalden and Davidoff, 2007)

Batalden (2018) has further developed the original improvement formula (shown in Figure 5.1) to highlight the importance of coproduction of healthcare services.

The domains of the updated improvement formula (see Figure 5.2) include:

- Patient Aim: Why is the patient seeking care? The help needed is grounded in the patient's reality.
- What is the science that can inform practice? Generalizable science includes observations and evidence from others and other contexts; adaptation may be needed.

FIGURE 5.1 THE ORIGINAL IMPROVEMENT FORMULA.

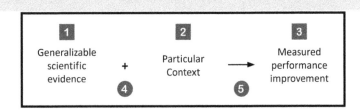

Characteristics of five knowledge systems involved in improvement	
Knowledge system	Illustrative features
1. Generalizable scientific evidence	Controls and limits context as a variable; tests hypotheses
2. Particular context awareness	Characterizes the particular physical, social, and cultural identify of local care settings (e.g., their processes, habits, and traditions)
3. Performance measurement	Assesses the effect of changes by using study methods that preserve time as a variable, use balanced measures (range of perspectives, dimensions), analyze for patterns
4. Plans for change	Describes the variety of methods available for connecting evidence to particular contexts
5. Execution of planned changes	Provides insight into the strategic, operational, and human resource realities of particular settings (drivers) that will make change happen

Source: Batalden and Davidoff, 2007. Used with Permission.

FIGURE 5.2 THE UPDATED IMPROVEMENT FORMULA.

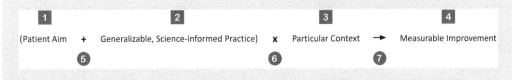

Source: Batalden, 2018. Used with permission.

- What is the particular context? Understanding the particular context is necessary to understand how a specific science-informed intervention can be adapted according to the context.
- What should be measured? Identify improvement measurements that can assess the degree to which the patient's aim was understood and achieved as well as what the effect of the intervention was. How do we connect the patient's aim and science-informed practice?
- How do we match possible interventions with the enabling and limiting features of the local setting, even as it changes?
- How will we test the change by mobilizing the strategic, operational, and human resources needed?

We will not go into the challenges of developing and disseminating evidence here (Neta and others, 2015; Woolf and others, 2015), but will assume for now that a proposed change has a strong evidence base. To effectively put this evidence into practice and improve care, we must understand the context – the clinical microsystem – where this evidence will be used. Avedis Donabedian, the founder of the study of quality in health care and medical outcomes research, referred to structures, processes, and outcomes to evaluate the quality of health care (Ayanian and Markel, 2016). We have further expanded his framework to be more specific to inquiry into the populations served, the professionals providing care, the habits, attitudes, communication and relationships, and the care processes in the microsystem.

It is also important that as we seek to make changes, we define how we will measure our success (Langley and others, 1996). The science of measurement in health care is still evolving (Woodcock, Liberati, and Dixon-Woods, 2019). We continue to seek robust ways to measure aspects of care that go beyond the clinical measures including *patient and family experience*, opportunities for *shared decision-making*, meaningful *functional outcomes*, and actual costs. In a world where care is coproduced, measuring what matters to patients is imperative. While strides have been made in this area (Black, Varaganum, and Hutchings, 2014; Gleeson and others, 2016; Gomes and others, 2016), widespread use of these metrics is not yet the norm.

Having decided how to measure success, the improver is now faced with the challenge of how to plan the improvement – how to adapt the generalizable evidence to a specific population and how to understand the effect of context on the ability to make changes (Kaplan and others, 2012). There are many examples of failed implementations including "toolkits" and *pathways* languishing on shelves, lack of staff engagement with a hoped-for change, and failure of sustained change (Senge and others, 1999). Without considering the nature of the system and how this particular evidence applies to that particular system, change efforts are likely to be an exercise in frustration. Finally, even with the best planning and attention to context, failure of execution is possible (Grol, 2001; De Allegri and others, 2011; Jabbour and others, 2018). The improver must determine how to best enact the plan and how to lead the system through change.

Reed and Card (2015) raise concerns that the oversimplification of the Plan-Do-Study-Act (PDSA) method from industry to health care has resulted in the loss of the originally intended rigor of improvement. They reflect that in many healthcare systems' efforts to "get on" with improvement and avoid lengthy planning phases, the results are often wasted PDSA cycles or failed improvements. McNicholas and colleagues (2019) further address the inconsistent fidelity of PDSA cycles, which impacts the scientific process of testing ideas. They report that quality improvement methods are challenging, although supportive strategies and resources will lead to increased understanding and increased fidelity of PDSA cycles.

The disciplined approach to increase microsystem members' understanding of the context is imperative because context is everywhere. Does the evidence apply in this particular context? What are the resources and abilities related to measurement, and what measurement will be useful in this particular setting? How does change occur in this microsystem? All are important questions (which are often not posed until after an improvement effort has failed) and should be explored to understand *in preparation* for conducting tests of change.

Case Study: Transforming from a Primary Care Clinic to an NCQA-Certified Patient-Centered Medical Home

This case study is an example of transforming a primary care practice to a *Patient-Centered Medical Home* using the clinical microsystem approach. The case exemplifies what it takes to provide patient-centered care using deep knowledge of a microsystem's patient populations, optimization of professional roles, and improvement of processes through the use of information and information technology and study of patterns including outcomes, variation, and trends in services and care. Supporting a primary care clinic in its transformation into a National Committee for Quality Assurance (NCQA)-recognized Medical Home (NCQA, 2014) can also develop improvement capability and set the stage for a culture of continual improvement.

While the NCQA provides a list of standards for recognition as a Medical Home, it is difficult if not impossible to sustainably meet those standards without fully understanding the context. To capitalize on these standards, a deep understanding of the systems and processes of care in a primary care clinic should be explored and understood as an interdisciplinary team. While a practice might choose to meet the

NCQA standards in a "checklist" fashion, taking a patient-centered quality improvement approach that engages staff, providers, and patients while leveraging information and information technology can engender a sense of ownership of the microsystem and improve the care team's communication, dynamics, and improvement capabilities. To achieve this, a focused, disciplined improvement strategy is necessary, blending NCQA standards with microsystem assessments, leading to improvement while achieving Patient-Centered Medical Home (PCMH) certification. Table 5.1 shows the blended PCMH and microsystem process.

The first activity for the organization was to create an interprofessional organizational oversight team to coordinate the strategy and timeline of PCMH program implementation in primary care (see Figure 5.3). This oversight team ensured that the quality improvement work done by individual clinic improvement teams met the relevant NCQA standards. The oversight team performed an initial assessment by comparing all the primary care clinics' processes of care to the NCQA standards to help identify where improvement was needed.

The second activity was the creation of individual primary care microsystem interdisciplinary improvement teams ($n=6$). The clinic improvement teams began their work by collecting the clinic 5Ps data: purpose, patients, professionals, processes, and patterns. The organizational oversight team facilitated completion of the core process survey to identify processes that were working well and processes that could be improved across all the primary care units in a standardized fashion.

All members of each primary care clinic completed the "Activity" survey to assess if their current role and functions in their own microsystem optimally leveraged their license, education, and training to identify mismatches and opportunities to enhance roles (see Figure 5.4; Godfrey and others, 2012).

Each microsystem improvement team then reviewed and analyzed their 5Ps data to identify improvement goals. Teams held weekly one-hour quality improvement meetings utilizing effective meeting skills including timed agendas, assigned meeting roles, and ground rules to ensure efficient and effective use of time. The organizational oversight team provided regular updates at all-staff microsystem meetings to keep everyone informed about improvement and progress toward the PCMH standards. This regular communication ensured that everyone was invited to the improvement process to offer individual perspectives, knowledge, and insights. In addition, when change was recommended, staff were not surprised and were more ready to be supportive.

The organizational oversight team regularly communicated with each clinic improvement team through weekly or biweekly meetings and huddles. This connection provided support and allowed the oversight team to be informed about emerging needs and challenges to alert the larger organization how it could help frontline improvement. The oversight team and the clinic improvement team kept track of

TABLE 5.1 PCMH SUCCESS ELEMENTS AND THEIR LINKS TO THE 5PS.

Success	Know Your Purpose	Know Your Patients	Know Your Professionals	Know Your Process	Know Your Patterns
Computer terminals are placed in every room to support scheduling, record, telephone triage, shared decision making, and patient education.		•		•	•
Staff use e-mail to communicate among themselves. There is open discussion about their shared work life, including improvement opportunities, difficult communications, conflicts, and celebrations of group successes.	•		•		•
Patients and providers use e-mail to communicate about medical problems, medication refills, referrals, test results, and other matters.		•	•	•	•
Patients complete a health status survey.		•			•
Specially-trained patient service triage patients using the Triage Coupler to support decision making.			•	•	
Staff training is ongoing and rigorously on performance and competency. Computer tools coupled with this training allow all staff to function at an advanced level with high morale and low turnover.			•	•	
After six to twelve months with the practice, employees enroll in a total quality management course at the local community college.			•	•	•
All staff are encouraged to use a standardized form to suggest practice. This form, based on the plan-do-study-act (PDSA) format, is designed to help the creation of a disciplined community of scientists. The form is circulated to all staff for input prior to the weekly staff meeting, where final revisions and decisions are made.				•	•

(continued)

TABLE 5.1 (*Continued*)

Success	Know Your Purpose	Know Your Patients	Know Your Professionals	Know Your Process	Know Your Patterns
The staff meet weekly to evaluate practice performance. They also attend a yearly off-site meeting for the purpose of team building.			•	•	•
Staff hold daily huddles to evaluate the prior day, the current day, and the future.				•	•
Problem-Knowledge Couplers (PKCs) couple patient-specific data with current biomedical knowledge to support evidence-based practice in routine care. The *couplers* are updated at 6-month intervals.			•	•	
The practice has an extensive data wall that is used daily to track numerous indicators such as Health Plan Employer Data and Information Set (HEDIS) technical quality metrics (Nelson, Splaine, Batalden, and Plume, 1998).		•		•	•
The data wall also displays statistical process control charts and measures of process and clinical outcomes as essential measures to manage and improve the practice (Langley, 1996).				•	•
The electronic medical record alerts staff to unique needs of patient sub-populations, such as the diabetic population, and tracks essential interventions that benefit those populations.		•	•	•	•

all the microsystems' progress and goals as well as the overall primary care improvement work plan utilizing a program *Gantt chart* (see Figure 5.5; Nelson and others, 2007).

The Gantt chart helped the oversight team track the improvement efforts of each microsystem team toward the NCQA standards. This also allowed the oversight team to identify any additional resources or support the microsystem teams needed to meet the deadlines from an organizational level.

FIGURE 5.3 TWO SYSTEM LEVELS OF ACTION TO PLAN FOCUSED AND DISCIPLINED IMPROVEMENT STRATEGY TO MEET PCMH STANDARDS.

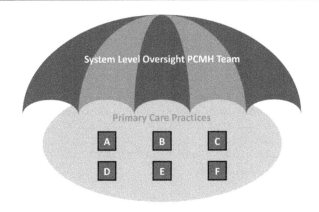

As the primary care improvement teams continued to review clinic data, develop specific aims, identify change ideas, perform small tests of change (PDSAs), and create *playbooks* (to standardize best practices) the team was simultaneously meeting the relevant NCQA Medical Home Standards. The primary care improvement teams continued these cycles until the oversight team confirmed that the identified processes and systems had been improved. The primary care clinic was now ready to complete the NCQA documentation to be submitted for review for PCMH certification.

The clinic was successful in obtaining NCQA PCMH certification, and the culture of the primary care practices had also changed. There was wide recognition by primary care clinics and leadership that the work of improvement is never done. The clinic had taken the first step in creating a "culture of improvement" and the start of a continuous quality improvement process that demonstrated ongoing, coordinated, and monitored improvement of care and processes to provide the high-value, high-quality care while creating a culture that supported an engaged and positive workplace.

Most healthcare professionals choose their career out of a desire to help people, not because of a deep desire to meet standards or check boxes. When skilled health professionals view their work as a process of meeting someone else's standards, morale can drop and a sense of ownership of the workplace can be lost (Hargis, Wyatt, and Piotrowski, 2011). When both the head and the heart of healthcare professionals are engaged by reframing the work in a way that encourages them to systematically take charge of their microsystem and improve the care they provide to

FIGURE 5.4 MEDICAL HOME ACTIVITY SURVEY.

Medical Home Activity Survey Sheet			
Position: MD	**% of Time**	**Position: RN**	**% of Time**
Activity: <u>Direct face-to-face contact with patient</u>		Activity: <u>Triage patient issues/concerns</u>	
Specific items involved:		• Phone	15%
• Review chart history	30%	• Face-to-face	
• Assess/diagnose patient		• Email/patient portal	
• Determine treatment plan		Activity: <u>Patient/family education</u>	
Activity: <u>Minor procedures</u>	9%	Specific items involved:	3%
•		•	
Activity: <u>See patients in hospital</u>	2%	Activity: <u>Direct patient care</u>	
•		Specific items involved:	
Activity: <u>Patient follow-up</u>		• Vaccines	
Specific items involved:		• Patient education	
• Answer patient messages and requests	10%	• Self-management education	25%
• Follow-up phone callas		• Independent visit for chronic disease follow-up	
• Respond to patient emails		• Blood draw	
• Team huddles/care management meetings		• Assist provider with unstable patient	
Activity: <u>Dictate/document patient encounter</u>		Activity: <u>Follow-up phone calls</u>	
• Dictate encounter	25%	Specific items involved:	
• Review transcriptions and sign off		• Answer patient phone call	
•		• Discuss patient with specialist	
Activity: <u>Complete form</u>		• Discuss patient with hospital	20%
Specific items involved:		• Discuss patient with VNA	
• Review transciption and sign off	5%	• Discuss patient with Pharmacy	
• Referrals		• Discuss patient with insurance company	
• Camp/school physicals		Activity: <u>Review and notify patients of lab resultss</u>	
Activity: <u>Write prescriptions/e-prescribe/call-ins</u>		Specific items involved:	5%
Specific items involved:	5%	• Normal with follow-up	
•		• Drug adjustments	
Activity: <u>Manage charts/EHR</u>		Activity: <u>Complete forms</u>	
Specific items involved:	5%	Specific items involved:	18%
•		• Referrals	
Activity: <u>Evaluate Results</u>		• Camp/school physicials	
Specific items involved:		Activity: <u>Call-in prescriptions</u>	
• Review results and determine next actions	5%	Specific items involved:	5%
•		•	
Activity: <u>See patients in nursing home</u>		Activity: <u>Team interactions</u>	
Specific items involved:	2%	Specific items involved:	
•		• Team huddles	7%
Activity: <u>Miscellaneous</u>		• Review cases w/PCP	
Specific items involved:	2%	Activity: <u>Miscellaneous</u>	
• CME; attend seminars; attend meetings		Specific items involved:	2%
•		• CME; attend seminars; attend meetings	
Total	**100%**	**Total**	**100%**

Source: Godfrey, M. M. and others, 2012, p. 23. Used with permission.

FIGURE 5.5 MEDICAL HOME GANTT CHART.

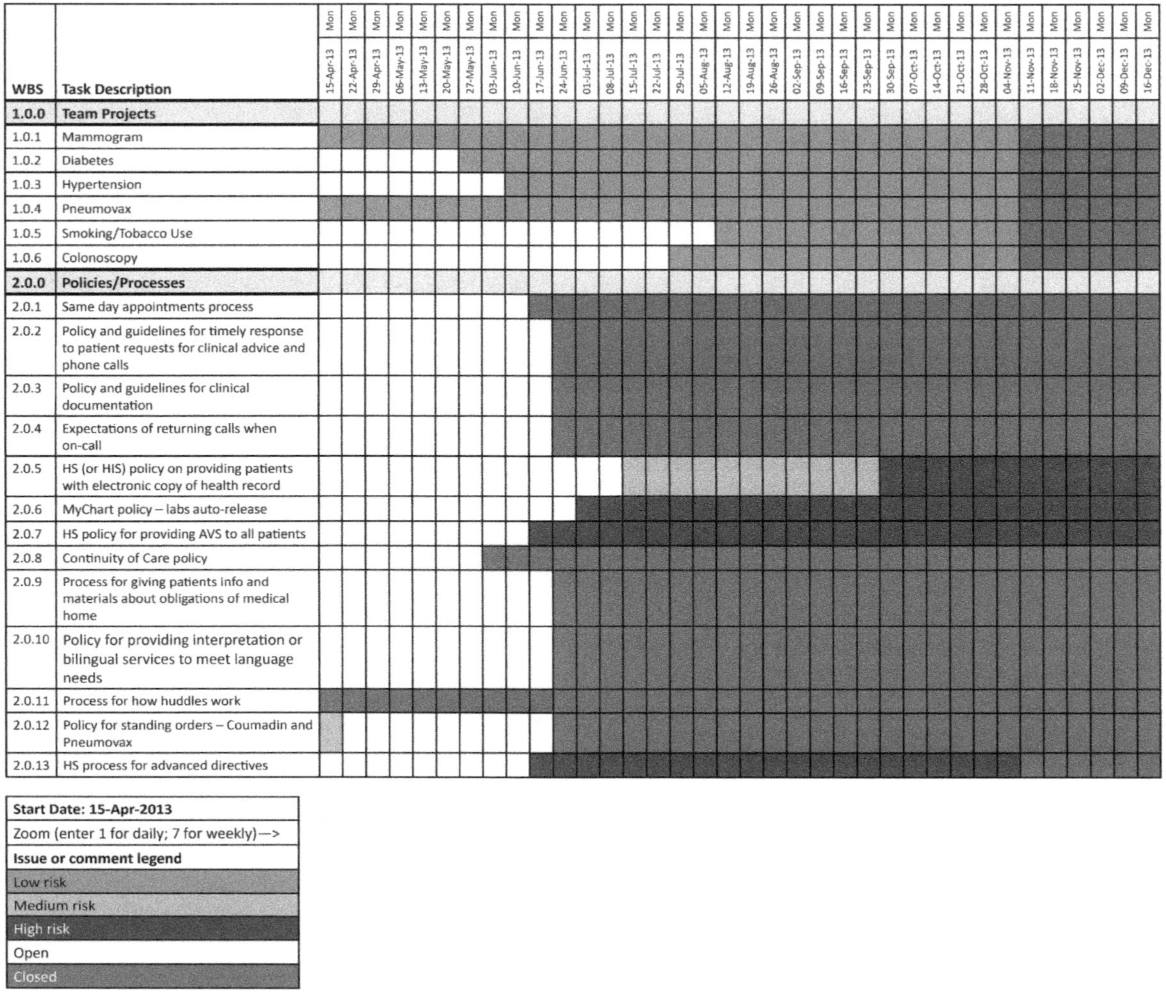

Column headers (weeks, each labeled "Mon"): 15-Apr-13, 22-Apr-13, 29-Apr-13, 06-May-13, 13-May-13, 20-May-13, 27-May-13, 03-Jun-13, 10-Jun-13, 17-Jun-13, 24-Jun-13, 01-Jul-13, 08-Jul-13, 15-Jul-13, 22-Jul-13, 29-Jul-13, 05-Aug-13, 12-Aug-13, 19-Aug-13, 26-Aug-13, 02-Sep-13, 09-Sep-13, 16-Sep-13, 23-Sep-13, 30-Sep-13, 07-Oct-13, 14-Oct-13, 21-Oct-13, 28-Oct-13, 04-Nov-13, 11-Nov-13, 18-Nov-13, 25-Nov-13, 02-Dec-13, 09-Dec-13, 16-Dec-13

WBS	Task Description
1.0.0	**Team Projects**
1.0.1	Mammogram
1.0.2	Diabetes
1.0.3	Hypertension
1.0.4	Pneumovax
1.0.5	Smoking/Tobacco Use
1.0.6	Colonoscopy
2.0.0	**Policies/Processes**
2.0.1	Same day appointments process
2.0.2	Policy and guidelines for timely response to patient requests for clinical advice and phone calls
2.0.3	Policy and guidelines for clinical documentation
2.0.4	Expectations of returning calls when on-call
2.0.5	HS (or HIS) policy on providing patients with electronic copy of health record
2.0.6	MyChart policy – labs auto-release
2.0.7	HS policy for providing AVS to all patients
2.0.8	Continuity of Care policy
2.0.9	Process for giving patients info and materials about obligations of medical home
2.0.10	Policy for providing interpretation or bilingual services to meet language needs
2.0.11	Process for how huddles work
2.0.12	Policy for standing orders – Coumadin and Pneumovax
2.0.13	HS process for advanced directives

Start Date: 15-Apr-2013
Zoom (enter 1 for daily; 7 for weekly) —>
Issue or comment legend
Low risk
Medium risk
High risk
Open
Closed

Source: Adapted from Nelson, E. C. and others, 2007, p. 367. Used with permission.

their patients as well as their work environment, ownership and cultural change can be fostered. This activation of the microsystem can engage all team members of the microsystem, increase the ownership of improvement, and at the same time meet all of the regulatory and reporting requirements that every area of health care now faces.

A Developmental Journey: Beginning to Assess, Understand, and Improve a Clinical Microsystem

Just as healthcare providers partner with patients and families to assess, diagnose, and treat when needed, microsystem members (including patients and families) can assess, diagnose, and treat their microsystem.

Assess and Diagnose

A clinical microsystem's developmental journey begins with the assessment of the unique context to make a "diagnosis." As context is explored with the involvement of all microsystem members, themes emerge and from those themes global and specific aims can be developed. This shared process of exploration is important for creating a sense of "ownership." While it is common to refer to "buy-in" of team members, ownership of the microsystem can result in improved relationships and support of shared goals that the members of the microsystem have developed (Lipmanowicz, 2010). A deeper understanding of context and systems will lead to better use of the improvement processes and tools, rather than just making changes without understanding the context and systems (Reed and Card, 2015).

The assessment process is designed to improve the microsystem's ability to identify and match the needs of distinct patient subpopulations with the resources available. If there is a mismatch, needed resources can be identified. The assessment process also helps to identify areas of unnecessary variation and promote efficiency by continuously removing waste and rework, creating processes and systems that support staff, and designing smooth, effective, and safe patient care services that lead to measurably improved patient outcomes. Along the way, improvement capability of those who work there will be increased through the process, and all members of the microsystem (including patients and families) will be engaged in the discovery and improvement process.

Improving the Microsystem with Patients, Families, and Interdisciplinary Teams

The planning of services that optimize coproduction requires knowledge of (1) the major patient subpopulations served by the clinical microsystem; (2) the ways microsystem members interact with one another, both in the execution of processes and through relationships and communications; and (3) the ways the members in the microsystem interact with the processes that unfold to produce critical outcomes. This knowledge comes from both formal analysis using the 5Ps framework as well as investigating the tacit understanding of the clinical unit's structure, its patients, its processes, and its daily patterns of work and interaction. It is important to make this tacit understanding explicit, as this will surface many assumptions and beliefs that are operating "below the surface." It is also essential to remember that patients and families are active members of the microsystem, not simply "customers" or "beneficiaries" of care.

Getting Started: Using the 5Ps to Explore Systems

Methods and tools have been developed for microsystem leaders and staff to use (and adapt as needed) to assess their microsystems and design tests of change for improvement and innovation. The aim is to increase each microsystem's capacity to better realize its potential and to better relate to other microsystems that work with it to form the service continuum or mesosystem. These tools are a helpful way to begin to understand the context of the microsystem, remembering that while there may be similarities across settings, every microsystem is unique. The questions in Table 5.2, the tools found in Part Two of *Quality by Design*, first edition (Nelson, Batalden, and Godfrey, 2007), and the workbooks at www.clinicalmicrosystem.org are intended to provide guidance and provoke thinking about information needed to improve a microsystem. They provide a framework for diagnosing the 5Ps of a microsystem – the purpose, patients, professionals, processes, and patterns – which are described next. Workbooks for a variety of microsystems including "supporting microsystems" such as pharmacy, laboratory, and diagnostic services are also available at www.clinicalmicrosystem.org.

The 5Ps framework is a tested and useful method for members of the microsystem to begin to see their practice in a new way to see new possibilities. Conducting a 5Ps assessment does not mean that improvement activities need to be postponed. Many clinical teams do their assessment before starting to make improvements, but some begin organizing improvement efforts and learning about their system's 5Ps simultaneously. Discoveries that occur in the 5Ps assessment process often make the needed improvements clear and ultimately inform improvement activities for now and in the future.

TABLE 5.2 KNOW THE PS FOR CLINICAL MICROSYSTEMS ACROSS THE HEALTH CONTINUUM.

Primary Care

Patients	Professionals	Processes	Patterns
• Age distribution and % of females?	• Who are the people in our clinical microsystem?	• Who are our supporting departments?	• What are our disease-specific health outcomes?
• Patient population with seasonal fluctuations?	• What roles and functions do we currently have, and how do they relate to our main aim or purpose?	• What are our key supporting processes?	• What is the number of out-of-practice visits?
• Most frequent diagnoses?	• What information technology do we depend on to support care?	• What is our interdependence (linkages) with other microsystems?	• What is our margin after costs?
• Frequent users of services?	• Where do our staff spend their time (for example: teaching or outreach)?	• What is our dependence on our macrosystem?	• What is the number of encounters per year?
• How satisfied are our patients with our services?	• What resources do we have available daily to provide patient care?	• What is our cycle time?	
	• What is the morale of our staff?	• Are staff knowledgeable about our key processes?	
	• Are health profession students part of our team?	• What is our demand?	
		• What are our indirect patient pulls?	

Inpatient Care

Patients	Professionals	Processes	Patterns
• Age distribution and % of females?	• Who are the people in our clinical microsystem?	• Who are our supporting departments?	• What are our census numbers by hour, day, and week, and what is the variation?
• Patient population with seasonal fluctuations?	• What roles and functions do we currently have, and how do they relate to our main aim or purpose?	• What are our key supporting processes?	• What is the number of discharges per day, per week, per month, and what is the variation?

Patients	Professionals	Processes	Patterns
• Most frequent diagnoses?	• What information technology do we depend on to support care?	• What is our interdependence (linkages) with other micro systems?	• What is the average length of stay?
• Frequent users of services?	• Where do our staff spend their time?	• What is our dependence on our macrosystem?	
• How satisfied are our patients with our services?	• What resources do we have available daily to provide patient care?		
	• What is the morale of our staff?		
	• Are health profession students part of our team?		

Home Health Care

Patients	Professionals	Processes	Patterns
• Age distribution and % of females?	• Who are the people in our clinical micro system?	• Who are our supporting departments?	• What are our census numbers by hour, day, and week, and what is the variation?
• Patient population with seasonal fluctuations?	• Where do our staff spend their time (for example: homes, driving, public transportation)?	• What are our key supporting processes?	• What is the number of discharges per day, per week, per month, and what is the variation?
• Most frequent diagnoses?	• What is the morale of our staff?	• What is our interdependence (linkages) with other microsystems?	• What is the average length of Stay?
• Frequent users of services?	• Are health profession students part of our team?	• What is our dependence on our macrosystem?	
• How satisfied are our patients with our services?			

(continued)

TABLE 5.2 (*Continued*)

Nursing Home Core

Patients	Professionals	Processes	Patterns
• Age distribution and % of females	• Who are the people in our clinical microsystem?	• Who are our supporting departments?	• What are our census numbers by hour, day, and week, and what is the variation?
• Patient population with seasonal fluctuations?	• What roles and functions do we currently have, and how do they relate to our main aim or purpose?	• What are our key supporting processes?	• What is the number of discharges per day, per week, per month, and what is the variation?
• Most frequent diagnoses?	• What information on technology do we depend on to support care?	• What is our interdependence (linkages) with other microsystems?	• What is the average length of stay?
• Frequent users of services?	• Where do our staff spend their time?	• What is our dependence on our macrosystem?	
• How satisfied are our patients with our services?	• What resources do we have available daily to provide patient care?		
	• What resources do we have available daily to provide patient care?		
	• What is the morale of our staff?		
	• Are health profession students part of our team?		

Specialty Care

Patients	Professionals	Processes	Patterns
• What are our most frequently referred patient types?	• Who are the people in our clinical micro system?	• What is the cycle time for usual episode of care?	• Who are the most frequent referring providers?
• What % of patients referred require the special skills and knowledge of our specialty?	• What roles and functions do we currently have, and how do they relate to our main aim or purpose?	• Who are our supporting departments?	• What is the satisfaction rating of our referring providers?
• Number of patients returned to referring providers per week?	• What information technology do we depend on to support care?	• What are our key supporting processes?	• What are the services of satisfaction and of dissatisfaction for our referring providers?
	• Where do our staff spend their time?	• What is our interdependence (linkages) with other micro systems?	
	• What resources do we have available daily to provide patient care?	• What is our dependence on our macrosystem?	
	• What is the morale of our staff?		
	• Are health profession students part of our team?		

It is important to understand that the 5Ps are always evolving. The 5Ps baseline assessment is a starting point and additional information, data, and facts should be added as improvement work uncovers and creates new data and information.

Know Your Purpose. Being clear about the purpose of the microsystem guides the relationship between the microsystem's work processes and the population's need. The purpose describes the microsystem's orientation – its true north – for improvement and development of the work processes and systems. Remember that this purpose must be relevant to the population the microsystem seeks to serve. The purpose of a microsystem is not the larger organization's vision or mission or a specific improvement goal. Rather, the conversation about purpose is intended to gain insight into what the microsystem means to each member.

Some helpful questions about purpose include:

- As we think of the people we care for and what we are trying to create, what is our intention?
- What brings meaning to our daily work?
- Why does our microsystem exist?

Avoid the temptation to refer to organizational demands such reducing costs, reducing length of stay, hitting a specific target, and so on. These are performance goals and not the reasons why the microsystem exists.

Know Your Patients. Relentless pursuit of patient knowledge is a cornerstone in connecting the populations served to the microsystem's work – what patients need, what they bring, what they get, and how they fare. With rare exceptions, such as the pioneering work of Ernest A. Codman and John E. Wennberg, most practitioners have lacked data on the vital details of the patient populations they care for (Gittelsohn and Wennberg, 1973; Donabedian, 1989; Wennberg and others, 1989; Codman, 1996; Millenson, 1997; Neuhauser, 2002). Further, they know even less about distinct subpopulations of patients. Clinical microsystems also need to be acutely aware of patients' and families' actual experience of care. Although patient satisfaction surveys are common, the results are often returned to the microsystem months after the survey administration, which makes it difficult to take timely action to improve services. A brief, point-of-service patient satisfaction survey, such as that shown in Figure 5.6 (Godfrey, Nelson, and Batalden, 2005), can be used to provide timely, patient-based feedback. A growing trend is to gather patient and family experience of care (as opposed to simple "satisfaction") through surveys (Homa and others, 2013). The Cystic Fibrosis Foundation care centers across the United States are using the experiences of people with CF and their family members increasingly to inform improvement and redesign of the care and services provided. (See Sidebar "Moving from Satisfaction to Patient and Family Experience of Care.")

FIGURE 5.6 PATIENT VIEWPOINT SURVEY.

PATIENT VIEWPOINT SURVEY*

Today's Office Visit.   Date _____

Here are some general questions about the visit you or the patient just made to this practice. We would like to know how you would rate each of the following.

	Excellent	Very Good	Good	Fair	Poor
1. Length of time you waited to get an appointment	☐	☐	☐	☐	☐
2. Convenience of the location of the office	☐	☐	☐	☐	☐
3. Getting through to the office by phone	☐	☐	☐	☐	☐
4. Length of time waiting at the office	☐	☐	☐	☐	☐
5. Time spent with the person you saw	☐	☐	☐	☐	☐
6. Explanation of what was done at the office	☐	☐	☐	☐	☐
7. The technical skills (thoroughness, carefulness, competence) of the person seen	☐	☐	☐	☐	☐
8. The personal manner (courtesy, respect, sensitivity, friendliness) of the person seen	☐	☐	☐	☐	☐
9. The clinician's sensitivity to special needs or concerns.	☐	☐	☐	☐	☐
10. The satisfaction with getting the help and information that you or the patient needed	☐	☐	☐	☐	☐
11. The quality of the visit overall	☐	☐	☐	☐	☐

General Questions

Here are some general questions about your or the patient's satisfaction with this practice.

12. If you or the patient could go anywhere to get health care, would you choose this practice or would you prefer to go someplace else?

☐ Would choose this practice   ☐ Might prefer someplace else   ☐ Not sure

13. "I am delighted with everything about this practice because my expectations for service and quality of care are exceeded."

☐ Agree   ☐ Disagree   ☐ Not sure

14. In the past 12 months, how many times have you or the patient gone to the emergency room for care?

☐ None   ☐ One time   ☐ Two times   ☐ Three or more times

15. In the past 12 months, was it always easy to get a referral to a specialist when one was needed?

☐ Yes   ☐ No   ☐ Does not apply to me

16. In the past 12 months, how often did you or the patient have to see someone else when you wanted to see a personal doctor or nurse?

☐ Never   ☐ Sometimes   ☐ Frequently

17. Are you or the patient able to schedule appointments when you choose?

☐ Never   ☐ Sometimes   ☐ Frequently

18. Is there anything our practice can do to improve the care and services?
☐ No, everything is satisfactory
☐ Yes, some things can be improved (please specify): _____
_____
_____
☐ Yes, lots of things can be improved (please specify): _____
_____
_____
_____

19. Did you or the patient have any good or bad surprises while receiving care?

☐ Good   ☐ Bad   ☐ No Surprises

Please describe: _____
_____
_____

About You or the Patient

20. In general, how would you rate your overall health or the health of the patient?

☐ Excellent   ☐ Very Good   ☐ Good   ☐ Fair   ☐ Poor

21. What is your age or the age of the patient?

☐ Under 18 years   ☐ 18 - 29 years   ☐ Over 30 years

22. What is your gender or the gender of the patient?   ☐ Male   ☐ Female

OPTIONAL As we continue to strive to improve health care, would you be interested in serving as an advisor to the practice?

☐ Yes   ☐ No   ☐ Maybe

Name _____

Phone _____

E-mail _____

See the Hospital CAHPS survey (www.cms.hhs.gov) for other questions that ask the patient's perspective on care.

* This survey is from the Medical Outcomes Study (MOS) Visit-Specific Questionnaire (VSQ), 1993 Patient Utilization, Dartmouth Medical School.

Moving from Satisfaction to Patient and Family Experience of Care

In 2012, the Cystic Fibrosis Foundation supported the development and validation of the CF Patient and Family Experience of Care (PFEC) survey (Homa and others, 2013). Between 2012 and 2014, the survey was deployed at cystic fibrosis (CF) programs having a reaccreditation site visit from the CF Foundation. The survey was updated in 2015 to reflect the new infection prevention and control guidelines and to change the data collection from a one-time event to a continuous data collection in which people with CF are asked twice a year to complete a survey (for children with CF, the survey is completed by parent or caregiver).

The PFEC survey contains questions about observations of care, not the level of satisfaction with the care. A sample question from the observed experience of care specific to infection control is, "Were you brought to the exam room as soon as you arrived for your appointment?"

Included response choices are "Yes, definitely," "Yes, somewhat," and "No." If the question were framed from a satisfaction perspective, the question could be worded as, "Were you satisfied with the time you waited to see the first CF team member?" Experience of care hinges on learning whether a need or clinical guideline was met or not and the satisfaction perspective learns about "happiness" with an aspect of care.

Interprofessional improvement teams in microsystems are using the PFEC survey around the USA and using patient experiences to inform improvement activities. Survey results have led to improvement in infection prevention and control practices, new supplies and equipment purchases to prevent the spread of pathogens between people with CF, and new process designs to enhance electronic medical record alerts.

Some helpful questions for the microsystem to ask about patients and families include:

- Who do we care for?
- Are there subpopulations for whom we should plan services differently?
- What are the most common patient diagnoses and conditions in our practice?
- What is the experience of patients and families in our microsystem?
- What are usual outcomes for our population and subpopulations?

Know Your Professionals. Often, members of clinical microsystems do not see their own work and the roles and functions of others (including patients and families) as interdependent. The true work of the microsystem is a collaborative effort supported by a shared aim and a system for providing care to distinct subpopulations of patients. The professionals are essential for good system functionality. Managing staff as vital resources and basing decisions on detailed data on patients' needs and demand for services are essential. The whole of the practice can be only as good as its individual components. Staff are often so busy trying to do "the job" that they have no time to reflect on the work they do, how they do it, and what the outcomes of their efforts are. Rework and workarounds are often the result of inabilities and opportunities to improve processes and systems. Involvement of all members of the microsystem is essential to render the best patient services.

Some helpful questions about professionals include:

- Who provides patient care, and who are the people supporting the clinical care team?
- What skills and talents do staff members need to provide the right service and right care at the right time?
- What are the activities of each member of the microsystem? Do education, licensure, and training of members match what they are actually doing?
- Does the microsystem use temporary staff?
- What is the role of information and information technology as a "microsystem member" such as an electronic medical record that contributes important information about care?
- What are the morale and the level of stress in your microsystem?
- What is the turnover rate?
- Would staff members recommend working in your microsystem?
- What are the roles in care and services that occur outside traditional visits?

Know Your Processes. Processes are how systems do their work. The interprofessional members of a microsystem participate in many processes to provide care and services to patients and families. Unfortunately, many health professionals are "process illiterate" (Batalden and Stoltz, 1994) and do not know the steps or details of how care and services are provided. The best way to eliminate process illiteracy is to use flowcharting or process mapping. Often microsystem members have never had the opportunity to meet together to review specific processes of care and learn the different views and perspectives of each member using the flowcharting process. Identifying core processes of the microsystem and engaging all members in the flowcharting process builds relationships and knowledge of each other's contributions. Flowcharting also enhances understanding of the interdependence that exists in the microsystem. Variation in clinical services is often related to an individual's preference about the way things are done rather than a decision about the best process for the patient. Table 5.3 provides an assessment tool to help clinical microsystems evaluate the services they provide.

All staff members (1) complete the assessment tool; (2) determine which process to improve (the highest-ranked problem process); and (3) begin to test changes by modifying the current process using small tests of change.

TABLE 5.3 PRACTICE CORE AND SUPPORTING PROCESSES ASSESSMENT.

Process	Works Well	Small Problem	Real Problem	Totally Broken	Cannot Rate	We're Working on it	Source of Patient Complaint
Appointment system							
Answering phones							
Messaging							
Scheduling procedures							
Reporting diagnostic test results							
Prescription renewals							
Making referrals							
Preauthorization for services							
Billing and coding							
Phone advice							
Assignment of patients to our practice							
Orientation of patients to our practice							
New patient workups							
Education for patients and families							
Prevention assessment and activities							
Chronic disease management							

Note: Each of the processes is rated by each staff member using the categories shown. If the process is a source of patient complaint, that is also noted.

Some helpful questions about processes include:

- How do we deliver care and services to meet our patients' needs?
- What are our core and supporting processes?
- How do core and supporting processes get accomplished?
- Who does what in our microsystem?
- Are they done in the same way by every member of the team?
- How do we depict these key processes with a flow chart?
- How does technology support our processes?
- How does technology support workflow and care delivery?
- How much time does it take for patients to receive services?

- How much undesirable variation in processes exists?
- How much waste and rework occurs, making the day more frustrating?
- Are patients assessed in a standard way?
- Do clinical support staff perform activities that anticipate the arrival of patients?
- What other microsystems does your microsystem "hand off" patients to and receive patients from?

Analysis and Improvement of Processes

A general internal medicine practice analyzed current processes and identified improvements that could lead to better efficiencies and reductions in waste. Every member of the practice – including physicians, nurse practitioners, nurses, and secretaries completed the Practice Core and Supporting Processes Assessment (see Table 5.4). This revealed that the diagnostic test reporting process needed to be improved by shortening the time taken to report results to providers and patients. After flowcharting the process – which revealed rework, waste, delay, and long cycle times – the group brainstormed change ideas and then rank-ordered the ideas. The group decided to test the idea of holding a huddle at the beginning of each day to review diagnostic test results and to specify actions for specific individuals. The aim was to eliminate extra phone calls from the patients and delays in taking action as a result of waiting for the provider to respond. With the process, all group members would know the action plan after the huddle.

Using the plan-do-study-act (PDSA) method, the team conducted its small test of change. Within two weeks patient phone calls for laboratory results had decreased, reflecting the fact that staff were now calling patients in a timely manner about their results. (For more information about analysis and improvement see Langley and others, 1996; Nelson and others, 1998a; Nelson and others, 1998b).

Know Your Patterns. Each microsystem's particular combination of patients, professionals, and processes creates patterns that reflect routine ways of thinking, feeling, and behaving on the part of both patients and staff in the system. Patterns are also related to the typical results and outcomes the system achieves. Some patterns will be well known and talked about (for example, hours of service, busy times of the day or week, common hassles, and bottlenecks). Some patterns may be well known but never discussed, such as hierarchy, unwarranted variation, and special considerations for certain staff members. Some patterns may be unrecognized by staff and patients but nevertheless have powerful effects (for example, mistrust stemming from a local culture dominated by historical divides that separate staff with different educational backgrounds, such as nurses, receptionists, physicians, and technicians). Other patterns might relate to the degree of psychological safety in the microsystem. Do all staff feel safe reporting safety issues or concerns in their daily work (Edmondson, 2018)? Leadership may also be reflected in important patterns. Is the leadership a command-and-control model or a more distributed leadership model? Some patterns are not known and not discussed, such as certain outcomes for a defined subpopulation of patients. It can be helpful to think of patterns as including both outcomes for individuals and populations as well as patterns of behavior, action, communication, and relationships.

Some helpful questions about patterns include:

- What are the health outcomes we produce?
- Are outcomes different across different subpopulations?
- Do we meet regularly to discuss how care and services are provided and patient safety?
- What are the regularly recurring associated or sequential work activities?
- What are the costs of care? What are the costs of delivering that care?
- How do we interact with each other in our microsystem?
- What are the usual communication patterns within the microsystem?
- How is our communication with surrounding or supporting microsystems?
- Is there a shared purpose and mutual respect in our microsystem?
- What are the relationships like within and across workgroups (such as with the nurse workgroups, physician workgroups, and administrative workgroups)?
- What does it feel like to work here?
- Do we regularly engage in social activities outside the workplace?
- How do we celebrate our work together?
- How do we stay mindful of the possibility of our efforts failing?

Jody Hoffer Gittell has developed the theory of *relational coordination* and a survey instrument to assess it to further explore communication and relationships within and between microsystems. The activities of creating a relational map and assessing the seven dimensions of relational coordination can make significant contributions to understanding the patterns of a microsystem. Abstract comments about "how we get along" and "who we talk to" become more tangible and actionable through the use of the relational coordination mapping and survey.

Relational Coordination

Relational coordination (RC) is a theory pioneered by Jody Hoffer Gittell that has been successfully adapted and applied in healthcare settings and researched around the world to improve care and outcomes. Through heightened team awareness of communications and relationships within and between workgroups and within and between microsystems, teams can test interventions targeted at structural, relational, and mechanical processes (Gittell and others, 2000; Gittell, 2011). Relational coordination is communicating and relating for the purpose of task integration. More specifically, it is coordinating work through communication that is frequent, timely, accurate, and problem-solving, supported by relationships of shared goals, shared knowledge, and mutual respect.

Seven Dimensions of RC

The seven dimensions of RC span relationships and communication, and include:

- Shared goals
- Shared knowledge
- Mutual respect
- Frequent communication
- Timely communication
- Accurate communication
- Problem-solving communication

Clinical microsystem members can begin the exploration of communication and relationship patterns specific to work processes by creating a relational coordination map (RC map). The RC map as depicted in Figure 5.7 is a result of a microsystem group considering the RC seven dimensions across their

FIGURE 5.7 RC MAP.

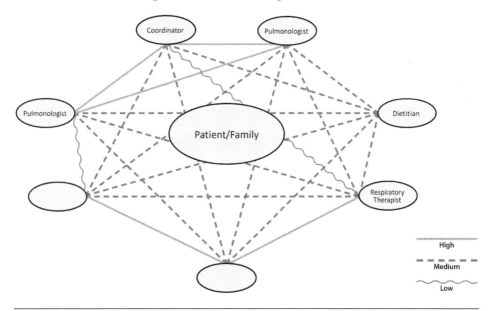

workgroups in their clinical microsystem specific to a defined work process. As the key shows, the total perceived RC between the workgroups can be rated as strong, moderate, or weak. The act of defining the workgroups and creating the RC map together begins to place a spotlight on communication and relationship challenges specific to work processes to begin to identify interventions to improve them. The RC mapping engages the members in simple discussions about the dimensions and how they are perceived within the microsystem. It is important that RC mapping be undertaken with a particular process in mind; it is not an exercise to learn if workgroups "like each other;" it is an exercise to learn how the dimensions of RC play out in specific work. The validated Relational Coordination Survey (Gittell, 2002) can be used for a formal assessment of RC at the microsystem level. Functional workgroups are designated by the microsystem, and RC assessment within and between these workgroups is measured (Gittell, 2016).

Putting it all Together: Co-Designing and Planning Services

Based on the 5Ps assessment, a microsystem can now help itself in a more informed way to identify opportunities to do things better for patients, families, and staff. Planning services are designed to do the following:

- Decrease unnecessary variation.
- Build feed-forward and feedback mechanisms for informed decision-making.
- Enable coproduction.
- Promote efficiency by continuously removing waste and rework.
- Create processes and systems that support staff to be the best they can be.
- Specify core and supporting processes and use flowcharts to design smooth, effective, and safe patient care that leads to measurably improved patient outcomes flow.

Figure 5.8 offers a panoramic view of a primary care clinical microsystem. It suggests the interplay of patients with practice staff and with processes, which in turn produces patterns that characterize the microsystem's performance. Managing these patterns can result in the best health care for patients and for microsystem staff. In addition to the core processes of the microsystem (such as an acute care visit), typical supporting processes in a primary care practice include such activities as renewing prescriptions, reporting diagnostic test results to patients, and making referrals.

FIGURE 5.8 HIGH-LEVEL VIEW OF A PRIMARY CARE CLINICAL MICROSYSTEM.

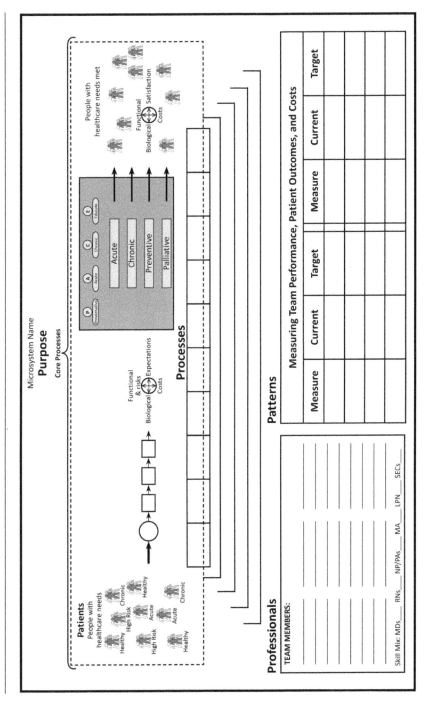

Source: Adapted from Nelson, E. C. and others, 2011, p. 30. Used with permission.

Using Process Knowledge to Redesign Care

Flowcharts can be used to diagram and diagnose each process to learn how to redesign it to maximize efficiency. This tool is particularly valuable with core or supporting processes whose patterns are characterized by hassles, bottlenecks, and mistakes (see Table 5.3). Many clinical microsystems have used the methods in Part Two of *Quality by Design* first edition for guided discovery and for taking actions to redesign their services; some examples of their work are provided in Table 5.4.

A review of some of the microsystem improvement efforts to which we have contributed has uncovered many common sources of waste. Table 5.5 summarizes some of these sources and recommends ways to reduce waste and improve efficiency.

High-performing clinical microsystems have learned to reap the benefits of daily meetings, or huddles, to plan the day and weekly or monthly meetings to strategize and manage improvement, as described by the plastic surgery team in the boxed example that follows. Holding regular sessions to advance patient-centered care and services has several benefits. It can:

- Promote collegiality and create an environment of equality.
- Improve communications.
- Make visible the team of interdisciplinary professionals engaged in planning and providing care for patients and families.
- Keep staff members *patient-focused*.

A clinical microsystem might ultimately build its own playbook – an organized collection of flowcharted processes that can be used for training, performance management, and improvement. The playbook can be used for educating new staff, cross-training staff, managing performance, and troubleshooting because it describes how processes should work.

Redesigning the Microsystem to Improve Quality of Care for Hospitalized Patients

Kevin O'Leary, Julie K. Johnson, Jason Stein, Milisa Manojlovich

Most adults requiring hospitalization are admitted for medical conditions (NCHS, 2015; Pfuntner, Wier, and Stocks, 2013), yet the optimal model of care for these patients is yet to be established (Pannick and others, 2014). Teams caring for medical patients are often large, with membership that continually evolves, and the team is seldom in the same place at the same time (O'Leary and others, 2009). Physicians are spread across multiple units and floors giving them little opportunity to develop relationships with nurses and other professionals who work on designated units (O'Leary and others, 2010b). Nurse and physician leaders commonly operate in silos, limiting their ability to address challenges collaboratively (O'Leary and others, 2010a). Patients and family members are generally poorly informed and lack opportunities to engage in decision-making and coproduction of their care (Batalden and others, 2016; O'Leary and others, 2010d). As a result, medical services lack the structure and professionals lack the shared accountability necessary to optimally coordinate care on a daily basis and improve performance over time.

A growing body of research has tested interventions to redesign aspects of care delivery for hospitalized medical patients (O'Leary and others, 2009; Kim and others, 2012; Singh and others, 2012; Fanucchi, Unterbrink, and Logio, 2014; Kim and others, 2014; Pannick and others, 2015; Bhamidipati and others, 2016; Mueller and others, 2016). These interventions include localization of physicians to specific units, unit nurse-physician co-leadership, interdisciplinary rounds, performance dashboards, and patient-engagement strategies. Studies show that these interventions improve processes and culture, but the evidence that patient outcomes have improved is equivocal. Importantly, most studies have examined the effect of single interventions in isolation, yet these interventions are better conceptualized as complementary and mutually reinforcing components of a redesigned clinical microsystem.

Research into clinical microsystems identified five overarching characteristics associated with success – local leadership, focus on the needs of staff, emphasis on the needs of patients, attention to performance, and a rich information environment (Nelson and others, 2002). Hospital medicine services provide an ideal opportunity to study the impact of redesigning clinical microsystems because challenges exist in each of these five areas (Table 5.6). Furthermore, improvements in these areas may impact care across a range of conditions, not just for a particular diagnosis.

The few studies in which interventions have been implemented as components of a larger effort to redesign clinical microsystems appear to show a positive impact on patient outcomes. For example, Stein and colleagues (2015) implemented an Accountable Care Unit (ACU) model, consisting of unit-based teams, structured interdisciplinary bedside rounds, unit-level reporting data, and unit-level nurse and physician co-leadership on a medical unit at Emory University Hospital. Although not rigorously assessed, the interventions appeared to reduce length of stay and mortality. Kara and colleagues implemented a similar model, the Accountable Care Team (ACT) model, including *geographic cohorting* of patients and providers, interprofessional bedside rounds, and monthly review of unit level data, on 11 units at Indiana University Health Methodist Hospital (Kara and others, 2015). The degree to which units implemented components of the intervention was associated with improved length of stay and costs, but not patient satisfaction scores. O'Leary and colleagues have sequentially implemented similar interventions, including geographic localization of physicians, unit nurse-physician co-leadership, structured interdisciplinary rounds (SIDR), and unit-level performance reports at Northwestern Memorial Hospital (O'Leary and others, 2010a–d, 2011a, 2011b). These interventions were associated with improvements in teamwork climate and a reduction in adverse events.

Larger-scale studies are needed to determine whether the use of complementary interventions anchored in a clinical microsystem framework is associated with improved patient outcomes. In light of the challenges related to systems redesign, further research should also elucidate strategies to successfully adapt interventions in the local context to optimize implementation and impact.

TABLE 5.4 ASSESSING YOUR PRACTICE DISCOVERIES AND ACTIONS: THE PS.

Know your Patients	Discoveries	Actions Taken
1. Age distribution	30% of our patients are > 66 years old	Designed special group visits to review specific needs of this age group, including physical limitations, dietary considerations.
2. Disease identification	We do not know what percentage of our patients have diabetes.	Team-reviewed coding and billing data to determine approximate numbers of patients with diabetes.
3. Health outcomes	Do not know what the range of HbA1c is for our patients with diabetes, or if they are receiving appropriate ADA-recommended care in a timely fashion.	Team conducted a chart audit with 50 charts during a lunch hour. Using a tool designed to track outcomes, each member of the team reviewed 5 charts and noted the findings on the audit tool.
4. Most frequent diagnosis	We learned we had a large number of patients with stable hypertension and diabetes seeing the physician frequently. We also learned that during certain seasons we had huge volumes of pharyngitis and poison ivy.	Designed and tested a new model of care delivery for stable hypertension and diabetes, optimizing the RN role in the practice using agreed-upon guidelines, protocols, and tools.
5. Patient satisfaction	We don't know what patients think unless they complain to us.	Implemented the point of service patient survey, patients completed and left in a box before leaving the practice.

Know your Professionals	Discoveries	Actions Taken
1. Provider FTE	We were making assumptions about provider time in the clinic without really understanding how much time providers are out of the clinic with hospital rounds, nursing home rounds, and so on.	Changed our scheduling process; utilized RNs to provide care for certain subpopulations.
2. Schedules	Several providers are gone at the same time every week, so one provider is often left and the entire staff work overtime that day.	Evaluated the scheduling template to even out each provider's time to provide consistent coverage of the clinic.
3. Regular meetings	The doctors meet together every other week. The secretaries meet once a month.	Began holding an entire practice meeting every other week on Wednesdays to help the practice become a team.
4. Hours of operation	The beginning and the end of the day are always chaotic. We realized we are on the route for patients between home and work and they want to be seen when we are not open.	Opened one hour earlier and stayed open one hour later each day. The heavy demand was managed better and overtime dropped.

TABLE 5.4 (*Continued*)

Know your Professionals	Discoveries	Actions Taken
5. Activity surveys	All roles are not being used to their maximum. RNs only room patients and take vital signs, medical assistants doing a great deal of secretarial paperwork, and some secretaries are giving out medical advice.	Roles have been redesigned and matched to individual education, training, and licensure.

Know your Processes	Discoveries	Actions Taken
1. Cycle time	Patient lengths of visits vary a great deal. There are many delays.	The team identified actions to eliminate and steps to combine and learned to prepare the charts for the patient visit before the patient arrives. The team also holds daily huddles to inform everyone on the plan of the day and any issues to consider throughout the day.
2. Key supporting processes	None of us could agree on how things get done in our practice.	Detailed flowcharting of our practice to determine how to streamline and do in a consistent manner.
3. Indirect patient pulls	The providers are interrupted in their patient care process frequently. The number one reason is to retrieve missing equipment and supplies from the exam room.	The team agreed on standardization of exam rooms and minimum inventory lists that were posted on the inside cabinet doors. A process was also determined for who would stock exam rooms regularly and how the rooms would be stocked, and through the use of an assignment sheet, people for this task were identified and held accountable.

Know your Patterns	Discoveries	Actions Taken
1. Demand on the practice	There are peaks and lows for the practice, depending on day of the week, session of the day or season of the year.	The team identified actions to eliminate and steps to combine, and learned to prepare the charts for the patient visit before the patient arrives. The team also holds daily huddles to inform everyone on the plan of the day and any issues to consider throughout the day.
2. Communication	We do not communicate in a timely way, nor do we have a standard forum in which to communicate.	Every other week practice meetings are held to help communication and e-mail use by all staff and to promote timely communication.
3. Cultural	The doctors don't really spend time with nondoctors.	The team meetings and heightened awareness of behaviors have helped improve this.

(continued)

TABLE 5.4 (*Continued*)

Know your Patterns	Discoveries	Actions Taken
4. Outcomes	We really have not paid attention to our practice outcomes.	Began tracking and awareness and posting results on a data wall to keep us alert to outcomes.
5. Finances	Only the doctors and the practice manager know about the practice money	Finances are discussed at the team meetings and everyone is learning how all of us make a difference in practice financial performance.

Note: HbA1c = glycosylated hemoglobin; ADA = American Diabetes Association; URI = upper respiratory infection.

Conclusion

Knowledge of the purpose, patients, professionals, processes, and patterns of a clinical microsystem drives the design, redesign, and creation of patient-centered services, ideally coproduced services. The process of convening an interprofessional improvement team to explore the context using the disciplined 5Ps structure further develops team relationships and a sense of ownership to identify and lead improvements. The design of services leads to critical analysis of the resources needed for the right person to deliver the right care, in the right way, at the right time. Tools and methods to support the transformation of clinical microsystems so they yield better results for patients and staff have been described here and offered for widespread use and adaptation.

Mesosystem Considerations

Every mesosystem (two or more clinical or supporting microsystems) will benefit from exploring and understanding their context of care across multiple microsystems to create a system of care for the identified population of patients. Adapting the 5Ps to a mesosystem pathway of care of multiple microsystems requires each microsystem in the mesosystem to consider the identified population and each of the 5Ps in their own microsystem. The mesosystem workbook in Part Two of this book outlines additional considerations for a mesosystem including the shared purpose of the mesosystem that all the individual microsystems can commit to and communication considerations between the microsystems to ensure smooth transition

TABLE 5.5 ASSESSING YOUR PRACTICE DISCOVERIES AND ACTIONS: COMMON OVERSIGHTS AND WASTES.

Common High-Yield Wastes	Recommended Methods to Reduce Waste	Traps to Avoid
1. Exam rooms not stocked or standardized: missing equipment or supplies.	• Create standard inventory of supplies for all exam rooms. • Design process for regular stocking of exam rooms, with accountable person. • Standardize and utilize all exam rooms.	• Don't assume rooms are being stocked regularly — track and measure. • Providers will use only "their own" rooms. • Providers cannot agree upon standard supplies — suggest "testing."
2. Too many appointment types, which creates chaos in scheduling.	• Reduce appointment types to 2 to 4. • Use standard building blocks to create flexibility in schedule.	
3. Poor communication among the providers and support staff about clinical sessions and patient needs.	• Conduct daily morning huddles to provide a forum to review the schedule, anticipate the needs of patients, and plan supplies and information needed for a highly productive interaction between patient and provider.	• People are not showing up for the scheduled huddle — gain the support of providers who are interested; test the idea and measure the results. • Huddle lasts longer than 15 minutes — use a worksheet to guide the huddle.
4. Missing information or chart for patient visits.	• Conduct daily morning huddles to provide a forum to review the schedule, anticipate the needs of patients, and plan supplies and information needed for a highly productive interaction between patient and provider.	• Avoid doing chart review when patient is present. • If you have computerized access to test results, don't print the results.

(continued)

TABLE 5.5 (Continued)

Common High-Yield Wastes	Recommended Methods to Reduce Waste	Traps to Avoid
5. Confusing messaging system.	• Standardize messaging process for all providers. • Educate and train on messaging content. • Use a process with a prioritization method, such as a bin system in each provider office.	• Providers may want their own way — this adds confusion for supply staff and decreases cross-coverage capacity. • Content of message can't be agreed upon — test something!
6. High number of prescription renewal requests via phones.	• Anticipate needs of the patients. • Create reminder systems in the office, such as posters, screen savers. • Standardize the information support staff obtain from patients before the provider visit — include prescription information and needs.	• It doesn't need to be the RN who takes the call — medical assistants can obtain this information.
7. Staff frustrated in roles and unable to see new ways to function.	• Review current roles and functions, using activity survey sheets. • Match education, training, licensure to function. • Optimize every role. • Eliminate functions.	• Be sure to focus on talent, training, and scope of practice, not on individual people.
8. Appointment schedules have limited same-day appointment slots.	• Evaluate follow-up appointment and return visit necessity. • Extend the intervals of standard follow-up visits. • Consider RN visits. • Evaluate the use of protocols and guidelines to provide advice for home care — www.icsi.org	• Do not set a certain number of same-day appointments without allowing for variations through-out the year.

9. Missed disease-specific or preventive interventions and tracking.	• Use flowcharts to track preventive activities and disease-specific interventions. • Be alert to creating a system for multiple diseases, and do not use many stickers and many registries. • Use "stickers" on charts to alert staff to preventive or disease-specific needs. • Review charts before patient visit.
10. Poor communication and interactions between members.	• Hold weekly team meetings to review practice outcomes, staff concerns, improvement opportunities.	• Hold weekly meetings on a regular day and at a regular time and place. • Do not cancel — make the meeting a new habit.
11. High no-show rate among patients.	• Consider improving same-day access.	• Automated reminder telephone calls are not always well received by patients.
12. Patient expectations for visit not met, resulting in phone calls and repeat visits.	• Use CARE vital sign sheet. • Evaluate patient at time of visit to determine whether their needs were met.	• Use reminders to question patients about needs being met. • New habits not easily made.

Mesosystem Questions

Important questions for the mesosystem include:

- How many CF lung transplantations are done a year?
- What is the experience of people with CF who seek lung transplantation?
- Who are the professionals involved?
- How do the referral, transfer, and transition processes occur between microsystems?
- What are their communication processes?
- What are the clinical outcomes?

TABLE 5.6 CHALLENGES ON MEDICAL SERVICES BY MICROSYSTEM DOMAIN.

Domains	Challenges
Local Leadership	• Nursing and physician leaders often operate in silos. • Physician leadership at the unit level may not exist. • Formal training of unit leaders is often lacking.
Focus on Needs of Staff	• Dispersion of physicians limits their connection to any particular unit. • Team members inconsistently given orientation to units/services. • Team member roles and expectations not defined.
Emphasis on Needs of Patients	• Patients have poor comprehension of plan of care. • Limited opportunities exist for patients and families to partner in care.
Attention to Performance	• Performance data often unavailable at the unit level. • Limited data to prompt changes during patients' hospitalizations.
Rich Information Environment	• Few opportunities for team members to share information and collaborate on better decisions. • Technology not leveraged to identify opportunities to improve care.

Source: Adapted from Bhamidipati and others, 2016; Fanucchi and others, 2014; Kim and others, 2012; Kim and others, 2014; Mueller and others, 2016; O'Leary and others, 2009; Pannick and others, 2015; Singh and others, 2012.

FIGURE 5.9 CF LUNG TRANSPLANT MESOSYSTEM 5PS.

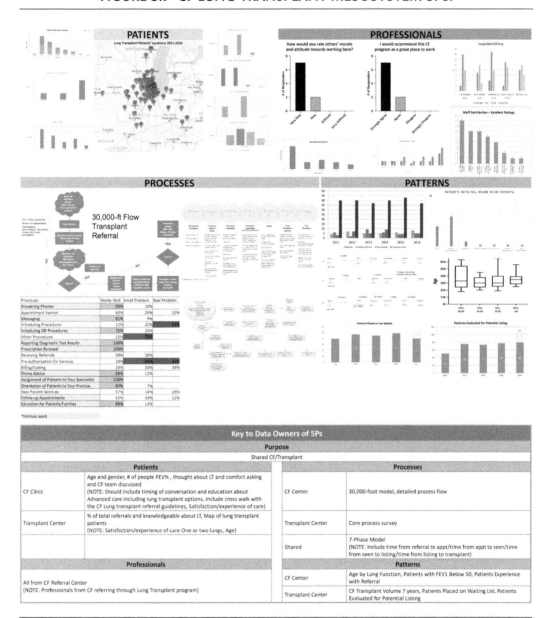

of the population from microsystem to microsystem. An example of mesosystem 5Ps assessment (shown in Figure 5.9) shows the 5Ps specific to the CF lung transplant population. Important questions for the mesosystem to answer include, how many CF lung transplantations are done a year? What is the experience of people with CF who seek lung transplantation? Who are the professionals involved? How do the referral, transfer, and transition processes occur between the microsystems? What are their communication processes? What are the clinical outcomes?

Summary

To be able to intentionally plan services and care for populations of patients and individual patients, high-performing clinical microsystems meet regularly to review current processes and outcomes to match with patient needs. These efforts should be supported by a continuous flow of data (for example, data can be produced throughout the day to identify unfilled appointment slots) to inform every member of the microsystem, to drive corrective actions (any staff person can schedule patients into unfilled slots anytime during the day), and to spawn improvements (at monthly all-staff meetings and annual retreats).

The service sector has many examples of people coming together to plan the services they deliver. In good restaurants waiters, cooks, and hostesses preview the menus for the day and review strategies to ensure that the meal service is flawless. Plans are made to cover breaks, and what-if scenarios are rehearsed. Flight crews routinely preview the flight plan, use checklists to prepare for take-off, and review flights after their completion, because they know all of this contributes to a culture of trust, reliability, and safety. Huddles to plan care and services and to share information have become more commonplace in healthcare settings. Examples include huddles before a primary care morning session and huddles before a hospital shift held at a white board reviewing safety concerns, patient and family concerns, some outcomes of current interest, concerns and challenges, and reminders of the microsystem goals (Barve and Kruer, 2018).

Focusing attention first and foremost on the patient and family and how they present their health needs to the system makes it relatively easy to identify the needed services and to determine how the best services can be designed within each microsystem and how these services can be best linked together. Coproduction of health care and services is based on the interdependent work of patients, families, and professionals who create, design, produce, deliver, assess, and evaluate the relationships and actions that contribute to the health of individuals and populations (Elwyn and others, 2019). Convening interdisciplinary members including patients and families regularly and using effective meeting skills, relationships can be enhanced and lead to ideal care services that meet everyone's needs.

The staff in many microsystems work in a complex environment characterized by competing interests, inefficiencies, hassles, and frustrations due to poorly operating processes. They may feel helpless or that they cannot make the system work correctly because the system is run by outsiders. As shown in this chapter's case study, this feeling can be counteracted by working from the inside out, meaning that staff learn about their own patients and their microsystem – and then make improvements – as they go about their work, rather than being told what to do by those outside the microsystem.

Review Questions

1. What are the 5Ps of a clinical microsystem?
2. What are some examples of patterns in a clinical microsystem?
3. What are the seven dimensions of relational coordination?
4. How would you plan to assess a pathway of care for a population in a mesosystem using the 5Ps?

Discussion Questions

1. As you consider the transformation described in the first case study, what was most important in enabling that transformation? What more would you want to know to confirm your hunch?
2. Give examples of the significance of context when leading change.
3. Consider the challenges described in Table 5.6 in the sidebar on improving inpatient care. Are these specific to the inpatient setting? How might you test a change to address one of them?

Additional Activities

1. Identify a microsystem and with an interprofessional improvement team assess the 5Ps to identify strengths and improvement opportunities.
2. Convene an interdisciplinary group of a mesosystem and help them assess the 5Ps of the mesosystem. What strategy can be used to get the microsystem members to support and improve a mesosystem?

References

Agency for Healthcare Research and Quality. *What is Patient Experience?* Rockville, MD: Agency for Healthcare Research and Quality. [https://www.ahrq.gov/cahps/about-cahps/patient-experience/]. Mar. 2017.

Ayanian, J. Z., and Markel, H. "Donabedian's Lasting Framework for Health Care Quality." *The New England Journal of Medicine*, 2016, 375(3), 205-207. doi: 10.1056/NEJMp1605101

Barve, K., and Kruer, R. "Using Daily Management and Visual Boards to Improve Key Indicators and Staff Engagement." *NEJM Catalyst*, 2018 May 15, 4(3).

Batalden, M., Batalden, P., Margolis, P., and others. "Coproduction of Healthcare Service." *BMJ Quality & Safety*, 2016, 25(7), 509-517. doi: 10.1136/bmjqs-2015-004315

Batalden, P., and Stoltz, P. "Fostering the Leadership of a Continually Improving Healthcare Organization." *Quality Letter for Healthcare Leaders*, 1994, 6(6), 9-15.

Batalden, P. B., and Davidoff, F. "What Is 'Quality Improvement' and How Can It Transform Healthcare?" *Quality and Safety in Health Care*, 2007, 16(1), 2-3. doi: 10.1136/qshc.2006.022046

Batalden, P. B. "Getting More Health from Healthcare: Quality Improvement Must Acknowledge Patient Coproduction – an Essay by Paul Batalden." *BMJ*, 2018, 362, k3617. doi: 10.1136/bmj.k3617

Bhamidipati, V. S., Elliott, D. J., Justice, E. M., and others. "Structure and Outcomes of Interdisciplinary Rounds in Hospitalized Medicine Patients: A Systematic Review and Suggested Taxonomy." *Journal of Hospital Medicine*, 2016, 11(7, Jul), 513-523. doi: 10.1002/jhm.2575

Black, N., Varaganum, M., and Hutchings, A. "Relationship Between Patient Reported Experience (Prems) and Patient Reported Outcomes (Proms) in Elective Surgery." *BMJ Quality & Safety*, 2014, 23, 534-542. doi: 10.1136/bmjq1s-2013-002707

Codman, E. A. *A Study in Hospital Efficiency: As Demonstrated by the Case Report of the First Five Years of a Private Hospital.* Oakbrook Terrace, IL: Joint Commission on Accreditation of Healthcare Organizations, 1996. (Originally published in 1914.)

De Allegri, M., Schwarzbach, M., Loerbroks, A., and Ronellenfitsch, U. "Which Factors Are Important for the Successful Development and Implementation of Clinical Pathways? A Qualitative Study." *BMJ Quality & Safety.* 2011, 20(3), 203-208. doi: 10.1136/bmjqs.2010.042465

Dixon-Woods, M. "The Problem of Context in Quality Improvement." In *Perspectives on Context: A Selection of Essays Considering the Role of Context in Successful Quality Improvement.* London: The Health Foundation, 2014 Mar., 87-101.

Dixon-Woods, M., and Martin, G. P. "Does Quality Improvement Improve Quality?" *Future Hospital Journal*, 2016, 3(3), 191-194. doi: 10.7861/futurehosp.3-3-191

Donabedian, A. "The End Results of Health Care: Ernest Codman's Contribution to Quality Assessment and Beyond." *Milbank Quarterly*, 1989, 67(2), 233-256.

Edmondson, A. *The Fearless Organization: Creating Psychological Safety in the Workplace for Learning, Innovation, and Growth.* Hoboken, NJ: John Wiley & Sons, 2018.

Elwyn, G., Frosch, D., Thomson, R., and others. "Shared Decision Making: A Model for Clinical Practice." *Journal of General Internal Medicine*, 2012, 27(10, Oct), 1361-1367. doi: 10.1007/s11606-012-2077-6

Elwyn, G., Nelson, E. W., Hager, A., and Price, A. "Coproduction: When Users Define Quality." *BMJ Quality & Safety*, 2019, 0, 1-6. doi: 10.1136/pmjqs-2019-009830

Fanucchi, L., Unterbrink, M., and Logio, L. S. "(Re)turning the Pages of Residency: The Impact of Localizing Resident Physicians to Hospital Units on Paging Frequency." *Journal of Hospital Medicine*, 2014, 9(2), 120-122. doi: 10.1002/jhm.2143

Gittell, J. H., Fairfield, K. M., Bierbaum, B., and others. "Impact of Relational Coordination on Quality of Care, Postoperative Pain and Functioning, and Length of Stay: A Nine-Hospital Study of Surgical Patients." *Medical Care*, 2000, 38(8), 807-819.

Gittell, J. H. "Coordinating Mechanisms in Care Provider Groups: Relational Coordination as a Mediator and Input Uncertainty as a Moderator of Performance Effects." *Management Science*, 2002, 48(11), 1408-1422.

Gittell, J. H. *The Oxford Handbook of Positive Organizational Scholarship*. New York, NY: Oxford University Press, 2011.

Gittell, J. H. *Transforming Relationships for High Performance: The Power of Relational Coordination*. Stanford, CA: Stanford University Press, 2016.

Gittelsohn, A., and Wennberg, J. "Small Area Variations in Health Care Delivery: A Population-Based Health Information System Can Guide Planning and Regulatory Decision-Making." *Science*, 1973, 182(4117), 1102-1108. doi: 10.1126/science.182.4117.1102

Gleeson, H., Cauldron, A., Swami, V., and others. "Systematic Review of Approaches to Using Patient Experience Data for Quality Improvement in Healthcare Settings." *BMJ Open*, 2016, 6:e011907, 1-11. doi: 10.1136/bmjopen-2016-011907

Godfrey, M. M., Nelson, E. C., and Batalden, P. B. *Clinical Microsystems: A Path to Healthcare Excellence: Improving Care Within Your Inpatient Units and Emergency Department*. Workbook. Hanover, NH: Dartmouth College, 2005.

Gomes, M., Gutacker, N., Bojke, C., and Street, A. "Addressing Missing Data in Patient-Reported Outcome Measures (Proms): Implications for the Use of Proms for Comparing Provider Performance." *Health Economics*, 2016, 255, 515-528. doi: 10.1002/hec.3173

Grol, R. "Successes and Failures in the Implementation of Evidence-Based Guidelines for Clinical Practice." *Medical Care*, 2001, 39, 46-54. doi: 10.1097/00005650-200108002-00003

Hargis, M. B., Wyatt, J. D., and Piotrowski, C. "Developing Leaders: Examining the Role of Transactional and Transformational Leadership Across Contexts Business." *Organization Development Journal*, 2011, 29(3), 51-66.

Homa, K., Sabadosa, K. A., Nelson, E. C., and others. "Development and Validation of a Cystic Fibrosis Patient and Family Member Experience of Care Survey." *Quality Management in Health Care*, 2013, 22(2), 100-116. doi: 10.1097/QMH.0b013e31828bc3bc

Jabbour, M., Newton, A. S., Johnson, D., and Curran, J. A. "Defining Barriers and Enablers for Clinical Pathway Implementation in Complex Clinical Settings." *Implementation Science*, 2018, 13(139), 1-13. doi:10.1186/s13012-018-0832-8

Kaplan, H. C., Provost, L. P., Froehle, C. M., and Margolis, P. A. "The Model for Understanding Success in Quality (MUSIQ): Building a Theory of Context in Healthcare Quality Improvement." *BMJ Quality & Safety*, 2012, 21(1), 13-20. doi: 10.1136/bmjqs-2011-000010

Kara, A., Johnson, C. S., Nicley, A., and others. "Redesigning Inpatient Care: Testing the Effectiveness of an Accountable Care Team Model." *Journal of Hospital Medicine*, 2015, 10(12), 773-779. doi: 10.1002/jhm.2432

Kim, C. S., Calarco, M., Jacobs, T., and others. "Leadership at the Front Line: A Clinical Partnership Model on General Care Inpatient Units." *American Journal of Medical Quality*, 2012, 27(2), 106-111. doi: 10.1177/1062860611413257

Kim, C. S., King, E., Stein, J., and others. "Unit-Based Interprofessional Leadership Models in Six US Hospitals." *Journal of Hospital Medicine*, 2014, 9(8), 545-550. doi: 10.1002/jhm.2200

Kringos, D. S., Sunol, R., Wagner, C., and others. "The Influence of Context on the Effectiveness of Hospital Quality Improvement Strategies: A Review of Systematic Reviews." *BMC Health Services Research*, 2015, 15, 277. doi 10.1186/s12913-015-0906-0

Langley, G. J., Nolan, K. M., Norman, C. L., Provost, L. P., and Nolan, T. W. *The Improvement Guide: A Practical Approach to Enhancing Organizational Performance*. San Francisco, CA: Jossey-Bass, 1996.

Lawal, A. K., Rotter, T., Kinsman, L., and others. "What is a Clinical Pathway? Refinement of an Operational Definition to Identify Clinical Pathway Studies for a Cochrane Systematic Review." *BMC Medicine*, 2016, 14(35), 1-5. doi: 10.1186/s12916-016-0580-z

Lipmanowicz, H. *"Buy-in Versus Ownership."* Liberating Structures. [http://www.liberating-structures.com/hl-articles/]. 2010

McNicholas, C., Lennox, L., Woodcock, T., and others. "Evolving Quality Improvement Support Strategies to Improve Plan–Do–Study–Act Cycle Fidelity: A Retrospective Mixed-Methods Study." *BMJ Quality & Safety*, 2019, 28, 356-365.

Millenson, M. *Demanding Medical Excellence*. Chicago, IL: University of Chicago Press, 1997.

Mueller, S. K., Schnipper, J. L., Giannelli, K., and others. "Impact of Regionalized Care on Concordance of Plan and Preventable Adverse Events on General Medicine Services." *Journal of Hospital Medicine*, 2016, 11(9, Sep), 620-627. doi: 10.1002/jhm.2566

National Center for Health Statistics. *Health, United States, 2014: With Special Feature on Adults Aged 55-64*. Hyattsville, MD: National Center for Health Statistics; 2015.

National Committee for Quality Assurance. *PCMH 2014 Standards and Guidelines*. Washington, DC: National Committee for Quality Assurance, 2014.

Nelson, E. C., Batalden, P. B., Mohr, J. J., and Plume, S. K. "Building a Quality Future." *Frontiers of Health Service Management*, 1998a, 15(1), 3-32.

Nelson, E. C., Splaine, M. E., Batalden, P. B., and Plume, S. K. "Building Measurement and Data Collection into Medical Practice." *Annals of Internal Medicine*, 1998b, 128(6), 460-466.

Nelson, E. C., Batalden, P. B., Huber, T. P., and others. "Microsystems in Health Care: Part 1. Learning from High-Performing Front-Line Clinical Units." *Joint Commission Journal on Quality Improvement*, 2002, 28(9), 472-493.

Nelson, E. C., Batalden, P. B., and Godfrey, M. M. (eds.). *Quality by Design: A Clinical Microsystems Approach*. San Francisco, CA: Jossey-Bass, 2007.

Neta, G., Glasgow, R. E., Carpenter, C. R., and others. "A Framework for Enhancing the Value of Research for Dissemination and Implementation." *American Journal of Public Health*, 2015, 105(1), 49-57. doi:10.2105/AJPH.2014.302206

Neuhauser, D. "Heroes and Martyrs of Quality and Safety – Ernest Amory Codman." *Quality and Safety in Health Care*, 2002, 11, 104-105.

O'Leary, K. J., Wayne, D. B., Landler, M. P., and others. "Impact of Localizing Physicians to Hospital Units on Nurse-Physician Communication and Agreement on the Plan of Care." *Journal of General Internal Medicine*, 2009, 24(11), 1223-1227.

O'Leary, K. J., Kulkarni, N., Landler, M. P., and others. "Hospitalized Patients' Understanding of Their Plan of Care." *Mayo Clinic Proceedings*, 2010a, 85(1), 47-52.

O'Leary, K. J., Ritter C. D., Wheeler H., and others. "Teamwork on Inpatient Medical Units: Assessing Attitudes and Barriers." *Quality and Safety in Health Care*, 2010b, 19(2), 117-121.

O'Leary, K. J., Thompson, J. A., Landler, M. P., and others. "Patterns of Nurse-Physician Communication and Agreement on the Plan of Care." *Quality and Safety in Health Care*, 2010c, 19(3), 195-199.

O'Leary, K. J., Wayne, D. B., Haviley, C., and others. "Improving Teamwork: Impact of Structured Interdisciplinary Rounds on a Medical Teaching Unit." *Journal of General Internal Medicine*, 2010d, 25(8), 826-832.

O'Leary, K. J., Buck, R., Fligiel, H. M., and others. "Structured Interdisciplinary Rounds in a Medical Teaching Unit: Improving Patient Safety." *Archives of Internal Medicine*, 2011a, 171(7), 678-684.

O'Leary, K. J., Haviley, C., Slade, M. E., and others. "Improving Teamwork: Impact of Structured Interdisciplinary Rounds on a Hospitalist Unit." *Journal of Hospital Medicine*, 2011b, 6(2), 88-93.

Øvretveit, J. "Understanding the Conditions for Improvement: Research to Discover Which Context Influences Affect Improvement Success." *BMJ Quality & Safety*, 2011, 20(S1), i18-i23. doi: 10.1136/bmjqs.2010.045955

Pannick, S., Beveridge, I., Wachter, R. M., and Sevdalis, N. "Improving the Quality and Safety of Care on the Medical Ward: A Review and Synthesis of the Evidence Base." *European Journal of Internal Medicine*, 2014, 25(10), 874-887.

Pannick, S., Davis, R., Ashrafian, H., and others. "Effects of Interdisciplinary Team Care Interventions on General Medical Wards: A Systematic Review." *JAMA Internal Medicine*, 2015, 175(8), 1288-1298.

Pfuntner, A., Wier, L. M., and Stocks, C. *Most Frequent Conditions in U.S. Hospitals, 2010.* Rockville, MD: Agency for Healthcare Research and Quality, 2013.

Reed, J. E., and Card, A. J. "The Problem with Plan–Do–Study–Act Cycles." *BMJ Quality & Safety*, 2015, 0, 1-6. doi: 10.1136/bmjqs-2015-005076

Senge, P. M., Kleiner, A., Roberts, C., and others. *The Dance of Change: The Challenges of Sustaining Momentum in Learning Organizations*, 1st edition. New York, NY: Currency/Doubleday, 1999.

Singh, S., Tarima, S., Rana, V., and others. "Impact of Localizing General Medical Teams to a Single Nursing Unit." *Journal of Hospital Medicine*, 2012, 7(7), 551-556.

Stein, J., Payne, C., Methvin, A., and others. "Reorganizing a Hospital Ward as an Accountable Care Unit." *Journal of Hospital Medicine*, 2015, 10(1), 36-40.

Wennberg, J., Freeman, J., Shelton, R., and Bubolz, T. "Hospital Use and Mortality Among Medicare Beneficiaries in Boston and New Haven." *New England Journal of Medicine*, 1989, 320, 1183-1211.

Woodcock, T., Liberati, E. G., and Dixon-Woods, M. "A Mixed Methods Study of Challenges Experienced by Clinical Teams in Measuring Improvement." *BMJ Quality & Safety*, 2019, 0, 1-10. doi: 10.1136/bmjqs-2018-009048

Woolf, S. H., Purnell, J. Q., Simon, S. M., and others. "Translating Evidence into Population Health Improvement: Strategies and Barriers." *Annual Review of Public Health*, 2015, 36, 463-482. doi: 10.1146/annurev-publhealth-082214-110901

Additional Resources

Patient-Centered Medical Home (PCMH), http://www.ncqa.org/programs/recognition/practices/patient-centered-medical-home-pcmh

Relational Coordination, https://heller.brandeis.edu/relational-coordination/

Sheffield Teaching Hospitals Microsystem Coaching Academy,
     https://www.sheffieldmca.org.uk/
Clinical Microsystems, http://www.clinicalmicrosystem.org/

Key Words/Terms

Clinical pathways (CPWs). A common component in the quest to improve the quality of health. CPWs are used to reduce variation, improve quality of care, and maximize the outcomes for specific groups of patients (Lawal and others, 2016).

Context: The circumstances that form the setting for an event, statement, or idea, and in terms of which it can be fully understood and assessed.

Functional outcomes: One of the four clinical value compass measures (clinical, functional, cost, and satisfaction) including physical function, emotional status, social/role function, and health risk status.

Gantt chart: A horizontal bar chart developed by Henry L. Gantt, frequently used to manage overall improvement work. A Gantt chart provides a graphical illustration of the improvement activity schedule, helping to plan, coordinate, and track specific tasks.

Geographic cohorting: Unit-based assignments of providers in hospital medicine.

National Committee for Quality Assurance (NCQA): An independent 501(c)(3) nonprofit organization in the United States that works to improve healthcare quality through the administration of evidence-based standards, measures, programs, and accreditation.

Pathways: See *Clinical pathways.*

Patient and family experience: The patient [and family] experience encompasses the range of interactions that patients have with the healthcare system, including their care from health plans, and from doctors, nurses, and staff in hospitals, physician practices, and other healthcare facilities. As an integral component of healthcare quality, patient [and family] experience includes several aspects of healthcare delivery that patients value highly when they seek and receive care, such as getting timely appointments, easy access to information, and good communication with healthcare providers (AHRQ, 2017).

Patient-centered medical home (PCMH): A team-based healthcare delivery model led by a healthcare provider to provide comprehensive and continuous medical care to patients with the goal to obtain maximal health outcomes.

Playbooks: A collection of core and supporting processes used routinely by the microsystem including flowcharts and diagrams of processes that have been tested using improvement science and represent the way the microsystem wants things done.

Relational coordination: Is a mutually reinforcing process of communicating and relating for the purpose of task integration. It captures the relational dynamics of coordinating work.

Shared decision-making: An approach where clinicians and patients share the best available evidence when faced with the task of making decisions, and where patients are supported to consider options to achieve informed preferences (Elwyn and others, 2012).

CHAPTER SIX

PARTNERSHIP WITHIN THE CLINICAL MICROSYSTEM'S FRAMEWORK: COPRODUCING GOOD OUTCOMES WITH PATIENTS AND FAMILIES

Maren Batalden, Julie K. Johnson, Cristin Lind, Helena Hvitfeldt, Paul B. Batalden, Tina C. Foster, Marjorie M. Godfrey

AIM

The aim of this chapter is to define the role of coproduction in healthcare services and to explore how the clinical microsystem framework can be helpful in supporting patients and health professionals as partners to coproduce better outcomes.

LEARNING OBJECTIVES

By the end of this chapter the reader will be able to:

1. Recognize the degree to which all healthcare services are inevitably coproduced and explore coproduction as an explicit strategy for improving healthcare service outcomes.

Quality by Design: A Clinical Microsystems Approach, Second Edition. Edited by Marjorie M. Godfrey, Tina C. Foster, Julie K. Johnson, Eugene C. Nelson and Paul B. Batalden.
© 2025 John Wiley & Sons, Inc. Published 2025 by John Wiley & Sons, Inc.

2. Review a framework for coproducing healthcare services within the individual clinical encounter at the level of the clinical micro-, meso-, and macrosystems and across the life cycle of a change project.
3. Explore tools for enhancing coproduction at every step along the Clinical Microsystem Improvement Ramp.

Introduction

> "For better or worse, I have come to believe that we – patients, families, clinicians, and the healthcare system as a whole – would all be far better off if we professionals recalibrated our work such that we behaved with patients and families not as hosts in the care system, but as guests in their lives" (Berwick, 2009, p. w559).

In every clinical encounter between a patient and healthcare professional, good and bad healthcare outcomes are coproduced within the context of a clinical micro-, meso-, and macrosystem. And, as detailed in this chapter, we believe that it is possible for healthcare professionals, patients, and patients' families to be intentional about their coproductive partnership. This chapter posits that cultivating intentional coproductive partnerships – at the level of the individual clinical encounter and in the design and evaluation of the healthcare system – will result in better healthcare service value. Cultivating coproduction, then, is about professionals and citizens making better use of one another's assets, resources, and contributions to improve outcomes and efficiency (Governance International, 2017).

This chapter revisits the 5Ps framework for assessing the clinical microsystem using a coproductive lens and it travels the clinical microsystem improvement ramp with new tools intended to facilitate a coproductive approach to healthcare service design and improvement at each step along the way.

Over the past decade, frameworks for understanding the role of the patient and family in healthcare services and clinical microsystems have evolved. The Institute of Medicine (2001) identified "patient-centeredness" as one of the six dimensions of quality in health care in the summer of 2000. Since that time, many have been working to craft frameworks and tools to catalyze improvement in that domain. Much of our dialogue, however, has remained stubbornly health profession centric. Too often patients are envisioned as passive recipients of health professional services, satisfied or dissatisfied with the work of their healthcare team, as though healthcare services were "products" manufactured by health professionals for the benefit of patients. Emerging literature suggests that a product-dominant paradigm for understanding healthcare service is flawed.

More than 50 years ago, economist Victor Fuchs observed that making a service was different from making a product. A service, he said, always requires two parties –

a service professional of some sort and a service user (or beneficiary or customer). The outcome of a service, he noted, is always coproduced (Fuchs, 1968). This is not an aspirational statement that distinguishes good service from bad service, but rather an observation about the way a service works. For example, a person with diabetes and her health professional team coproduce diabetes outcomes. Members of the health professional team draw blood, prescribe medications, make referrals to specialists, and provide education and counseling. But a person with diabetes makes the everyday choices that determine their health outcomes – what to eat, how and whether to exercise, how and how often to check blood sugars, how and whether to take medications and keep appointments, how to engage family and friends in the illness, and when to seek professional help. Both the health professional team and the person with diabetes can play their roles poorly or well, but the health outcomes that result – good or bad – will inevitably be coproduced.

The degree to which people coproduce health outcomes with members of their health professional team varies widely. Chronic health conditions are different than acute illness or injury; healthcare service provided in the operating room, intensive care unit, or emergency department is different than healthcare service provided in an ambulatory clinic. People seeking healthcare service differ in their capacity and desire for self-care and active partnership with the healthcare system. An inherent asymmetry in expertise challenges this partnership. Health professionals have special expertise in human biology, pathophysiology, evidence-based evaluation, and management of clinical conditions; people seeking help from health professionals bring unique expertise in the complexity of their lives – that includes personal histories, relationships, values, strengths and vulnerabilities, fears, insights into their illness burden, and the resources within their reach. Increasingly, in the context of a digital revolution that has proliferated access to information, some patients also bring expert knowledge about their disease and its treatments, including awareness of contradictions among healthcare professionals and lack of coordination between team members.

Although the idea that health outcomes are inevitably coproduced by patients and health professionals is simple, we have perhaps inadvertently migrated away from this basic truth in the way we design and improve healthcare services. Our dominant paradigm asserts that healthcare professionals create services and "deliver" them (like packages) to customers or patients. We talk about patient engagement, patient activation, and the need to focus on the patient experience as though we, as health professionals, are inviting patients into our work rather than starting from the recognition that maintaining and restoring the health of individuals and communities is shared work. In fact, we probably need to acknowledge that the work disproportionately belongs not to health professionals but to individuals and communities seeking well-being. Best estimates suggest that healthcare services might modify the risk of premature death by about 10 percent; health behaviors and social and environmental factors account for 40 percent and 20 percent of the risk, respectively (Braverman and Robert, 2014; Bradley and others, 2016). The right question regarding health-related value is how the healthcare system can contribute most to the work that individuals and communities are already doing (and/or need to do) to create health-related value for themselves.

Improvement Science and Relationship-Centered Care

The core tools of improvement science articulated in the clinical microsystem framework – setting clear aims, understanding root causes to problems, mapping processes, using measurement effectively, and implementing small serial tests of change using iterative PDSA cycles – remain vital to making meaningful change in health care. Many of these tools, however, have been adapted from approaches to performance improvement that have their roots in manufacturing and have the goal of streamlining the process, reducing variation, and improving efficiency. Increasingly in health care – as in other service industries – improvers seek to supplement these classic tools of improvement science with approaches that highlight the power and importance of relationships. Car parts on an assembly line have no opinions or preferences with regard to the processes that transform them into vehicles; however, people entering as patients into a relationship with a clinical microsystem have thoughts, feelings, stories, and a significant amount of agency that they bring to bear on their health-related goals and challenges. At every step in the life cycle of an improvement initiative – choosing aims, identifying change ideas, and selecting measures that matter – a partnership between health professionals and patients and families is critical.

Creating a culture of partnership in healthcare service design, delivery, and improvement is a paradigm shift for all participants – clinicians, patients and families, administrators, and payors. The work invites us to adopt different roles that require new knowledge, behaviors, values, and dispositions. This is adaptive, not technical change. It requires courage and risk-taking, trust and forgiveness. Several decades of change-making with the tools of improvement science have taught us that something new will likely emerge through experimentation in multiple small cycles of change at the level of individual patients and clinicians in clinical encounters and at the level of clinical micro-, meso-, and macrosystems.

A Framework for Patient Professional Partnership

First-generation efforts to develop a greater patient-professional partnership in quality improvement most often invited patients to react to health professionals, health system activities, and priorities. Efforts to gather information about the patient and family experience in the care system – through post-encounter surveys – have become not only routine but also a part of the regulatory and accreditation framework for healthcare systems. This attention to patient and family or "consumer" experience has helped to catalyze a necessary paradigm shift. As is often the case, however, the stepping stones of culture change at one stage can inadvertently become stumbling blocks in the next stage. For example, as patients rate their satisfaction with health professional work, the focus shifts to improving patient satisfaction ratings, which may inadvertently limit our ability to engage more deeply with patients and families. As we expand beyond the role of patient as reactor or evaluator of healthcare services, we benefit from new frameworks. Phrases such as "patient engagement" and "involvement" reveal the healthcare system's implicit view of itself as the center of health creation. Other industries are showing us new collaboration methods and approaches that call into question the healthcare system's formulation privilege, that is, the tacit right of health professionals and health system leaders to set the agendas, generate the questions, and initiate efforts. New methods aim to facilitate reciprocity and equality for all stakeholder groups as a means to generate healthcare services that meet the needs of patients and families, populations, and the healthcare system.

Leaning on the good work of Carman and colleagues (Carman and others, 2013), we offer a framework for conceptualizing partnership in healthcare improvement (see Table 6.1).

TABLE 6.1 A FRAMEWORK FOR PATIENT–PROFESSIONAL PARTNERSHIP.

		Phase		
		Diagnose: Assess and set aims	**Treat: PDSA and SDSA**	
		Initiation	**Planning**	**Implementation**	**Evaluation**
		identifying areas of one's health that one would like to address	*coordinating one's overall health and care*	*taking medication; self care; making lifestyle choices that support health*	*tracking the effects of treatment and lifestyle choices*
Place	Clinical encounter Microsystem Mesosystem Macrosystem				

Degree of parity in relationship between patients and professionals

The Framework for Patient-Professional Partnership includes three factors:

1. Place – the level in which the partnership occurs within the system.
2. Phase – the phase of a change initiative's life cycle in which collaboration begins.
3. Parity – the degree of reciprocity present in the partnership.

Place

Where within the health system does the patient-professional partnership occur? What level of the healthcare system is targeted for improvement? For example, a partnership can take place at the level of the clinical encounter – the face-to-face meeting or telephone call or virtual connection between a patient and a health professional. The partnership within the clinical encounter can be deepened and strengthened intentionally through many mechanisms – communication skills training for both patients and health professionals, *"speak up" campaigns* for patients and families, shared goal setting, and the use of decision aids and teach-back strategies. A partnership might also be explicitly enhanced within the context of a clinical microsystem by a variety of means – increasing transparency about performance, opening medical records, maximizing continuity in the relationship between health professional and patient through staffing or scheduling, and inviting patients to serve on improvement teams. At the meso- and macrosystem level, similar opportunities exist for engaging people more fully, as patients, consumers, and citizens, in the commissioning and governance of healthcare services, setting priorities, allocating resources, designing and evaluating services, and solving problems.

Place from the patient perspective. Many patients describe an advocacy journey that begins with gaining mastery over one's health situation and continues by expanding to larger and larger spheres of influence to improve health care for others. As breast cancer survivor and advocate Musa Mayer writes:

> The path of healthcare advocacy usually begins with a devastating illness or condition, our own, or that of someone we love. Fear, grief, and helplessness are transformed through learning into action. As we become "experienced" patients, moving past our initial coping with diagnosis, symptoms, and treatments, many of us are motivated to reach out to others who are coping with our condition, to give back as we've been given to. In an effort to make a broader impact, some of us then begin a lengthy process of self-education so as to understand the medical aspects of our disease and science behind the condition and its treatments more fully. If research becomes a particular interest, we then undertake training to learn about scientific methodology and evidence-based health care, research design, basic statistics, and epidemiology.

What begins as difficult personal experience is eventually transformed into an avocation and a mission to be of help to others. Often, we discover in our advocacy a chance to pursue undeveloped interests and skills. But we always begin with the authenticity of our own experience [Mayer, 2012, p. 72].

Place from the professional perspective. For most clinicians, an understanding of the power of partnership also begins in the clinical encounter. Most health professionals begin their professional journey with a deep desire to meet and help a fellow human being who is suffering. Professional socialization and the development of a particular kind of professional expertise sometimes inadvertently distances professionals from the people they seek to help. Features of the clinical micro-, meso-, and macrosystems that interfere with the partnership between clinicians and patients – operational inefficiencies and dysfunction, productivity pressures, and external regulatory mandates – also contribute to health professional burnout and dissatisfaction. Many health professionals feel ill-equipped for leadership and change-making at the level of the clinical micro-, meso-, and macrosystem. Inviting patients into partnership as systems improvers – a domain where many health professionals themselves feel uncertain – can sometimes challenge health professional identity.

Phase

Returning to Figure 6.1, the columns of the framework invite us to consider "phase," that is, when in the developmental life cycle of an improvement initiative collaboration begins. (The same temporal framework might be considered in the context of an individual clinical encounter as well.) The execution of a project or the development of a healthcare system innovation may be considered along a timeline from *initiation, planning, implementation,* and *evaluation* (Figure 6.1). The clinical microsystem improvement ramp emphasizes that planning, implementation, and evaluation are recursive processes that occurs through serial small tests of change (PDSA cycles) until a system develops enough confidence in a change that it becomes a sustainable hard-wired change in practice or routine operations.

FIGURE 6.1 THE PHASES OF PROJECT EXECUTION/SYSTEM DEVELOPMENT LIFE CYCLE.

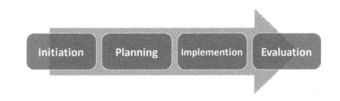

Initiation refers to the selection of a problem, the commissioning of a solution, and the designation of the necessary problem-solving resources within a larger system. In health care, health professionals have typically held the role of initiator exclusively. Increasingly, health systems now convene advisory boards and use them as a mechanism to solicit patient and family perspectives on change ideas at the level of the micro-, meso-, and macrosystem. It remains rare, however, for advisory boards to engage with a high degree of parity in the earliest design phases of initiatives when priorities are being set and scoped. As a result, patients and families sometimes perceive that by the time they are invited to participate, initiatives have a too narrow focus or a relatively low priority. Projects that include patients and families in the early initiation phase may be more likely to address more complex issues, such as multiple chronic conditions, social determinants of health, whole person health and well-being, and public/community health. Often the mandate for improvement originates external to the healthcare system at the level of a regulatory body or payer; consequently, degrees of freedom for choosing focus are sometimes constrained. Even at the level of the clinical encounter we recognize significant opportunities for enhancing the degree to which patients and families are engaged early in setting visit agendas.

Planning involves determining what will be done, by whom, and by when. At the level of the clinical encounter, patients and families may be more frequently engaged collaboratively in choosing and planning treatment options; however, if treatment goals are not set collaboratively, true partnership in choosing and planning treatment options is difficult. Several people have articulated useful conceptual frameworks to support shared decision-making in planning (Elwyn, 2012). Critical to effective partnership at this stage at the level of the micro- and mesosystem is having effective patient and family member participation on improvement teams. In many healthcare systems, patients and families are beginning to take on planning and leadership roles on project teams, and emerging literature defines best practices for this sort of collaboration (Crawford and others, 2002; Armstrong and others, 2013; Pomey and others, 2015; Renedo and others, 2015). Effective collaboration on improvement teams requires preparation and orientation for both patients and families and health professionals. As noted above, building improvement teams that invite and fully engage the assets of patient and family team members requires time, iteration, and a mature culture of continuous improvement and reflection.

Implementation is the actual conduct of planned activities. At the level of the clinical encounter in the context of chronic disease management, it is the patient and/or carer who assumes primary responsibility for the work of daily care as soon as the clinical visit is over. As we expand our degree of collaboration at this level, healthcare professionals might improve their ability to understand and mitigate the burden of treatment on the patient's life and actively work to enhance patient and family ability to monitor health status and health behaviors. At the level of the micro- and mesosystem, patients and families have historically played a less prominent role in implementing change ideas; they are often volunteering and have limited time to invest in the slow and complex work of making healthcare systems change. However, patients and families increasingly engage in formal efforts to gather ongoing information from other patients and families through interviews and observation, develop educational and self-management material, support peers in physical and virtual networks, work as patient navigators or care coordinators, teach and coach healthcare professionals, and much more.

Evaluation is a reflection on how well the project was executed (process) and whether it met its objectives (outcomes) after project completion. As noted above, many initial efforts to develop a partnership with patients and families in health care belong to this phase in the form of post-encounter patient satisfaction surveys. The US *Hospital Consumer Assessment of Healthcare Providers and Systems (HCAHPS)* is just one example in which healthcare consumers are invited to describe their experience with a healthcare service encounter on a variety of domains (Centers for Medicare and Medicaid Services, 2017). Both quantitative and qualitative data from the survey can be used to improve care. *Pay-for-performance* incentives from payers linked to measured patient experience have heightened attention to the importance of attending to the quality of the partnership between health professionals and patients and families.

Of note, soliciting patient and family perspectives on evaluation of changes introduced at the level of the micro- and mesosystem is less common. Existing data sources are limited, and improvement teams often have limited bandwidth for primary data collection from patients and families. Sometimes system improvement efforts that begin collaboratively by inviting patient and family engagement in design evolve over time to be more health-professional-centric as health professionals assume primary leadership responsibilities for change efforts. Sustained engagement of patients and families over the lifespan of a project requires continued investment and regular recommitment. The presence or absence of patient and family voices in a project or program evaluation is a clear signal regarding the health system's priorities.

In the context of healthcare improvement, making increasingly intentional decisions about when patients and professionals come together to engage as partners is critical. A health system that demonstrates robust partnership will have opportunities for dialogue and engagement across all levels of place and phase. Engaging patients and families at the end of a project to seek evaluative feedback can be powerful, but seeking patient and family perspective and engagement at the beginning and at every twist and turn along the way holds the most profound potential for supporting transformative change.

Early and sustained partnership is difficult. Most healthcare institutions have limited infrastructure to support these partnerships and underdeveloped practices and policies for shared governance and decision-making. Healthcare professionals sometimes worry that genuine partnerships in early-phase improvement decisions will invite patients and families to make unreasonable demands or develop unrealistic expectations. The necessary degree of transparency about constraints and competing agendas feels new and uncomfortable. True partnership is time consuming. Recruiting patients and families who can be effective team members in an improvement effort requires investment; both patients and families and health professionals need orientation and education and practice before they can work together effectively. Timelines – due dates for grant applications and deadlines for achieving pay-for-performance outcomes – often mitigate against the slow growth of relational trust that makes partnership possible.

Parity

The third dimension in the partnership framework is parity in power. Implicit and explicit hierarchies within healthcare constrain the capacity to coproduce outcomes effectively. At their human core, illness and injury are states of vulnerability. The traditional word *patient* means "one who suffers"; the term connotes passivity and the need for help, not active agency. To adopt the role of the patient at the level of the individual clinical encounter is traditionally associated with putting oneself in the hands of an expert, a professional who will offer care. A call for "parity" or "reciprocity" of power in this relationship is complex. When we are healthy, seeking support for our wellness, we are consumers (not patients) and it feels natural that we should claim our power to use, design, and evaluate healthcare services as equals. When we are desperately ill, seeking help for overwhelming pain and acute shortness of breath, we feel anything but powerful. Whenever we engage the healthcare system, we engage in some capacity on a spectrum from consumer to patient. Living with chronic illness and disability of any duration requires daily work and becomes integrally intertwined with our personal identities. Claiming our rightful and necessary agency for our well-being is a developmental journey.

A call for parity in partnership within the clinical encounter must recognize and respect what each partner brings. The health professional's years of formal training and experience are critical to the relationship; so too, is the lived experience of the patient and family. The patient-health professional partnership is, of course, not just a relationship. It is also a transaction in which one party is paying – directly or indirectly – and the other party is getting paid to participate. Full reciprocity of relationship within the dynamics of the transaction is not possible. But equity in the dynamics of power is different than equality. Each partner has a responsibility to facilitate shared knowledge of the situation and one another's perspective, to work toward the establishment of shared goals, and to cultivate deep mutual respect for one another. All patients and health professionals that have intentionally embarked on this journey toward greater parity in partnership have stories to tell. Although the stories sometimes tell of rocky roads as partners renegotiate their roles, the stories also tell of discovery in which patients and families find greater agency and authority, and health professionals learn to let go of their assumptions about their centrality a little.

With respect to parity in partnership for improvement at the level of the micro-, meso-, and macrosystem, we have a long road ahead. Often in efforts to partner with patients and families, an invitation to serve on a team is extended to a single representative. While this is a powerful and important first step, it is usually difficult for a single patient or family member to find his/her voice in the unfamiliar lexicon of a health professional world. It is rare for patients and families and health professionals to have proportionally equal representation. Dynamics change dramatically when there are as many patients and family members as health professionals in the room.

The question of parity in micro-, meso-, and macrosystem efforts opens difficult debates that we are only just beginning to engage in. Health professionals, of course, engage in improvement work as part of their jobs for which they receive wages. Must patients and families engage in this improvement work as volunteers? If they are to be paid, what business model would support health systems to engage in this work at scale? What about the distribution of benefits that accrues from successful partnerships? Surely, both patients and families and health professionals might benefit from improved workflows that produce better health outcomes. But if there are pay-for-performance financial rewards or cost savings that accrue to the health system as a consequence of the improvement partnership, should they be shared? If we share collectively in these rewards, how might we consider sharing risk and responsibility when we coproduce undesired outcomes?

Many frameworks have been articulated to describe a continuum of parity in relationships between service user and service provider, between citizen and government. We like the diagram from the Canadian Department of Public Health (Figure 6.2). We might imagine our journey as one in which we intentionally work to move the line of interaction between patient and health professional from left to right.

We might imagine the larger sphere in Figure 6.2 to be a representation of the health professional and the smaller spheres to represent patients and families, a graphic description of the traditional assumptions about hierarchy of power and expertise. The first step toward partnership might be an effective explanation, depicted as single-headed arrows going from health professional to patient and family. As partnership deepens, so too does communication with improved listening and eventually genuine bidirectional conversation. At the next stage, however, the diagram

FIGURE 6.2 COPRODUCTION CONTINUUM: HEALTH PROFESSIONALS AND PATIENTS.

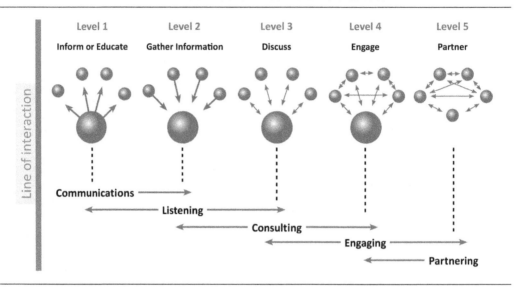

Source: Adapted from *Health Canada Policy Toolkit for Public Involvement in Decision Making.* Health Canada, 2000. Adapted from Patterson Kirk Wallace. Reproduced with permission from the Minister of Health, 2017.

hints at something very powerful as arrows connect many more spheres to one another. Here we unleash the power of networks and teams and no longer rely on a single source of expertise. In the last image, we see a genuine collaboration where mutual respect has grown enough that parity in power and reciprocity is possible.

Methods for Partnering with Patients and Families

For quality improvement professionals who want to partner with patients and families in their work across place and phase with increasing parity, the questions very quickly become practical. What tools might we use? How might we modify any existing tools from the microsystem approach and improvement science to enhance partnership? What additional tools are needed?

The wide spectrum of methods to enhance partnership takes inspiration from many disciplines – anthropology and ethnography, design thinking in business and architecture, community organizing for political change, and critical theories in educational pedagogy. There are few "one size fits all" best practices for partnership in healthcare improvement. The appropriateness of any approach depends on a variety of factors, not least of which is the microsystem's readiness to partner meaningfully with patients. Some methods require significant expertise, time, and financial resources, while others require only a posture of openness and curiosity and a willingness to try something new.

The purpose of each tool is distinct. Some are useful in facilitating deeper understanding of an individual's experience, while others aggregate data from a group. Selecting an approach depends on the aim and on available resources. Employing a variety of methods makes it possible for patients to contribute in the way that works best for them, and therefore often results in greater diversity of input. At the heart of any method is a desire for increased collaboration, enhanced mutual respect, and patient empowerment. Care should be taken to avoid assuming a solely mechanistic mindset regarding partnership, as it can lead to tokenism or other symbolic forms of patient involvement, which will be frustrating for patients and of limited value to the improvement initiative.

Expanding the 5Ps Framework

In Chapter Six of the first edition of this text (Godfrey and others, 2007), we noted that the planning of patient-centered services requires knowledge of:

1. The needs of the major patient subpopulations served by the clinical microsystem.
2. The ways the people in the microsystem interact with one another.
3. The ways the people in the microsystem interact with the processes that unfold to produce critical outcomes.

This knowledge comes from both formal analysis and tacit understanding of the clinical unit's structure, its patients, its processes, and its daily patterns of work and interaction. When planning services for their patients, members of the microsystem benefit from building comprehensive knowledge of the 5Ps in their clinical microsystem. When members of a clinical microsystem work together to gain information about their *purpose, patients, professionals, processes,* and *patterns,* they acquire knowledge that can be used to make long-lasting improvements in the clinical microsystem. This 5Ps framework has helped would-be health-professional improvers learn to see the systems they labor to improve. Worksheets and practical action guides developed for using a 5Ps framework support efforts to assess different clinical microsystems – primary care clinics, specialty clinics, acute care units, emergency departments, and long-term care settings. Understanding the component parts of the clinical microsystem is critical to understanding the context in which any intended improvement must take place.

In Table 6.2, we augment the original 5Ps clinical microsystem framework with a coproduction lens, suggesting new questions that might enhance our understanding of the system we seek to improve.

TABLE 6.2 THE 5PS CLINICAL MICROSYSTEM FRAMEWORK AUGMENTED WITH A COPRODUCTION LENS.

	Traditional microsystem learning questions	A coproduction lens on microsystem learning questions
Know your purpose	What is our aim? What do we actually intend to "make?" As we think of the people we care for and what we are trying to create, what is our intention?	How do different patients and families understand the aim of the microsystem? In what way does the microsystem add value to the health-related value creation that patients and families are already engaged in?
Know your patients	Whom are we caring for? Are there subpopulations we could plan services for differently? What are the most common patient diagnoses and conditions in our practice? What other microsystems support what we do to meet patients' needs? How satisfied are patients with our microsystem?	In keeping with the invitation from design thinking to build "empathy" with the end users of a service, improvers might work to dig more deeply in understanding patients' lived experience. What are patients' unmet, unspoken needs? What resources, assets, and strengths do they bring? What might we learn from taking an appreciative inquiry approach into those patients who are maintaining good health?
Know your professionals	Who provides patient care, and who are the people supporting the clinical careteam? What skills and talents do staff members need to provide the right service and care at the right time? What is the morale of our team? What is the role of information technology as a team member?	In what ways are patients and families regarded as members of the professional team? How are patients prepared and supported for their roles in self care, monitoring of processes and outcomes, and care coordination? How do professionals adapt their invitation to partnership to different patients?
Know your processes	How do we deliver care and services to meet our patients' needs? Who does what in our microsystem? Do our hours of operation match the needs of our patients? What are our core and supporting processes? How does technology support our processes? How do we learn from failures or near misses?	What role do we expect our patients to play in our care processes? In coordinating processes of care between microsystems? What are the core processes of self care and disease management in which patients and families engage outside of our microsystem? What value do our care processes add for our patients and families? What costs and burdens do they pose? How do our patients use technology to support their processes of care?

TABLE 6.2 (*Continued*)

	Traditional microsystem learning questions	A coproduction lens on microsystem learning questions
Know your patterns	What are the health outcomes of our patients? What are the costs of care? How do we interact within our microsystem? What are the regularly recurring associated or sequential work activities? What does it feel like to work here? What are the costs in our microsystem? Do information systems provide data and information in a timely way to inform us about the impact of our services? How do we stay mindful of the possibility of our efforts failing?	What microsystem outcomes matter most to patients and families? What is the relationship between the outcomes we routinely measure and outcomes that matter to patients and families? How does it feel to receive care in our microsystem? How do we collect information from patients about the impact of our work in their lives?

Expanding the Microsystem Improvement Ramp

Using the improvement ramp as an approach to framing improvement within the clinical microsystem, we can identify opportunities for enhancing partnership with patients and families at every step. Figure 6.3 shows the improvement ramp with suggestions for methods to employ. Methods listed to the left of the ramp offer support during specific stages in an initiative, while those listed to the right are used throughout. First, teams assemble, build knowledge of the system and processes they seek to change, and set an aim with iteratively sharper focus. Next, teams select a change idea and plan ways of measuring the impact of the change. Then, through serial small tests of change with embedded learning, teams implement and ultimately sustain successful change.

Shadowing/observation. Shadowing involves observing a healthcare visit or other process from the perspective of the patient or family member. By experiencing a healthcare visit alongside a patient or family member, health professionals can better understand the visit flow with delays, redundancies, and discontinuities; they can view signage and physical space layout through patients' eyes; they can listen with new ears to communication among staff and between staff and patients. The resulting insights can expose unmet needs and areas for improvement. One tool emerging from a compendium of human-centered design tools is called "empathy mapping." This tool invites an observer to pay attention to what users (or patients) see, hear, say, and do and to intuit what they feel and think (Cystic Fibrosis Foundation, 2017).

FIGURE 6.3 PATIENT–PROFESSIONAL PARTNERSHIP ALONG THE IMPROVEMENT RAMP.

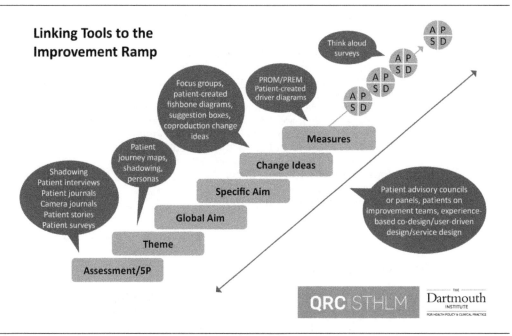

Source: The Dartmouth Institute Microsystem Academy, 2007. Adapted by QRC Stockholm, 2014.

Interviews. Interviewing patients involves a dialogue that can be quite different from the typical healthcare encounter. Through open-ended questions and deep listening, interviewers encourage patients to share what they themselves believe health professionals should know about their experience. Analysis of these interviews may yield new insights about patients' needs, feelings, expectations, and desires. Interviews may be conducted by health professionals, by patient and/or family members, learners, or independent staff. Many choices affect the utility and explanatory power of the interviews – who will conduct the interview, how patients and families are selected and invited to participate, the manner in which data is recorded, and the way in which themes are identified in analysis. Interviews that are audio or video recorded can be very powerful in communicating interview content with large groups (Cystic Fibrosis Foundation, 2017).

Patient journals. Several methods have been developed to help patients capture their experiences for the purpose of informing improvement efforts. Patients might be asked to keep a daily journal of their illness for a period of time, to make a video of their illness, or to take or draw a "picture" of their illness. As health professionals build deeper understanding of the lived experience of patients and carers, their ability to design and implement meaningful improvement initiatives grows.

Patient journey mapping. Process mapping – a core tool in improvement science – tends to produce descriptions of steps in a process from a health professional or health system-centric perspective. Journey mapping is a strategy for graphic capture of the specific events that occurred before, during, and after a patient's episode of care or a longitudinal experience with illness, as well as the positive or negative emotions experienced along the way. The result makes it possible to better understand and identify unmet needs as well as current strengths within the system. Journey mapping takes an explicitly patient-centric view. Another tool that has been described is service blueprinting, which can be considered an attempt to integrate a healthcare system-focused process map and a patient-focused journey map. A service blueprint captures both the concrete physical and temporal aspects of different components of a service as well as the actions and emotions of service providers and service users (Cystic Fibrosis Foundation, 2017).

Focus groups. Focus groups involve convening a group of patients and/or family members to discuss a theme, such as a broad exploration of the experience of living with a particular condition or more targeted discussion of a particular aspect of care. The conversational dynamics within a focus group can be generative, though must be moderated skillfully to minimize bias. Traditionally used for evaluation, they can also be a forum for in-depth discussions around health experiences and needs. Focus group conversations can also be useful in engaging specific improvement tasks such as creating fishbone or driver diagrams, generating improvement ideas, or prioritizing improvement efforts through facilitated processes, such as multi-voting.

Personas. A persona is a fictional representation of a patient based on real data regarding values, needs, behaviors, attitudes, expectations, and emotions. Though not intended to be a substitute for actual patient participation, a persona can be a prompt to keep patients' needs, capabilities, and priorities at the center of improvement work. Teams can create different personas to represent distinct subgroups of a patient population, which enables them to remain mindful of important differences between groups. Invoking the persona provides a rhetorical sounding board for a group to test ideas and challenge assumptions (see "Brandon" case study in Chapter Two).

Coproduction change concepts. A *change concept* is a general change principle that can be used to develop a specific change idea. Improvement change concepts include several suggestions for optimizing workflows – reduce wait time, increase standardization, match inventory to predicted demand, change the order of steps in a process, introduce parallel processing. A core list of change concepts for health system improvement – including many that have their roots in Lean frameworks – have been developed by Associates in Process Improvement and popularized by the Institute for Healthcare Improvement (Langley and others, 2009).

A subset of change concepts focuses on the relational aspects of a coproduced healthcare service – give people access to information, listen to customers, coach customers to use the service, develop alliances. A coproductive lens on improvement, however, invites us to consider additional change concepts that support the quality of the partnership among patients and families and health professionals and invites patient and family agency. For example, invite patients and families to network and share solutions, understand and limit barriers to the use of the service or products, understand and limit burdens caused by the service or product, and recognize and invite patient and family assets and capacities. Table 6.3 lists 36 change concepts that we like to call "coproduction change concepts."

Patient-reported outcome measures. With respect to measuring what matters to patients, our clinical performance measures sometimes miss the mark. Often, in measuring healthcare outcomes, we settle for measures that capture care processes – lab draws, prescription of medication, or performance of a diagnostic test – and fail to measure the impact of our efforts on patients' symptoms or overall functional status. The science of measuring patient symptoms and quality of life is advancing quickly. Perhaps most promising in this domain is an increasingly long list of available Patient-Reported Outcome Measures (PROMs), which use validated questionnaires to turn symptoms and functional limitations and overall quality of life into numerical scores. Developed initially for use in research, patient-reported outcome measures are increasingly used by health systems in quality improvement. *Digital interfaces* are making data more transparently available to all stakeholders (see Additional Resources at the end of the chapter for more information on PROMs and digital interfaces).

Think aloud surveys. Another strategy emerging from the domain of human-centered design invites users (including patients and families) to engage in an activity or task and narrate their thoughts and feelings in real time as they work. This is a simple, inexpensive way of building understanding about the process that is the target for improvement or testing proposed change ideas. The method enables improvers to learn about process design flaws as well as user perceptions and misconceptions; it is a pragmatic strategy for studying iterative small tests of change.

Experience-based codesign (EBCD). Experience-based codesign employs a variety of tools developed by design thinkers in an approach that enables patients and

TABLE 6.3 CHANGE CONCEPTS FOR COPRODUCTION.

Change Concepts for Coproduction

1. Use pull systems
2. Reduce choice of features
3. Increase choice of features
4. Give patients/users more access to information
5. Help patients/users understand information
6. Conduct training
7. Implement cross-training
8. Share risks and benefits
9. Emphasize natural and logical consequences
10. Develop alliances and cooperative relationships
11. Listen to patients/users; ask open-ended questions
12. Coach patients/users in how to use products or service
13. Focus on outcomes that matters to patients/users
14. Understand contribution made by product or service to outcome that matters to patient/user
15. Use a coordinator
16. Reach agreement on expectations
17. Standardize
18. Customize
19. Attend to emotion, aesthetic, and experience
20. Don't waste the patient/user's time
21. Provide exactly what is wanted
22. Provide what is wanted exactly where it is wanted
23. Provide what is wanted exactly when it is wanted
24. Ensure that goods and services work and that they work together
25. Aggregate solutions to reduce patient/user time and hassle
26. Recognize and invite individual patient/user agency and capacity
27. Invite patients/users to network and share solutions
28. Remove barriers to use of product or service
29. Understand and limit burdens created by product or service
30. Optimize information technology to enable partnership
31. Distinguish unique needs of different customers
32. Enable trust
33. Share power
34. Optimize time together
35. Eliminate aspects of the product or service that do not add value
36. Find and enable patient/user supports and resources outside of the healthcare system

providers to develop services together. The EBCD cycle, as described by Paul Bate and Glenn Robert, is divided into six stages:

1. Setting up the project.
2. Gathering staff experiences through observational fieldwork and in-depth interviews.
3. Gathering patient and carer experiences through observation and a collection of short, filmed, narrative-based interviews.
4. Bringing staff, patients, and carers together in a codesign event to share – prompted by an edited 20- to 30-minute "trigger" film of patient narratives – experiences of a service and identify priorities for change.
5. Sustained codesign work in small groups formed around those priorities (typically 4-6).
6. A celebration and review event (Bate and Robert, 2007; Robert and others, 2015).

A helpful tool kit that describes this process and a portfolio of distinct methods for facilitating experience-based codesign has been developed by King's College (https://www.pointofcarefoundation.org.uk/resource/experience-based-co-design-ebcd-toolkit/).

Another toolkit, developed by the National Health Service (https://improvement.nhs.uk/documents/1486/ebd_guide___toolkit.pdf), outlines a more flexible approach that suggests alternatives to video in capturing patient and carer experience.

Welcoming patient and family members on improvement teams. When patients join quality improvement teams as equal and active members, they can provide continuous input and help the entire project stay patient-centered. They also often bring unexpected, valuable personal and professional skills to the team. Their presence sends a strong signal to the team and the clinical practice that patients are collaborative partners. As noted above, successful engagement of patient and family members on improvement teams requires attention to several details – recruiting the right patient and family members, orienting patients and families and health professionals to their collaborative roles, supporting each in the evolution of their partnership, and ongoing evaluation of the shared work in the relationship. Helpful resources to support the integration of patient and family advisors have been developed by many, including the Institute for Patient and Family-Centered Care and the Agency for Health Care Quality.

The following case study is an example of how Cambridge Health Alliance improved care for patients using a coproduction lens.

Case Study: Example from Cambridge Health Alliance

In 2016, healthcare delivery system leaders at the Cambridge Health Alliance began work on improving care for patients with chronic obstructive pulmonary disease (COPD) with the intent of improving clinical outcomes, reducing cost and waste, and bettering patient and health professional experience. Evidence-based guidelines for this condition highlight the importance of several care system behaviors that might be included as part of a best-practice care bundle – appropriate staging of illness with baseline and interval pulmonary function testing, appropriate use of inhaled medications by stage of illness, smoking cessation counseling, use of supplemental oxygen as needed, referral to pulmonary rehabilitation and advanced care planning, and engagement of palliative care services for patients with late stage disease. Guidelines suggest systemic steroids and antibiotics for the management of disease flares. As traditional improvement science dictates, we began with review of the generalizable evidence on COPD care from the literature and sought to build understanding of the health system context in which we were trying to introduce improvements. But our efforts also included qualitative interviews of 10 patients with chronic obstructive pulmonary disease who had recently suffered an illness flare that led to a hospitalization.

In an effort to understand the lived experience with illness that leads to emergency department visits and hospitalizations, we invited patients to describe a "flare" of their illness. Patients told us of the terror associated with being unable to breathe, the relative powerlessness of prescribed inhalers and nebulizers in that moment, and desperate attempts to seek help and advice from adult children, spouses, and neighbors. A "911" emergency call seemed to many experiencing a disease flare like the only safe course of action. The interviews took the health professional team right into the emotional center of the illness experience that drives patients to seek costly care in the emergency department. The stories allowed the healthcare team to imagine the potential power of giving patients a new tool in their toolbox for responding more quickly and effectively to a disease flare. In collaboration with a small number of patient volunteers, we trialed a COPD "rescue kit" in which patients received an advance prescription for systemic steroids and antibiotics. Instead of calling their healthcare providers and waiting for their providers to prescribe medication for managing a flare, patients were instructed to recognize signs and symptoms of a disease flare and initiate medication independently before calling their provider.

Not all patients felt comfortable assuming responsibility for independently initiating therapy for a disease flare, but most were thrilled to have the opportunity. Not all primary care providers felt comfortable ceding responsibility to patients for initiating medical therapy for a disease flare and worried that patients might take too many antibiotics and steroids. Most, however, were willing to pursue the option for at least selected patients in their panel. After a few small serial tests of change, we engaged clinical pharmacists to provide formal education to all patients receiving COPD rescue packs. Although formal program evaluation is still in process, preliminary data suggests significant reductions in ED use and hospitalization following a prescription for a COPD rescue pack.

The change idea in this intervention emerged from a small number of interviews with patients who have lived experience with the problem that is the focus of the improvement effort. It is striking that the bundle of evidence-based care practices for standardizing care for patients with chronic obstructive pulmonary disease offers relatively little that speaks directly to the core experience of suffering a disease flare. Importantly, the change idea that emerged from these interviews recalibrates the balance of power between health professionals and patients and explicitly invites patients to take effective action as intentional coproducers of their health outcomes.

Conclusion

In summary, we recognize that the endeavor to improve health outcomes is work that is inevitably shared among health professionals and patients and families. Learning how to be good partners is fundamental to the success of this shared work. There is a moral argument for this partnership rooted in the importance of respect for persons. The argument, however, is also pragmatic. All too often, when health professionals take on the burden of improving healthcare services FOR patients and families and not WITH them, they miss the mark and invest significant resources in initiatives that do not effectively meet needs. In improving healthcare quality, we have opportunities to better our work through deepening partnerships between health professionals and patients and families. Using the framework provided in this chapter, we invite improvers to consider opportunities for stronger and more equitable partnerships at every level – from the individual clinical encounter to the clinical microsystem to the meso- and macrosystem – and across the life cycle of a change initiative from conceptualization and planning to implementation and evaluation. Tools from many disciplines – human-centered design, anthropology, and community organizing – augment the traditional toolbox in quality improvement to help us build a deeper understanding of one another and make better use of each other's assets, resources, and contributions to achieve better outcomes or improved efficiency.

Mesosystem Considerations

Individual microsystems within a mesosystem often differ in important ways, including the degree to which coproduction occurs. This presents an opportunity for cross-microsystem learning and sharing. Patients and families bring tremendous knowledge about the actual interactions and spaces between microsystems, and the work to be done to improve coordination and communication cannot be undertaken without them. Using *appreciative inquiry* to explore successes energizes both the high-performing microsystem and its neighbors. The framework to support microsystems (which may be connected via the patient's journey but not by any formal administration) must be developed and managed by the mesosystem. The "vertical" mesosystem dimension, aligning microsystem goals with those of the larger organization, is also crucial here. Microsystems will need support and encouragement from the larger organization to develop effective coproduction strategies; mesosystem leaders will also need to help microsystems develop new ways of working and a culture that embraces coproduction. Patient and family involvement in co-design may also look different at the micro- and mesosystem levels, but is crucial at both (as well as at the macrosystem level). There is much to learn from examples in other service sectors about effective coproduction; the mesosystem plays an important role in leading the learning and supporting authentic and meaningful invitations to all microsystem members to participate.

Summary

In this chapter, we introduced the idea that healthcare outcomes are not produced by health professionals or health systems alone, but rather coproduced by health professionals and patients working in the context of the healthcare system. Recognizing that all health outcomes – good and bad – are inevitably coproduced, we posit that improved partnerships between health professionals and patients are an important mechanism for healthcare service improvement. We offered a three-part framework for thinking about opportunities for coproductive partnership at different (1) places or levels from the individual clinical encounter to the clinical micro-, meso-, and macrosystem; at different (2) phases in the encounter or in the life cycle of a change project; and with different degrees of (3) parity and reciprocity in partnership. Using the clinical microsystem approach to improvement – with its initial commitment to understanding the 5Ps through setting aims, identifying changes to make, and choosing measures – we described tools and identified opportunities to cultivate more effective partnerships at every step.

Review Questions

1. What is meant by the term "coproduction" of healthcare service?
2. Identify five tools or strategies for strengthening partnership among patients and families and health professionals in healthcare quality improvement.

Discussion Questions

1. What does the term "coproduction" add to the list of other related terms such as patient engagement, patient-centered care, patient activation, and patient experience?
2. Consider a particular healthcare quality improvement initiative and use Figure 6.2 to describe activities along the partnership spectrum. When, during the improvement initiative in question, were health professionals engaged in behavior that mirrored the image of the large sphere with single-headed arrows directed at small spheres? When did the interaction have double-headed arrows? When were arrows pointing in multiple directions, engaging multiple stakeholders? When were all of the spheres of equal size?

Additional Activities

1. Using Table 6.1 as a brainstorming tool, choose an improvement initiative and consider ways of expanding partnership with patients and families on multiple levels across different points in the life cycle of the change initiative.
2. Choose a partnership tool described in this chapter and learn more about it. Experiment with using the tool in your improvement work and report on what you discover.

References

Armstrong, N., Herbert, G., Aveling, E., and others. "Optimizing Patient Involvement in Quality Improvement." *Health Expect,* 2013, 16, e36-e47.

Bate, S. P., and Robert, G. *Bringing User Experience to Healthcare Improvement: The Concepts, Methods, and Practices of Experience-Based Design.* Oxford: Radcliffe Publishing, 2007.

Berwick, D. M. "What 'Patient-Centered' Should Mean: Confessions of an Extremist." *Health Affairs*, 2009, 28(4, Jul./Aug.), w555-w565.

Bradley, E. H., Canavan, M., Rogan, E., and others. "Variation in Health Outcomes: The Role of Spending on Social Services, Public Health, and Health Care, 2000-09." *Health Affairs*, 2016, 35(5, May), 760-768. doi: 10.1377/hlthaff.2015.0814

Braverman, P., and Gottlieb, L. "The Social Determinants of Health: It's Time to Consider the Causes of the Causes." *Public Health Reports*, 2014, 129(S2), 19-31. doi: 10.1177/00333549141291S206

Carman, K. L., Dardess, P., Maurer, M., and others. "Patient and Family Engagement: A Framework for Understanding the Elements and Developing Interventions and Policies." *Health Affairs*, 2013, 32(2), 223-231. doi: 10.1377/hlthaff.2012.1133

Centers for Medicare and Medicaid Services. "HCAHPS: Patients' Perspectives of Care Survey." [http://www.cms.gov/Medicare/Quality-Initiatives-Patient-Assessment-Instruments/HospitalQualityInits/HospitalHCAHPS.html]. Dec. 2017.

Crawford, M. J., Rugger, D., Manley, C., and others. "Systematic Review of Involving Patients in the Planning and Development of Health Care." *BMJ*, 2002, 325(7375), 1263.

Cystic Fibrosis Foundation and The Dartmouth Institute Microsystem Academy. *Action Guide for Accelerating Improvement in Cystic Fibrosis Care*, 2nd edition. Bethesda, MD: Cystic Fibrosis Foundation, 2017.

Elwyn, G., Frosch, D., Thomson, R., and others. "Shared Decision Making: A Model for Clinical Practice." *Journal of General Internal Medicine*, 2012, 27(10, Oct), 1361-1367. doi: 10.1007/s11606-012-2077-6

Fuchs, V. R. *The Service Economy*. New York, NY: Columbia University Press, 1968.

Godfrey, M. M., Nelson, E. C., Wasson, J. H., and others. "Planning Patient-Centered Services." In E. C. Nelson, P. B. Batalden, and M. M. Godfrey (eds.), *Quality by Design*. San Francisco: Jossey-Bass, 2007, 125-126.

Governance International. [http://www.govint.org/]. Sep. 2017.

Health Canada. *Health Canada Policy Toolkit for Public Involvement in Decision Making*. Ottawa: Corporate Consultation Secretariat, 2000.

Institute of Medicine (U.S.), Committee on Quality of Health Care in America. *Crossing the Quality Chasm: A New Health System for the 21st Century*. Washington, DC: National Academies Press, 2001. doi: 10.17226/10027

Langley, G. L., Moen, R., Nolan, K. M., and others. *The Improvement Guide: A Practical Approach to Enhancing Organizational Performance*. San Francisco, CA: Jossey-Bass Publishers, 2009.

Mayer, M. "Seeking What Matters: Patients as Research Partners." *The Patient*, 2012, 5(2), 71–74. doi: 10.2165/11632370-000000000-00000

Pomey, M., Hihat, H., Khalifa, M., and others. "Patient Partnership in Quality Improvement of Healthcare Services: Patients' Inputs and Challenges Faced." *Patient Experience Journal*, 2015, 2(1), 29-42.

Renedo, A., Marston, C. A., Spyridonidis, D., and others. "Patient and Public Involvement in Healthcare Quality Improvement: How Organizations Can Help Patients and Professionals to Collaborate." *Public Management Review*, 2015, 17(1), 17-34.

Robert, G., Cornwell, J., Locock, L., and others. "Patients and Staff as Codesigners of Healthcare Services." *BMJ*, 2015, 350, g7714. doi: 10.1136/bmj.g7714

Additional Resources

Empathy Map Canvas (Updated), https://medium.com/the-xplane-collection/updated-empathy-map-canvas-46df22df3c8a

Institute for Healthcare Improvement mobile app portal, https://app.ihi.org/apps/

Institute for Patient- and Family-Centered Care, http://www.ipfcc.org/

iWantGreatCare Digital Data Interface, https://www.iwantgreatcare.org/search

King's College EBCD Toolkit, https://www.pointofcarefoundation.org.uk/resource/experience-based-co-design-ebcd-toolkit/

National Health Service EBCD Toolkit, https://improvement.nhs.uk/documents/1486/ebd_guide___toolkit.pdf

NEJM Catalyst Patient-Reported Outcome Measures (PROMs), http://catalyst.nejm.org/implementing-proms-patient-reported-outcome-measures/

Think Aloud Survey Tool, https://www.nngroup.com/articles/thinking-aloud-the-1-usability-tool/

Working with Patient and Families as Advisors Implementation Handbook, https://www.ahrq.gov/sites/default/files/wysiwyg/professionals/systems/hospital/engagingfamilies/strategy1/Strat1_Implement_Hndbook_508_v2.pdf

Key Words/Terms

Appreciative inquiry (AI): A change-management approach that focuses on identifying what is working well, analyzing why it is working well, and then doing more of it. The basic tenet of AI is that an organization will grow in whichever direction that people in the organization focus their attention.

Change concept: A stimulant for developing and designing detailed and specific change ideas to test.

Digital interfaces: The media by which humans interact with computers. Interfaces represent an amalgamation of visual, auditory, and functional components that people see, hear, touch, or talk to as they interact with computers.

Evaluation: A reflection on how well the project was executed (process) and whether it met its objectives (outcomes) after project completion.

Hospital Consumer Assessment of Healthcare Providers and Systems (HCAHPS): A survey instrument and data collection methodology for measuring patients' perceptions of their hospital experience. It is the first national, standardized, publicly reported survey of patients' perspectives of hospital care.

Implementation: The actual conduct of planned activities.

Initiation: The selection of a problem, the commissioning of a solution, and the designation of the necessary problem-solving resources within a larger system.

Patient reported outcome measures (PROMs): Patients' perception of their health status and experience of care such as the PHQ-9 (a self-report questionnaire completed by patients that measures the severity of depressive symptoms).

Pay-for-performance: A payment model that offers financial incentives to physicians, hospitals, medical groups, and other healthcare providers for meeting certain performance measures. Also known as "value-based purchasing."

Planning: Determining what will be done, by whom, by when.

Speak Up campaign: The Joint Commission's award-winning Speak Up™ program urges patients to take an active role in preventing healthcare errors by becoming involved and informed participants on their healthcare team.

CHAPTER SEVEN

IMPROVING PATIENT SAFETY AND RELIABILITY

Julie K. Johnson, Paul R. Barach, Gautham K. Suresh, Tanya Lord, Marjorie M. Godfrey, Tina C. Foster

AIM

The aim of this chapter is to link important elements of high-performing microsystems to specific design concepts and actions that can enhance patient safety and reliability of care.

LEARNING OBJECTIVES

By the end of this chapter, the reader will be able to:

1. Describe the frequency, scope, and impact of medical errors in healthcare systems.
2. Describe methods for identifying and measuring safety events.
3. Compare and contrast the personal approach versus the systems approach to patient safety in microsystems.
4. Describe how microsystem members should respond to medical errors and adverse events within their microsystem.
5. Discuss the role of apology and full disclosure of adverse events.
6. Describe the organizational, regulatory, and legal aspects of patient safety.

Quality by Design: A Clinical Microsystems Approach, Second Edition. Edited by Marjorie M. Godfrey, Tina C. Foster, Julie K. Johnson, Eugene C. Nelson and Paul B. Batalden.
© 2025 John Wiley & Sons, Inc. Published 2025 by John Wiley & Sons, Inc.

Introduction

In the quest to improve health care, increasing attention is being paid to gaining control over quality by making care safer, effective, timely, and centered on patient needs. Payers, regulators, and governments are seeking evidence of safe, high-quality care, yet public and fully transparent reporting that paints a meaningful picture open to sector-wide comparison does not yet exist.

In this chapter, we explore patient safety from a microsystem perspective as well as an injury epidemiology perspective and address the tensions that exist between the conceptual theories and the operational applications, tensions that raise such questions as how are we to embed safety into a microsystem's journey and can we promote system resilience, given the many trade-offs inherent in the delivery of complex care and the numerous transitions of care (gaps and hand-offs) among the many microsystems.

This chapter begins with a case study. The case study highlights many obvious points where the system failed, where it disrespected Noah's mother, and where it did not address Noah's or his family's needs. What are the ways to think about these system failures? Many valuable tools are available for analyzing medical errors and patient harm and we will present some common ones following the case study.

Safety, Medical Errors, and Patient Harm

Although the topics of safety, medical errors, and patient harm have been studied for decades (Brennan and others, 1991; Leape and others, 1991; Leape, 1994; Bates and others, 1997; Cook, Woods, and Miller, 1998; Berwick and Leape, 1999; Perrow, 1999), the release of the IOM report "To Err Is Human" brought the topic to national attention (Kohn, Corrigan, and Donaldson, 1999). The IOM report and its sister report updated in 2018, emphasized that medical errors continue to be the leading causes of death in the United States and that these errors are responsible for the deaths of 44,000 to 98,000 patients each year in U.S. hospitals (National Academies of Sciences, 2018). Human performance deficiencies and diagnostic errors (Singh, Meyer, and Thomas, 2014) have been identified in more than half of surgical adverse events, especially during care delivered by trainees (Singh and others, 2007), and are most commonly associated with cognitive error in the execution of care (Suliburk and others, 2019). Yet, there is little social agreement about how to reduce medical errors and improve patient safety. IOM reports call for an urgent and comprehensive approach to improving patient safety. The financial burden due to medical errors is enormous. For example, in Massachusetts, where the patient safety movement is considered to have started 25 years ago with the tragic death of Betsy Lehman, a recent report from the Betsy Lehman Center for Patient Safety identified 62,000 errors in Massachusetts over 12 months with excess claim costs attributed to errors of $617 million (Fain, 2019).

Clinical microsystems provide a conceptual and practical framework for thinking about the organization and delivery of care. Ideally, within clinical microsystems the building blocks of healthcare safety should be a precondition and should exist prior to the patient and family encounter. A patient entering a clinical microsystem to receive health care arrives with expectations about the type of care, level of respect, and services they are going to receive and about the desired results of their care and services. Patients arrive with an unstated, implicit trust that the healthcare system will help them and not harm them. Unfortunately, as our case study illustrates and numerous studies have shown, patients are often harmed by medical errors that occur within clinical microsystems (Johnson, Haskell, and Barach, 2016). Creating the precondition of safety is necessary to assess and reliably improve the processes at the microsystem, mesosystem, and macrosystem levels of the organization and ensure vigilance about safety hazards, tracking of near misses and medical errors, and also ensure the appropriate immediate and subsequent responses to patient harm.

Case Study: Noah

My son, Noah, was born in 1995 a healthy baby except for continual ear infections, which compromised his hearing and delayed his speech. When Noah was two years old, he had a set of ear tubes placed in his ears to allow fluid to drain and reduce the occurrence of ear infections. Noah's speech rapidly improved. In 1999 when Noah was four years old, his ear, nose, and throat (ENT) specialist recommended that Noah have a tonsillectomy and adenoidectomy.

I asked that we just remove Noah's adenoids and leave the tonsils, which is the treatment that I had done when I was a child. The specialist responded that there was an option to do that, but that he was sure that in six months Noah would need to have the tonsils removed and that it would be cruel to put Noah under anesthesia twice in one year. I agreed to the surgery. Noah's surgery was on a Friday morning. Following the surgery, we were told that the surgery was uneventful and Noah was in the recovery room. He was vomiting and they attributed that to the anesthesia. He was pretty lethargic and miserable, which they said was to be expected and though they had told me that Noah would be discharged when he was able to drink, they decided to send him home.

Noah continued to throw up at home all Friday, Saturday, and into Sunday. I called the hospital more than 10 times during the weekend. They asked me if he was vomiting blood and I continually told them no. He wasn't drinking at all and by Sunday he had stopped urinating. They had suggested Tylenol suppositories because he would not take any medication orally and they thought that the nausea was from pain. He continued to throw up all night. He was not recovering like they said he would. On Sunday morning, I called the on-call surgeon three or four times asking that Noah be seen because he was not getting any better and seemed to be quite a bit worse. We took Noah to the emergency department at the children's hospital. He was not admitted to the hospital but was observed for 23 hours in the extended emergency department (ED), which was a new unit and most of the nurses were float nurses from other departments. He was treated for dehydration and started on intravenous morphine as well as medication to stop his vomiting. His pain improved, but he still would not drink or eat. They tried to entice him with slushies and popsicles – anything they could think of, but he refused it all. He was extremely lethargic, and I was concerned, but they told me that the morphine was making him groggy and it was to be expected. Noah developed a cough that sounded like he was clearing his throat all the time. I went to the nurses' station to ask if this was normal and was told that this was okay and "not to worry."

It was a confusing 23 hours alone with Noah, punctuated by visits from hospital staff. I found it difficult to identify the roles of the people who came into his room. At one time, I voiced my concerns in great detail to a woman who came in. She smiled and apologized, then went to remove the trash from the room. Noah's surgeon consulted by phone – but never came to see us. At one point, an older gentleman poked his head in and said, "How's it going in here?" I responded automatically, "Okay," and then the man disappeared.

Monday morning, a nurse came in and announced that they had talked to Noah's surgeon, and that he wanted him sent home with an intravenous line (PICC line) to continue the fluids at home. A visiting nurse would come to our home during the evening so Noah could sleep with an IV. The nurse handed me a paper to sign, and I signed it. I was so exhausted that I just signed the paper without looking at it. The nurse left the room, and I waited for about three to four hours without seeing anyone else. I went to the nursing station and told them that I was really worried and needed to speak to Noah's doctor. The nurses responded, "You can't talk to a doctor; you have been discharged." This was the first time that I realized that I had signed his discharge paper. I told them that I still really needed to talk to a doctor, and that I did not feel comfortable taking Noah home. The nurse told me, "There is nothing we can do." Defeated, I called my husband who had gone home for a shower and told him we could go home. He heard the concern in my voice and reassured me that being discharged was a good thing.

Four hours after leaving the ED, Noah hemorrhaged from his tonsil surgical site. Although I performed CPR, he was gone before the paramedics made it to our home.

After Noah's death, the hospital stopped responding to our requests for information. The surgeon talked to us for a little while, but he became more and more frustrated with talking to me. At one point he said, "I do not understand what happened to your son and if I do not understand it then you're certainly never going to understand it." The lack of interest in speaking to us, the lack of information, and the lack of care sent us seeking answers through the legal system. The lawsuit was the second worst thing that happened to us.

Ten years later, I contacted the hospital where Noah had had his surgery. I was finishing a doctorate degree focused on patient safety at University of Massachusetts Medical School. I had been asked to present Noah's case to our third-year medical students. I wanted my presentation to be accurate and not based only on my memories. The hospital invited me back to spend a day meeting with the different providers who had taken care of Noah. Ten years of questions were answered that day. Solutions were discussed, including how to ask patients and families questions. Was Noah vomiting blood after surgery? Yes. Does blood that has been swallowed and thrown up look bright red? No. It is brown and granular like coffee grounds. I didn't know this, I saw "things" in his vomit but didn't know what I was seeing. Changing the question from "Is he vomiting blood?" to "What does his vomit look like?" might have provided information that would have changed Noah's care.

The older gentleman who stuck his head in Noah's room? Turned out that he was the ED attending and he remembered that day. He was dismayed at Noah's discharge process. He apologized and explained that no department ever took "ownership" of Noah. The ED saw him as a surgical patient, and surgery saw him as an ED patient. His apology and my discussions with the rest of the staff lifted a weight that I had been unaware I was carrying.

Learning from Errors and Adverse Events

For learning to occur in a healthcare system, there must be an agreement on definitions, which can help support the right metrics and indicators for patient safety. For example, iatrogenic injury originates from or is caused by a physician (*iatros*, Greek for "physician"; Simpson, 1989). However, the term has come to have a broader meaning and is now generally considered to include unintended or unnecessary harm or suffering arising from any aspect of healthcare management. Problems arising from acts of omission as well as from acts of commission are included. One of the more difficult problems in discussing patient or medication safety is imprecise taxonomy, since the choice of terms has implications for how problems related to patient safety and medication safety are addressed (Nebeker, Samore, and Barach, 2004). This makes the comparison of different studies and reports problematic. The lack of standardized nomenclature and a universal taxonomy for medical errors complicates the development of a response to the issues outlined in the IOM report.

The National Research Council defines a safety "incident" as an event that, under slightly different circumstances, could have been an accident. The word "accident" is intertwined with the notion that human error is responsible for most injuries (NRC, 1980). This notion can be challenging since judgments about human behavior retrospectively are strongly influenced by *hindsight bias*. As such, the ability to classify events into a safety framework requires a standard set of definitions to facilitate the analysis of events and the aggregation of data (Runciman, 2006a; Runciman and others, 2006b; Sherman and others, 2009; de Feijter and others, 2012). There remain major variations in nomenclature with no universally accepted definitions (Fischhoff, 1975). The International Classification for Patient Safety, developed by the World Health Organization's World Alliance for Patient Safety, offers definitions and concepts consisting of 11 major levels, including near misses where harm was avoided (see Table 7.1; WHO, 2009). Such a classification system facilitates learning across disciplines and organizations and should be more widely adopted.

Personal Versus Systems Approach

In a personal approach to medical error, when a medical error occurred and was called to the attention of others, the nurse, physician, or other health professional involved in caring for the patient was likely to be blamed for causing the error. This person would then be subjected to ridicule, punitive measures, or disciplinary action; perhaps forced to undergo retraining; and in severe cases terminated from the job.

When errors are exposed there is frequently a general resistance to transparency regarding the details and circumstances. The reason for this stems from the fact that the medical profession has generally adopted a personal approach to human error (Hickey and others, 2018). Accordingly, error is considered a shortcoming of a person or small group of individuals with whom responsibility is therefore deemed to rest. Consequently, blame is implied, if not stated. This personal approach to human error is satisfying in many respects; failures are "contained" and accounted for (Reason, 2000). It provides easy and direct causation for colleagues, patients, and their families.

Recently there has been increasing awareness among most healthcare institutions that (1) errors are usually caused by multiple factors related to the overall systems of care (including working conditions, human factors, and organizational culture); (2) individuals are not solely responsible for causing errors; and (3) blaming or punishing individuals for causing errors actually prevents the identification of the true set of underlying causes of errors. A fundamental flaw of the personal approach

TABLE 7.1 CLASSIFICATION OF PATIENT SAFETY EVENTS.

Safety	Freedom from accidental injuries
Error	The failure of a planned action to be completed as intended (i.e., error of execution) or the use of a wrong plan to achieve an aim (i.e., error of planning). Errors may be errors of commission or ommission and usually reflect deficiencies in the systems of care.
Adverse event	An injury related to medical management, in contrast to complications of disease. Medical management includes all aspects of care, including diagnosis and treatment, failure to diagnose or treat, and the systems and equipment used to deliver care. Adverse events may be preventable or non-preventable.
Preventable adverse event	An adverse event caused by an error or other types of systems or equipment failure.
"Near miss" or "close call"	Serious error or mishap that has the potential to cause an adverse event but fails to do so because of chance or because it is intercepted. Also called potential adverse event.
Adverse drug event	A medication-related adverse event.
Hazard	Any threat to safety, e.g., unsafe practices, conduct, equipment, labels, names.
System	A set of interdependent elements (people, processes, equipment) that interact to achieve a common aim.
Event	Any deviation from usual medical care that causes an injury to the patient or poses a risk of harm. Includes errors, preventable adverse events, and hazards (see also INCIDENT).
Incident (or adverse incident)	Any deviation from usual medical care that causes an injury to the patient or poses a risk of harm. Includes errors, preventable adverse events, and hazards.
Potential adverse event	A serious error or mishap that has the potential to cause an adverse event but fails to do so because of chance or because it is intercepted (also called "near miss" or "close call").
Latent error (or latent failure)	A defect in the design, organization, training, or maintenance in a system that leads to operator error and whose effects are typically delayed.

is that it ignores causal factors beyond the individuals; therefore, there is a high likelihood of error recurrence (Cassin and Barach, 2012). This systems approach (Reason, 2000) encourages a broad investigation of the multiple contributing factors to an error and looks beyond the immediately obvious causes. The basic premise in the systems approach is that humans are fallible, and errors are to be expected even in the best organizations staffed by the best people. Non-medical industries have all embraced a systems approach to error by focusing on preventing, predicting, recognizing, and rescuing the errors that they anticipate will occur. Human fallibility contributing to error causation is the result of intrinsic and unavoidable imperfections of human cognitive processes such as memory, vigilance, attention, concentration, and reasoning, as well as the tendency of human performance to degrade with fatigue, sleep-deprivation, distractions, excessive task demands, stress, and anxiety (Barach and Van Zundert, 2019). The WHO framework (Table 7.2)

TABLE 7.2 CONDITIONS THAT CONTRIBUTE TO ERRORS AND ADVERSE EVENTS AS SEEN THROUGH THE WHO FRAMEWORK.

Conditions that contribute to errors and adverse events as seen through the WHO framework

Work Conditions – W

- Inadequate staffing, excessive patient-nurse ratio, excessive workloads
- Undesirable shift patterns and work schedules that promote fatigue
- Equipment poorly designed, not available, or poorly maintained
- Poor ergonomic design of work area
- Lack of administrative and managerial support
- Protocols and standard procedures not available or hard to access
- Use of unclear written communication and verbal communication methods that are prone to misinterpretation; unclear task design and lack of clarity of the organizational structure and about when and how to seek help
- Inadequate supervision or backup
- Poor team structure, functioning and leadership

Human Conditions – H

- Mismatch between skills and healthcare worker and requirements of the job
- Healthcare worker lacks knowledge, is in poor physical or mental health, is in a highly emotional state, is under stress, or does not consistently adhere to safety standards
- Patient's condition is very complex or serious
- Patient has language problems or hearing impairments that make effective communication more difficult
- Patient personality and social factors make care more difficult

Organizational Conditions – O

- Financial constraints and economic pressures encourage production and efficiency over safety
- Equipment, personnel or other resources are either lacking or are not allocated to patient safety
- Lack of policies, standards, goals and regulations make it difficult to work safely
- Excessively stringent regulations encourage violations
- Medical-legal environment

Source: Adapted from Vincent and others. In Nelson and others, 2011, p. 98. Used with permission.

outlines work conditions (W), human conditions (H), and organizational conditions (O) that contribute to errors and adverse events.

Methods of Identifying and Measuring Safety Events

Although it is tempting to rely on one or two tools to simplify the complexity involved in understanding errors and patient harm, the challenge for healthcare professionals is to preface the search for root causes with an appreciation of the broader contextual factors of the error.

Many methods are available to explore the causal system at work (Reason, 1997; Dekker, 2002) and all suggest the importance of holding the entire causal system in the analytic frame, not just seeking a "root" cause. Errors and failures occur within the microsystem; and ultimately it is the well-functioning, resilient microsystem that can prevent or mitigate errors. One method that takes a broader look at error builds on William Haddon's overarching framework for injury epidemiology (Haddon, 1972). As the first director of the National Highway Safety Bureau (1966 to 1969), Haddon was interested in the broad issues of injury causes that result from the transfer of energy in such a way that inanimate or animate objects are damaged. Haddon (1973) identified 10 strategies for reducing losses:

1. Prevent the marshaling of the energy.
2. Reduce the amount of energy marshaled.
3. Prevent the release of energy.
4. Modify the rate or spatial distribution of release of energy.
5. Separate in time and space the energy being released and the susceptible structure.
6. Use a physical barrier to separate the energy and the susceptible structure.
7. Modify the contact surface or structure with which people can come in contact.
8. Strengthen the structure that might be damaged by the energy transfer.
9. When injury does occur, rapidly detect it and counter its continuation and extension.
10. When injury does occur, take all necessary reparative and rehabilitative steps.

It is more than 35 years since William Haddon, as president of the Insurance Institute for Highway Safety in Washington, DC, published his now classic paper, "Energy damage and the ten countermeasure strategies," in the *Journal of Trauma* (Haddon, 1973). The paper further developed ideas from his article "On the escape of tigers: an ecologic note" published three years earlier in the *American Journal of Public Health* (Haddon, 1970). In them, Haddon presents a conceptual framework that is not limited as a tool for injury prevention but can also be used successfully as

FIGURE 7.1 HADDON MATRIX ANALYZING AN AUTO ACCIDENT.

		Factors		
		Human	**Vehicle**	**Environment**
Phases	Pre-injury	Alcohol intoxication	Braking capacity of motor vehicles	Visibility of hazards
	Injury	Resistance to energy insults	Sharp or pointed edges and surfaces	Flammable building materials
	Post-injury	Hemorrhage	Rapidity of energy reduction	Emergency medical response

a way to identify preventive systemic interventions for almost all public health problems including reducing harm from medical errors (Runyan, 2003).

These interventions, or strategies, have a logical sequence that can be described in terms of pre-injury, injury, and post-injury. The Haddon framework is a 3 × 3 matrix in which the causal factors involved in an automobile injury (human, vehicle, and environment) head the columns, and the phases of the event (pre-injury, injury, and post-injury) head the rows. Figure 7.1 shows a completed *Haddon matrix*. It focuses the analysis on the interrelationships among the three factors and the three phases. A mix of *countermeasures* derived from Haddon's strategies is necessary to minimize harm and loss. Furthermore, countermeasures can be designed for each phase – pre-event, event, and post-event. This approach confirms what is known about adverse events in complex environments: it takes a variety of multi-level strategies to prevent or mitigate harm. Understanding injury in its larger context helps leaders and staff recognize the basic fragility of systems and the importance of mitigating inherent hazards by better preparedness and increasing the resilience of the system (Dekker, 2002).

Building on injury epidemiology, we can also use the Haddon matrix to think about analyzing medical injuries (Layde and others, 2002). To translate this tool from injury epidemiology to patient safety, we have revised the phase descriptions from pre-injury, injury, and post-injury to pre-event, event, and post-event. We have revised the factor descriptions from human, vehicle, and environment to provider, patient and family, and system and environment. In this latter factor, system refers to the processes and systems that are in place for the microsystem to perform; environment refers to the context within which the microsystem exists. We added system to recognize the significant contribution that systems make toward harm and error in a clinical microsystem. The next step in applying Haddon's matrix to analyzing medical injuries is to develop countermeasures to address the issues in each cell of the matrix (see Figure 7.2).

FIGURE 7.2 SAFETY MATRIX FOR ANALYZING PATIENT SAFETY EVENT.

		Factors		
		Provider	Patient and Family	System and Environment
Phases	Pre-event			
	Event			
	Post-event			

Diagnostic Errors

Diagnostic errors are extremely common; according to Graber, one in every ten diagnoses is probably wrong (Graber, 2013). Fortunately, the vast majority of diagnostic errors are inconsequential; the original problem resolves, the error is caught in time, the patient is resilient, or the treatment that was provided worked anyway (Graber, Sanchez, and Barach, 2017). For some fraction of patients, however, the error results in harm and death. One estimate places the annual toll of *diagnostic error* in the USA at 40,000 to 80,000 deaths per year (Leape, Berwick, and Bates, 2002). When timely surgical intervention is critical, misdiagnosing conditions such as spinal cord compression, necrotizing fasciitis, and acute myocardial infarction, among many others, can be lethal. The decision whether to operate on patients in whom these diagnoses are being considered is also a diagnostic decision, and the pressure and angst inherent in these situations is substantial and undeniable (Gawande, 2002).

Data compiled from malpractice claims have clarified the relative incidence of surgical errors and what conditions are most commonly encountered. Diagnostic error is in the number one or two categories of claims in all of these studies (Gawande and others, 1999; Gruen and others, 2006). More than half of the diagnostic errors originate in ambulatory settings. In one recent study of 2,531 cases of diagnostic error in ambulatory settings, 17 percent were surgery related, with orthopedics, urology, and general surgery being the leading categories (CRICO, 2014). Most of these cases involved patients with cancer, cardiovascular conditions, or various injuries, especially orthopedic injuries. In another study of 7,438 closed claims from 2007 to 2013, 1,877 were attributed to diagnostic error (Troxel, 2014). Of the 3,963 claims involving surgeons, 524 were related to issues in diagnosis. All system-related errors are considered preventable. The original IOM report, "To Err is Human," and the 2018 updated report both concluded that the repair of system-related flaws would be the most effective approach to improving safety in health care.

Creating a Culture of Safety

It is widely understood today that the first step toward improving the safety and quality of care is addressing the perceptions – the varying mental models held by care providers and state agencies – about care delivery (Senge, 1994). There has been an important re-conceptualization of clinical risk through emphasizing how upstream "latent factors" enable, condition, or exacerbate the potential for "active errors" and patient harm. Understanding the characteristics of a safe, resilient, and high-performing system requires research to optimize the relationship between people, tasks, and dynamic environments (Mohr and Barach, 2006). The *socio-technical* approach suggests that adverse incidents can be examined from both an organizational perspective that incorporates the concept of latent conditions and the cascading nature of human error commencing with management decisions and actions, and equally, inactions (Cassin and Barach, 2012). There are consequences for inaction in complex health delivery systems; inaction can lead to patient harm. Organizational resilience is found in the responsiveness of care delivery teams to an emerging hazard (Barach and Phelps, 2013). Some teams are more resilient – able to recover from errors reliably without leading to patient harm, while others do not learn, and repeat the same errors (Hollnagel, Woods, and Leveson, 2006).

Ineffective engagement and inauthentic partnering with clinicians remains one of the biggest obstacles globally in addressing the growing implementation gap in providing cost-effective quality care. Physician discontentment, cynicism, and the growing number of burnt-out clinicians all point to a serious trust gap (Jorm, 2012). Several studies have identified the need to "engage physicians" as the biggest challenge in healthcare reform, for example, in the efforts to mobilize key stakeholders to support hospital-based efforts to improve care transitions and reduce avoidable readmissions to hospital (Hesselink and others, 2013). Physician involvement in leading, facilitating, and participating in the adoption of new care models is key in large part because new care models require doctors to significantly change their behaviors.

Innovation in patient care is best designed in concert with those on the frontlines of healthcare delivery – patients and clinicians – and incorporates relevant knowledge from other scientific disciplines, such as operations research, organizational behavior, industrial engineering, and *human factors* psychology (Sanchez and Barach, 2012). To best engage with medical staff, the focus of improvement efforts should be on bringing even more scientific discipline and measurement to the design of healthcare delivery.

Acquiring a safety culture is a process of organizational learning that recognizes the inevitability of error and proactively seeks to identify latent threats. Characteristics of a strong safety culture include:

1. A commitment of the leadership to discuss and learn from errors.
2. Communications founded on mutual trust and respect.
3. Shared perceptions of the importance of safety.
4. Encouragement and practice of teamwork.
5. Incorporation of non-punitive systems for reporting and analyzing adverse events (Pronovost and others, 2003).

For any patient safety intervention to be successful, it is important for the right organizational culture to exist. A local culture of safety, where safety is valued above production and efficiency, is a key characteristic of industries where complex, high-risk activities are routinely undertaken under considerable time pressure with a very low frequency of errors and almost complete absence of catastrophic failures (Bognar and others, 2008). Examples of such organizations are nuclear power plants, naval aircraft carriers, and air traffic control centers, all which are often referred to as high-reliability organizations (HROs; Weick and Sutcliffe, 2001).

The five hallmarks of effective safety management systems in HROs are:

1. Preoccupation with failure
2. Reluctance to simplify interpretations
3. Sensitivity to operations
4. Commitment to resilience
5. Deference to expertise

Striving for a safety culture is a process of collective learning. When the usual reaction to an adverse incident is to write another procedure and to provide more training, the system will not become more resistant to future organizational accidents. In fact, these actions may deflect the blame from the organization as a whole. There is a long tradition in medicine of examining past practices to understand how things might have been done differently. However, morbidity and mortality conferences, grand rounds, and peer reviews share many of the same shortcomings, such as (1) a lack of human factors and systems thinking; (2) a narrow focus on individual performance that excludes analysis of the contributory team factors and larger social issues; (3) retrospective bias (a tendency to search for errors as opposed to the myriad system causes of error induction); and (4) a lack of multidisciplinary integration into the organization-wide culture (Small and Barach, 2002).

If clinicians at the sharp (microsystem) end are not empowered by the meso-system leaders to be honest and reflective on their practice, rules and regulations will have a limited impact on enabling safer outcomes. Health system leaders need to understand the fundamental dynamics that lead to adverse events. Employing tools such as root cause analysis and failure mode and effects analysis can help clinicians and others better understand how adverse events occur (Dekker, 2002).

In an organization with a strong safety culture and true *psychological safety*, the healthcare workers are willing to report errors and near misses, feel safe from punitive retaliation, willingly point out safety hazards, collaborate across different levels in the organization's hierarchy to reduce safety vulnerabilities, and consider protecting patient safety as an important part of their job (Edmondson, 2003).

A focus on learning from *near misses* offers several advantages (Barach and Small, 2000):

1. Near misses occur 3 to 300 times more often than adverse events, enabling quantitative analysis.
2. There are fewer barriers to data collection, allowing analysis of interrelations of small failures.
3. Recovery strategies can be studied to enhance proactive interventions and to deemphasize the culture of blame.
4. Hindsight bias is more effectively reduced.

High-performing microsystems draw on principles of both personal and social ethics. The traditional biomedical ethical base is important but not sufficient. To own the work in systems, including ownership of the performance of the system, invites attention to the precepts of social ethics. Hannah Arendt, a German American philosopher and political theorist, provides useful guidance. She believes individuals in a society must be able to make promises to one another. If we make promises, we must be able to seek forgiveness at times when our promises could not be kept (Arendt, 1958). Applying these principles to the clinical microsystem and to the behavior of patients and providers, we need to be able to make authentic promises about the performance of the microsystem, about our own role(s) in the microsystem, and about the roles of others involved in the work; and when those promises cannot be kept we need to be able to acknowledge the failure of the system to protect the patient and seek their forgiveness.

To create a culture of safety, leaders of microsystems and macrosystems should not just make safety a high priority; rather, patient safety should be a precondition. Paul O'Neill, an internationally renowned safety leader who served as the Secretary of the U.S. Treasury for two years under President George W. Bush, believed in the power of transparency and that to achieve an injury-free workplace, safety is "a precondition – not [merely] a priority" (O'Neill, 2011). Setting the limit at zero acceptable injuries to patients and staff requires strong leadership and a supportive board of directors (Millar, Freeman, and Mannion, 2015). Leaders who stimulate conversations about safety, mindfulness, promise making, and forgiveness; who allocate resources to patient safety; and who demonstrate their commitment to safety through activities such as executive walk rounds visibly demonstrate a deep commitment to creating a culture of safety.

Role of Risk Management and Patient Disclosure

When patients seek medical care, they entrust their health to us. Healthcare providers have a responsibility or "fiduciary duty" to act in the best interests of the patient (Kraman and Hamm, 1999). Properly assessing the type of procedure planned (for example, invasive versus noninvasive), patient risk factors, type of drug to use (for example, hypnotic versus analgesic), and type of team and level of support are all critical. When assessing the level of risk of the procedure, we should ask the following questions. What are the desired clinical effects? How quickly are effects desired? What is the desired duration of effects? Are there any adverse "other" clinical effects?

Organizational policies requiring that adverse events be disclosed to patients have been in existence for at least 20 years (Peterkin, 1990; Kraman and Hamm, 1999). However, in some places, such apology and disclosure policies are still considered a new, or even a radical idea. They hold clinicians and organizations to what may be perceived as a standard of extreme honesty (Wu, 1999). Many clinicians remain skeptical about policies requiring disclosure of adverse events. Moreover, some clinicians may fail to disclose adverse events to patients even though they believe that disclosure is the right thing to do (Sweet and Bernat, 1997). For example, in a study of clinicians' responses to a hypothetical case in which a drug error led to a patient's death, one-third of the clinicians said they would disclose only incomplete or inaccurate information to the patient's family (Chan and others, 2005). A study of house officers found that they seldom disclosed adverse events, especially if they believed the institution would be judgmental (Wu and others, 1991). Reluctance to disclose adverse events arises from a variety of psychological and cultural factors as well as both legitimate and unfounded concerns about legal and financial risks (Barach and Small, 2000; Gallagher and others, 2003). On the other hand, ethical and legal considerations argue strongly in favor of disclosure.

Injured patients and their families want to know the cause of their bad outcomes, especially if the adverse event was caused by an error (Singh and others, 2007). The most important factor in the decision to file lawsuits is not negligence but ineffective communication between patients and providers (Wu, 1999). Malpractice suits often result when an unexpected adverse outcome is met with no effort to apologize, with a lack of empathy from physicians, and a perceived or actual withholding of essential information (Wu and others, 1997).

Studies consistently show that healthcare providers are understandably reticent about discussing errors, believing they have no appropriate assurance of legal protection (LeBlang and King, 1984). This reticence, in turn, impedes systemic and programmatic efforts to prevent medical errors. A growing initiative in health care has been to encourage open and frank discussion with patients and their families after an adverse event; this initiative has met with salutary effects. The lack of evidence that disclosure adversely impacts claims, case resolution, and patient and family perceptions is changing organizational practices.

Not disclosing adverse events may permit clinicians to act as if an adverse event never occurred. Bosk (1979) has documented this phenomenon, noting that there is almost an above-the-fray "fighter pilot mentality" among surgeons. They do not want to admit to mistakes or adverse events because their mentality tells them that they cannot make mistakes (Tasker, 2000). There is also the potential of ridicule from peers and loss of reputation and income (Small and Barach, 2002).

Evidence from the University of Michigan supports an aggressive disclosure policy (Clinton and Obama, 2006). In 2002, the University of Michigan Health System launched a program with three components: (1) acknowledge cases in which a patient was hurt because of medical error and compensate these patients quickly and fairly; (2) aggressively defend cases that the hospital considers to be without merit; and (3) study all adverse events to determine how procedures and systems can be improved.

Disclosing an adverse event should occur when the adverse event (1) has a perceptible effect on the patient that was not discussed in advance as a known risk; (2) necessitates a change in the patient's care; (3) potentially poses an important risk to the patient's future health, even if that risk is extremely small; and (4) involves providing a treatment or procedure without the patient's consent

(Cantor and others, 2005). From an ethical perspective, the disclosure process should begin at the time of discussing the consent form and interventions with the patients.

Public, Regulatory, and Legal Aspects

The increasing mistrust among the public and healthcare organizations and providers around the true preventable harm caused by health care is occurring around the world, including in Australia (Garling, 2008), the US (Berwick, 2013), and the UK (Francis, 2013). This is fueling call for more regulation and legal oversight of healthcare providers. The mistrust in the US is being fueled by the widespread knowledge among the public that healthcare costs are twice those in other leading Western countries, that out-of-pocket costs have doubled for many people, and that outcomes are nevertheless highly variable and are generally not as good as those in other developed countries. The public is confronted with media reports about large variations in healthcare safety (Frankel, Tilden, and Suchman, 2019), high-visibility public outcries for more transparent regulatory oversight of healthcare services (Shammas, 2015; Gabler, 2019; McGrory and Bedi, 2019; Sievers, 2019), and major investigations around unsafe pediatric cardiac surgery centers that have shut down hospital services (for example, investigations into Saint Mary's Medical Center in West Palm Beach; Johns Hopkins All Children's Hospital; Saint Christopher's Hospital for Children in Philadelphia; Bristol Royal Infirmary, UK; the Bristol Royal Hospital for Children, UK; and more generally, at Mid Staffordshire Hospital, UK).

Public reporting of outcomes data is increasingly accepted as a reality, but it is not without controversy and challenges. Research from various non-healthcare industries indicates that the decision to change systems or processes (performance improvement) often depends on the perceptions of the individuals who must implement the change. Increasing evidence suggests that public reporting improves healthcare delivery and patient outcomes and that patients and providers are slowly changing their behavior (Werner and Bradlow, 2010). Public reporting systems can improve system performance when they are designed for learning as opposed to compliance (Anoushiravani and others, 2018). For example, incident investigation and public reporting are integral features of pediatric cardiac care and are likely to be fundamental in directing future initiatives. However, incident investigations of quality and safety departments can differ from those in clinical practices that have increasingly complex procedures. Resolving these differences requires clear communication and deep engagement on the issues, which means involving clinicians, professional bodies, and consumers in the spirit of transparency and adjusting to changes in the workplace.

As the healthcare environment continues to change, and as *public reporting* expands to include new areas, the trade-offs and tensions highlighted above must be carefully monitored and addressed. Surgeon-specific data reporting, such as the UK Cardiac Surgery Database, although well-intentioned, endorses the personal approach to error management by implying individual accountability and disregarding nonsurgical and institutional factors that affect patient outcome (Bridgewater and others, 2003). Successful public reporting will need to balance the tensions of how to protect patients and the public interests against creating an overly risk-averse environment driven by medicolegal fears and risk-averse providers. Balancing and addressing these tensions by following the principles below may help move health care toward more reliable performance and reduce the potentially unintended consequences of public reporting (Barach and Lipshultz, 2016).

Microsystem Safety Principles

Drawing on the authors' three decades of combined experience in managing, analyzing, and working with multiple microsystems across diverse health settings and countries, and our understanding of the patient safety literature, we offer the following safety principles, which may be used as a framework for adapting and sustaining patient safety concepts into clinical microsystems.

Principle 1: Errors Are Human Nature and Will Happen Because Humans Are Not Infallible. Errors are not synonymous with negligence. Medicine's ethos of infallibility leads, wrongly, to a culture that sees mistakes as individual problems or weaknesses and remedies them with blame and punishment. Instead, people should be looking for the multiple contributing factors, which can be resolved only by improving systems. Develop specific interventions to mitigate the well-known hazards and harm associated with patient hand offs, medication errors, *CLABSI*, *CAUTI*, wrong-sided procedure, etc.

Principle 2: The Microsystem Is the Key Unit of Measurement, Analysis, and Learning. Organizations can train microsystem staff to include safety principles in their daily work through huddles, rehearsing scenarios, conducting simulations, and role play. The goal is for the microsystem to behave as a robust, high-reliability organization – an organization that is preoccupied with the possibility of failure or with chronic unease about safety breaches (Wickens, Gordon, and Liu, 1998). At the heart of the microsystem is the team. Turning healthcare experts into expert teams requires substantial planning and practice (Cosman, Pramudith, and Barach, 2017). There is a natural resistance to move beyond individual roles and accountability to the team mindset. One can facilitate this commitment by (1) fostering a shared awareness of each member's tasks and role on the team through cross-training and other team-training modalities; (2) training members in specific teamwork skills such as communication, situation awareness, leadership, followership, resource allocation, and adaptability; (3) conducting team training in simulated scenarios with a focus on both team behaviors and technical skills; (4) training team leaders in the necessary leadership competencies to build and maintain effective teams; and (5) establishing and consistently utilizing reliable methods of team performance evaluation and rapid feedback.

Principle 3: Use Reliable Methods to Identify Events and Monitor Their Frequency. Leading healthcare organizations measure quality relentlessly with systematic reporting and monitoring, real-time feedback, and regular benchmarking against peers and industry best practices. This inquisitiveness extends to understanding the drivers behind low- or high-scoring measures. Staff at all levels are encouraged not just to measure, but to measure the outcomes that matter most to patients and to themselves. Once a standardized database has a critical mass, it can be a big catalyst for improvement as clinicians see what works and what doesn't. Continuously seek ways to risk-adjust measurements and to improve benchmarking (Solomon, Gusmano, and Maschke, 2016). Accountability and quality improvement measures are not the same; they were designed for different purposes and suffer when one is confused with the other. Use external measures to identify opportunities for improvement, but turn to robust, lean, statistical process control charts, run charts, and other tools to actually discover and alter workflows and care processes. Beware of introducing metrics that may inspire "gaming" of reported measurements and that encourage "normalized deviance" by healthcare providers and managers (Hannan and others, 2012).

Principle 4: Design Systems to Identify, Prevent, Absorb, and Mitigate Errors. Identify errors by establishing effective, sustainable reporting systems that encourage and support transparency and freedom from punitive actions and empower workers to feel comfortable with speaking up, even if that means they will challenge the authority gradient. Design work, technology, and work practices to uncover, mitigate, or attenuate the consequence of error reactively as well as proactively. There are many approaches that reduce the impact of errors by simplifying and standardizing the systems and processes people use. For example, tools such as checklists, flowcharts, and ticklers compensate for deficiencies in vigilance and memory.

Principle 5: Recognize the Effect of Culture as a Key Enabler for Change and Improvement. Patient safety is everyone's job. The culture of a care-giving unit underpins all processes and all improvements to care. A safety culture is one that recognizes that the most important part of making health care safer is a transparent climate that supports reporting errors, near misses, and adverse events and treats these events as opportunities for learning and improving (Westrum, 1992; Reason, 1997). Embrace and celebrate patient and clinician storytelling, which may provide opportunities for learning where safety is ensured and where it is breached.

Changing established behavior of any kind is difficult. It is particularly challenging in complex, critical healthcare settings because of the varied relationships between a wide range of organizations, professionals, patients, and carers (Amalberti and others, 2005). When implementing change in clinical practice, it can take a long time to overcome the barriers to change. For example, a clinical guideline can take from three to five years to be fully vetted and implemented. Certain trust-building factors may help to foster an environment that is conducive to behavior change. An organization where there is strong leadership, authentic communication, and transparent governance has a much greater chance for success. No matter how necessary change seems to upper management, the barriers must be authentically acknowledged and not swept under the carpet if a strategic change is to be implemented successfully. The key to successful change is in the planning, messaging, and implementation. However, barriers to changing established practice may prevent or impede progress in all organizations, whatever the culture.

Principle 6: Talk To, Listen To, and Involve Patients in Preventing Errors. Patients have much to say about safety. Involve the patients and their families early and often in preventing errors. Meaningful co-design with patients means appreciating that patients spend much more time thinking about their bodies and health than you do and have much to offer (Batalden and others, 2016).

Principle 7: Integrate Practices from Human Factors Engineering into Microsystem Functioning and System Physical Design. Design patient-centered healthcare environments that are based on human factor principles that can mitigate interruptions and distractions. The physical environment has a huge impact on providers' and patient's attention, satisfaction, safety, and emotional support (Mohr and Barach, 2006; Debajyoti, Harvey, and Barach, 2012). Design systems for human cognitive failings and the impact of performance-shaping factors such as fatigue, poor lighting, and noisy settings (Debajyoti, Harvey, and Barach, 2012).

Principle 8: Develop Tools to Make Information Readily Accessible and Transparent. Recognize that consumers want information relevant to them, not necessarily what experts think they should want. Engage patients, families, and community members in all efforts to improve public reporting of health outcomes. Developing and maintaining decision aids requires an investment of effort and money. There may be a tendency to bypass such information documentation activities if easier avenues for securing information can be identified. Well-designed, ergonomic solutions and consistent policies on the use of these resources increase the chances that such tools will be successfully adopted. A standardized database with a critical mass can be a big catalyst for improvement as clinicians see what changes work, and what do not. Sharing data and metrics using established collaborative learning tools will go a long way toward building trust and learning.

Principle 9: Identify the Clinical Leadership Required to Improve Safety. Healthcare leaders whose organizations are in control and strive for exceptional outcomes must seek the best statistical, lean, six sigma, and other improvement tools (Popovich, Wiggins, and Barach, 2019). We mean that they plan and execute to (1) methodically measure care outcomes; (2) understand the key drivers of these outcomes; (3) understand how to make these outcomes best of class; and (4) systematically prevent avoidable harm to patients. Effective leadership (at microsystem, organizational, and national levels) is crucial for addressing systems issues and for creating the kind of "learning" organization that is necessary for providing safer care from the sharp end of the operating room to the boardroom (Mohr, Abelson, and Barach, 2002).

Principle 10: When Harm Happens, Disclose Early and Apologize. Early disclosure of adverse events is increasingly recognized as an important aspect of providing care of patients. When a patient is harmed by health care, a sincere apology should be made, and all details of the event pertaining to the patient should be disclosed to the patient and his or her family. This disclosure should include:

- An apology.
- A prompt and compassionate explanation of what is understood about what happened and the probable effects to the patient.
- An assurance that a full analysis will take place to reduce the likelihood of a similar event happening to another patient.
- An assurance that there will be a follow-up based on the analysis.

Clinicians and organizations have clear ethical obligations to tell the truth about what happened, make a sincere apology, and to do it in a way that is sensitive, yet informative and clear. A growing body of evidence demonstrates that the benefits of disclosure outweigh the burdens, and that effective disclosure can reduce costs and improve patient safety and quality of care. Although the ultimate goal is to avoid and eliminate adverse events, it is important to have mechanisms to mitigate the damage caused by these events, and disclosure is an important strategy for mitigation and improvement. Finally, we need to ensure providers are supported during and after this disclosure.

Principle 11: Improve Access to and Quality of Clinical Information Systems (CIS). Information systems are the central core of an effective microsystem and require careful planning, continuous resources, and dedicated attention. Information systems designed for and by a clinical team using a technology that enables real-time adaptation provides much greater efficiency for the staff in decreasing the time to complete standard tasks (Patrick, Barach, and Besiso, 2017). Engaging and supporting clinical staff in the design and testing processes of CIS, in a manner that reflects their local workflow processes, ensures it is better suited to their needs and will be a better aid to their work. Additionally, it creates a continuous process improvement environment that enables the workflow processes to be adapted dynamically to optimize the efficiency improvement, and the technology enables measurement and recoupment of the costs of supporting the ongoing adaptation of these processes.

Principle 12: Relentlessly Seek Out Assurance of Organizational Quality Via Internal and External Audits. Many lead healthcare executives are skeptical if they are capturing the right data for safe outcomes and also expressed concerns about the reliability of the data they are reporting. Seek independent assurance about the reliability of your quality measures and focus your external reporting on important patient outcomes rather than on detailed processes and protocols. Providers will have to balance the need for assured data reliability with the resources required to achieve such a goal. One way to achieve greater efficiency is to concentrate on those outcome measures that matter most to patients. Accreditors need to rethink new ways to support and encourage self-monitoring and use novel ways to engage patients and users, including using patient surveyors and guidance teams (Brubakk and others, 2015).

A discussion of patient safety in clinical microsystems cannot be complete without acknowledging how characteristics of high-performing microsystems can be used in shaping any microsystem's response to the challenge of embedding safety into the daily work of caring for patients. Table 7.3 lists primary and additional success characteristics of high-performing microsystems (identified in Chapter One) and provides specific actions for patient safety that can be further explored in your own clinical microsystems. This list of actions is not intended to be exhaustive but rather should be seen as a starting point when applying patient safety concepts to your microsystems.

TABLE 7.3 LINKAGE BETWEEN MICROSYSTEM CHARACTERISTICS AND PATIENT SAFETY.

Microsystem Characteristic	Specific Actions for Patient Safety
Leadership	• Define the safety vision of the organization. • Identify existing constraints in the organization. • Allocate resources for safety plan development, implementation, and ongoing monitoring and evaluation. • Build in microsystem participation and input to plan development. • Align organizational quality and safety goals. • Provide updates to the board of trustees.
Organizational support	• Work with clinical microsystems to identify patient safety issues and make relevant local changes. • Put the necessary resources and tools into the hands of individuals; this action needs to be real, not superficial.
Staff focus	• Assess current safety culture. • Identify the gap between the current culture and the safety vision. • Plan cultural interventions. • Conduct periodic assessments of culture.
Education and training	• Develop a patient safety curriculum. • Provide training and education of key clinical and management leadership. • Develop a core of people with patient safety skills who can work across microsystems as a resource.
Interdependence of the Care Team	• Build the plan-do-study-act (PDSA) or standardize-do-study-act (SDSA) approaches into debriefings. • Use daily huddles for after-action reviews, and celebrate identifying errors.
Patient focus	• Use daily huddles for after-action reviews, and celebrate identifying errors. • Support disclosure and truth around medical error.
Community and market focus	• Analyze safety issues in the community, and partner with external groups to reduce risk to populations.
Performance results	• Develop key safety measures. • Create the business case for safety.

(continued)

TABLE 7.3 (*Continued*)

Microsystem Characteristic	Specific Actions for Patient Safety
Process improvement	• Identify patient safety priorities based on assessment of key safety measures.
	• Address the safety work that will be required at the microsystem level.
	• Establish patient safety demonstration sites.
	• Transfer the learning across microsystems.
Information and information technology	• Enhance error-reporting systems.
	• Build safety concepts into information flow (for example, checklists, reminder systems and the like)

Conclusion

As healthcare organizations strive to gain control over their quality and their costs, they can expect the journey toward "high reliability" to take them through various stages, with the pursuit of excellence and safety gradually becoming systematic, almost second nature, toward a culture obsessed with outcomes, safety, and measurement. Safety is a dynamic property of each clinical microsystem. An understanding of local conditions that jeopardize safety and reliability can be acquired by using a variety of powerful tools and techniques. However, improvements in safety will not happen absent courageous and intelligent leadership and systemic change.

Responsibility for quality will likely become less reliant on individuals and more on teams. Staff should learn to embrace standardized processes trading individual for collective autonomy, leading to improved outcomes and a sharp decline in harm rates. Regulatory demands are expected to change significantly as providers, payers, and governments acknowledge the need to converge internal and external measurements and reporting around the key outcomes that matter most to the patient and the community (population health). Quality audits will likely become the norm and adopt the same standards as financial assurance, to give regulators, patients, and other stakeholders confidence that reports accurately reflect real performance.

Mesosystem Considerations

The case study in this chapter describes a number of events at the microsystem level; however, behind each of these frontline events, there are antecedents at the meso- and macro-levels. The mesosystem plays a key role in safety. Practitioners at the sharp end need support when adverse events occur; at the same time, a culture of accountability must be maintained. While each microsystem may have its own culture, cultural norms are supported and enacted at the mesosystem level, reflecting the crucial role of the mesosystem (with microsystem support) in developing and maintaining a culture of safety. As seen in the case study's description of the disconnect between the surgical and emergency department services, poor communication between microsystems often plays a major role in adverse events. Effective handovers, respectful and clear communication, and relational coordination between microsystems are essential for safety. These are all developed at the mesosystem level. In sum, from macro- to microsystem levels, safety considerations are paramount and must be thoughtfully attended to.

Summary

Despite spectacular progress in the diagnosis and treatment of diseases over the past century, real-world care remains suboptimal and is characterized by considerable variation in outcomes, persistent disparities, and too often, preventable defects causing harm to patients. The complexity of contemporary healthcare delivery results in care that is often fragmented, unnecessarily costly, and often not based on evidence. Additionally, it is clear that patients are exposed to preventable harm as a result of poor coordination and communication, inconsistent processes and practices, and poorly designed systems.

This chapter explored patient safety from a microsystem and an injury epidemiology perspective and demonstrated how to embed safety into a microsystem's operations.

Review Questions

1. What is the frequency and scope of medical errors in healthcare systems?
2. What is the difference between medical error and adverse events?
3. How would you describe the difference between the person approach versus the systems approach to patient safety in microsystems? Can you offer examples of each approach?
4. What are the methods used to identify medical errors and adverse events in a microsystem?

Discussion Questions

1. How should microsystem members respond to medical errors and adverse events within their microsystem?
2. Discuss the various safety activities, processes, and operational systems within a microsystem that you are aware of. What activities, processes, and operational systems might you develop to further increase safety and reliability?
3. How might you keep safety awareness alive and active in your microsystem?
4. Discuss medical errors and adverse events and cite clear examples of their differences.
5. Once you design a new process in your microsystem, how might you identify potential errors before incorporating your process into daily practice?

Additional Activities

1. Review the case study about Noah and discuss these questions in a small group setting:
   a. What were the barriers that prevented Noah from receiving effective care in the emergency department?
   b. What communication failures were apparent in Noah's care?
   c. Where were the system failures in Noah's care?
   d. Where in the process of care did incidents (errors, near misses, adverse events, and harm) occur?
   e. What are the key learning points and how do we learn from this incident to proactively prevent similar incidents from occurring in the future?

References

Amalberti, R., Auroy, Y., Berwick, D. M., and Barach, P. "Five System Barriers to Achieving Ultra-Safe Health Care." *Annals of Internal Medicine*, 2005, 142(9), 756-764.

Anoushiravani, A., Seyeed, Z., Padela, M., and others. "Quality Improvement Through Public Reporting: The Surgeon Scorecard – Are We There Yet?" *Journal of Hospital Administration*, 2018, 7(4), 27-35.

Arendt, H., *The Human Condition*. Chicago, IL: University of Chicago Press, 1958.

Barach, P., and Small, S. D. "Reporting and Preventing Medical Mishaps: Lessons from Non-Medical Near Miss Reporting Systems." *BMJ*, 2000, 320(7237), 759-763.

Barach, P., and Phelps, G. "Clinical sensemaking: A Systematic Approach to Reduce the Impact of Normalised Deviance in the Medical Profession." *Journal of the Royal Society of Medicine*, 2013, 106(10), 387-390. doi: 10.1177/0141076813505045

Barach, P., and Lipshultz, S. "The Benefits and Hazards of Publicly Reported Quality Outcomes." *Progress in Pediatric Cardiology*, 2016, 42, 45-49.

Barach, P., and Van Zundert, A. "The Crucial Role of Human Factors Engineering in the Future of Safe Perioperative Care and Resilient Providers." *ESA Newsletter*, 2019, 76, 1-5.

Batalden, M., Batalden, P., Margolis, P., and others. "Coproduction of Healthcare Service." *British Medical Journal Quality & Safety*, 2016, 25, 509-517.

Bates, D., Spell, N., Cullen, D. J., and others. "The Costs of Adverse Drug Events in Hospitalized Patients." *Journal of the American Medical Association*, 1997, 277(4), 307-311.

Berwick, D., and Leape, L. "Reducing Errors in Medicine." *British Medical Journal*, 1999, 319, 136-137.

Berwick, D. *A Promise to Learn – A Commitment to Act: Improving the Safety of Patients in England.* London: Department of Health, 2013.

Bognar, A., Barach, P., Johnson, J., and others. "Errors and the Burden of Errors: Attitudes, Perceptions and the Culture of Safety in Pediatric Cardiac Surgical Teams." *Annals of Thoracic Surgery*, 2008, 4, 1374-1381.

Bosk, C. *Forgive and Remember: Managing Medical Failure.* Chicago, IL: The University of Chicago Press, 1979.

Brennan, T., Leape, L. L., Laird, N. M., and others. "Incidence of Adverse Events and Negligence in Hospitalized Patients: Results of the Harvard Medical Practice Study I." *New England Journal of Medicine*, 1991, 324(6), 370-376.

Bridgewater, B., Grayson, A. D., Jackson, M., and others. "Surgeon Specific Mortality in Adult Cardiac Surgery: Comparison Between Crude and Risk Stratified Data." *BMJ*, 2003, 327, 13-17.

Brubakk, K., Vist, G., Bukholm, G., and others. "A Systematic Review of Hospital Accreditation: The Challenges of Measuring Complex Intervention Effects." *BMC Health Services Research*, 2015, 15(280), 1-10. doi: 10.1186/s12913-015-0933

Cantor, M. D., Barach, P., Derse, A., and others. "Disclosing adverse events to patients." *The Joint Commission Journal on Quality and Patient Safety*, 2005, 31(1), 5-12. doi: 10.1016/S1553-7250(05)31002-6

Cassin, B., and Barach, P. "Making Sense of Root Cause Analysis Investigations of Surgery-Related Adverse Events." *Surgical Clinics of North America*, 2012, 1-15. doi: 10.1016/j.suc.2011.12.008

Chan, D. K., Gallagher, T. H., Reznick, R., and Levinson, W. "How Surgeons Disclose Medical Errors to Patients: A Study Using Standardized Patients." *Surgery*, 2005, 138(5), 851-858. doi: 10.1016/j.surg.2005.04.015

Clinton, H., and Obama, B. "Making patient safety the centerpiece of medical liability reform." *The New England Journal of Medicine*, 2006, 354, 2205-2208. doi: 10.1056/NEJMp068100

Cook, R. I., Woods, D. D., and Miller, C. *A Tale of Two Stories: Contrasting Views of Patient Safety.* Chicago, IL: National Patient Safety Foundation, 1998.

Cosman, P., Pramudith, S., and Barach, P. "Building Surgical Expertise Through the Science of Continuous Learning and Training." In J. Sanchez, P. Barach, H. Johnson, and J. Jacobs (eds.), *Perioperative Patient Safety and Quality: Principles and Practice.* Cham, Switzerland: Springer, 2017, 185-204.

CRICO Strategies. "Malpractice risks in the diagnostic process." *Annual benchmarking report*, 2014.

Debajyoti, P., Harvey, T. E., and Barach, P. "Case 20: The Houston Medical Center Bed Tower: Quality and the Built Environment." In C. P. McLaughlin, J. K. Johnson, and W. A. Sollecito (eds.), *Implementing Continuous Quality Improvement in Health Care: A Global Casebook.* Sudbury, MA: Jones & Bartlett Learning, 2012, 349-362.

de Feijter, J. M., de Grave, W. S., Muijtjens, A. M., and others. "A Comprehensive Overview of Medical Error in Hospitals Using Incident-Reporting Systems, Patient Complaints and Chart Review of Inpatient Deaths." *PLoS One*, 2012, 7(2), e31125.

Dekker, S. *The Field Guide to Human Error Investigations.* Burlington, VT: Ashgate, 2002.

Edmondson, A. C. "Speaking Up in the Operating Room: How Team Leaders Promote Learning in Interdisciplinary Action Teams." *Journal of Management Studies*, 2003, 40, 1419-1452.

Fain, B. *The Financial and Human Cost of Medical Error.* Boston, MA: Betsy Lehman Center for Patient Safety, 2019.

Fischhoff, B. "Hindsight Does Not Equal Foresight: The Effect of Outcome Knowledge on Judgment Under Uncertainty." *Journal of Experimental Psychology: Human Perception and Performance*, 1975, 1, 288-299.

Francis, R. *Report of the Mid Staffordshire NHS Foundation Trust Public Inquiry.* London: House of Commons, 2013.

Frankel, R. M., Tilden, V.P., and Suchman, A. "Physicians' Trust in One Another." *JAMA.* 2019, 321(14),1345-1346. doi: 10.1001/jama.2018.20569

Gabler, E. "UNC Children's Hospital Suspends Most Complex Heart Surgeries." *The New York Times.* [https://www.nytimes.com/2019/06/17/us/heart-surgery-children-unc.html]. Jul 29, 2019.

Gallagher, T. H., Waterman, A. D., Ebers, A. G., and others. "Patients' and Physicians' Attitudes Regarding the Disclosure of Medical Errors." *JAMA*, 2003, 289(8), 1001-1007.

Garling, P. *Final Report of the Special Commission of Inquiry: Acute Care Services in NSW Public Hospitals.* Special Commission of *Inquiry*, 2008.

Gawande, A. A., Thomas, E. J., Zinner, M. J., and Brennan, T. A. "The Incidence and Nature of Surgical Adverse Events in Colorado and Utah in 1992." *Surgery*, 1999, 126(1), 66-75. doi: 10.1067/msy.1999.98664

Gawande, A. A. *Complications: A Surgeon's Notes on an Imperfect Science.* New York, NY: Picador, 2002.

Graber, M. L. "The Incidence of Diagnostic Error." *BMJ Quality & Safety*, 2013, 22(part 2), ii21-27.

Graber, M. L., Sanchez, J. A., and Barach, P. "Diagnostic Error in Surgery and Surgical Services." In J. Sanchez, P. Barach, H. Johnson, and J. Jacobs (eds.), *Surgical Patient Care: Improving Safety, Quality and Value.* Cham, Switzerland: Springer International Publishing, 2017, 397-412.

Gruen, R. L., Jurkovich, G. J., McIntyre, L. K., and others. "Patterns of Errors Contributing to Trauma Mortality: Lessons Learned from 2,594 Deaths." *Annals of Surgery*, 2006, 244(3), 371-380.

Haddon, W. "On the Escape of Tigers: An Ecologic Note." *American Journal of Public Health*, 1970, 60, 2229-2234. doi: 10.2105/AJPH.60.12.2229-b

Haddon, W. "A Logical Framework for Categorizing Highway Safety Phenomena and Activity." *Journal of Trauma*, 1972, 12(3), 193-207.

Haddon, W. "Energy Damage and the Ten Countermeasure Strategies." *Journal of Trauma*, 1973, 13(4), 321-331. doi: 10.1097/00005373-197304000-0001

Hannan, E. L., Cozzens, K., King, S. B., and others. "The New York State Cardiac Registries: History, Contributions, Limitations, and Lessons for future Efforts to Assess and Publicly Report Healthcare Outcomes." *Journal of the American College of Cardiology*, 2012, 59(25), 2309-2316.

Hesselink, G., Vernooij-Dassen, M., Barach, P., and others. "Organizational Culture: An Important Context for Addressing and Improving Hospital to Community Patient Discharge." *Medical Care*, 2013, 51, 90-98.

Hickey, E. J., Halvorsen, F., Laussen, P. C., and others. "Chasing the 6-Sigma: Drawing Lessons from the Cockpit Culture." *Journal of Thoracic and Cardiovascular Surgery*, 2018, 155(2), 690-696. doi: 10.1016/j.jtcvs.2017.09.097

Hollnagel, E., Woods, D. D., and Leveson, N. G. (eds). *Resilience Engineering: Concepts and Precepts.* Aldershot, UK: Ashgate, 2006, 238-256.

Johnson, J. K., Haskell, H., and Barach, P. (eds). *Case Studies in Patient Safety: Foundations for Core Competencies.* Burlington, MA: Jones & Bartlett Learning, 2016.

Jorm, C. *Reconstructing Medical Practice: Engagement, Professionalism and Critical Relationships in Health Care.* Aldershot, UK: Gower Publishing, 2012.

Kohn, L. T., Corrigan, J. M., and Donaldson, M. S. (eds). *To Err is Human: Building a Safer Health System.* Washington, DC: National Academies Press, 1999.

Kraman, S. S., and Hamm, G. "Risk Management: Extreme Honesty May Be the Best Policy." *Annals of Internal Medicine*, 1999, 131, 963-967.

Layde, P., Cortes, L. M., Teret, S. P., and others. "Patient safety Efforts Should Focus on Medical Injuries." *Journal of the American Medical Association*, 2002, 287(15), 1993-1997.

Leape, L. L., Brennan, T. A., Laird, N., and others. "The Nature of Adverse Events in Hospitalized Patients: Results of the Harvard Medical Practice Study II." *New England Journal of Medicine*, 1991, 324(6), 377-384.

Leape, L. L. "Error in Medicine." *Journal of the American Medical Association*, 1994, 272(23), 1851-1857.

Leape, L., Berwick, D., and Bates, D. "Counting Deaths from Medical Errors." *JAMA*, 2002, 288(19), 2405.

LeBlang, T. R., and King, J. L. "Tort Liability for Nondisclosure: The Physician's Legal Obligations to Disclose Patient Illness and Injury." *Dickinson Law Review*, 1984, 89(1), 1-52.

McGrory, K., and Bedi, N. "New Federal Report Details Widespread Problems at All Children's." *Tampa Bay Times*. [https://www.tampabay.com/investigations/2019/02/22/federal-investigators-found-systemic-failures-at-all-childrens/]. Feb. 22, 2019.

Millar, R., Freeman, T., and Mannion, R. "Hospital Board Oversight of Quality and Safety: A Stakeholder Analysis Exploring the Role of Trust and Intelligence." *BMC Health Services Research*, 2015, 15, 196. doi: 10.1186/s12913-015-0771-x

Mohr, J. J., Abelson, H., and Barach, P. "Leadership Strategies in Patient Safety." *Journal of Quality Management in Health Care*, 2002, 11(1), 69-78.

Mohr, J. J., and Barach, P. "The Role of Microsystems." In P. Carayon (ed.), *Handbook of Human Factors and Ergonomics in Health Care and Patient Safety.* Boca Raton, FL: CRC Press, 2006, 95-107.

National Academies of Sciences, Engineering, and Medicine. *Crossing the Global Quality Chasm: Improving Health Care Worldwide.* Washington, DC: The National Academies Press, 2018. doi: 10.17226/25152

National Research Council (U.S.), Assembly of Engineering, Committee on FAA Airworthiness Certification Procedures. *Improving aircraft safety: FAA certification of commercial passenger aircraft.* Washington, DC: National Academy of Sciences, 1980.

Nebeker, J., Samore, M., and Barach, P. "Clarifying Adverse Drug Events: A Clinician's Guide to Terminology, Documentation, and Reporting." *Annals of Internal Medicine,* 2004, 140(10), 1-8.

O'Neill, P. "Paul O'Neill on Patient Safety." Podcast. [https://www.leanblog.org/2011/07/podcast-124-paul-oneill-on-patient-safety/]. Jul. 2011.

Patrick, J. D., Barach, P., and Besiso, A. "Information Technology Infrastructure, Management, and Implementation: The Rise of the Emergent Clinical Information System and the Chief Medical Information Officer." In J. A. Sanchez, P. Barach, J. Johnson, and J. P. Jacobs (eds.), *Surgical Patient Care: Improving Safety, Quality, and Value.* New York, NY: Springer, 2017.

Perrow, C. *Normal Accidents: Living With High-Risk Technologies.* Princeton, NJ: Princeton University Press, 1999.

Peterkin, A. "Guidelines Covering Disclosure of Errors Now in Place at Montreal Hospital." *Canadian Medical Association Journal,* 1990, 142(9), 984-985.

Popovich, E., Wiggins, H., and Barach, P. "The Patient Flow Physics Framework." In W. Sollecito and J. Johnson (eds.), *Continuous Quality Improvement in Health Care: Theory, Implementations, and Applications,* 5th edition. Burlington, MA: Jones & Bartlett, 2019, 143-174.

Pronovost, P. J., Weast, B., Holzmueller, C. G., and others. "Evaluation of the culture of safety: Survey of clinicians and managers in an academic medical center." *Quality & Safety in Health Care,* 2003, 12(6, Dec), 405-410. doi: 10.1136/qhc.12.6.405

Reason, J. *Managing the Risks of Organizational Accidents.* Burlington, VT: Ashgate, 1997.

Reason, J. "Human Error: Models and Management." *BMJ,* 2000, 320, 768-770.

Runciman, W. B. "Shared Meanings: Preferred Terms and Definitions for Safety and Quality Concepts." *Medical Journal of Australia,* 2006, 184(10), s41-s43.

Runciman, W. B., Williamson, J. A., Deakin, A., and others. "An Integrated Framework for Safety, Quality and Risk Management: An Information and Incident Management System Based on a Universal Patient Safety Classification." *Quality & Safety in Health Care,* 2006, 15(s1), i82-i90.

Runyan, C. W. "Back to the Future: Revisiting Haddon's Conceptualization of Injury Epidemiology and Prevention." *Epidemiological Review,* 2003, 25, 60-64. doi: 10.1093/epirev/mxg005

Russ, A. L., Fairbanks, R. J., Karsh, B. T., and others. "The Science of Human Factors: Separating Fact from Fiction." *BMJ Quality & Safety,* 2013, 22(10), 802-808. doi: 10.1136/bmjqs-2012-001450

Sanchez, J., and Barach, P. "High Reliability Organizations and Surgical Microsystems: Re-Engineering Surgical Care." *Surgical Clinics of North America,* 2012, 92, 1-14.

Senge, P. *The Fifth Discipline Fieldbook: Strategies and Tools for Building a Learning Organization.* New York, NY: Knopf Doubleday Publishing Group, 1994.

Shammas, B. "St. Mary's Medical Center Ends Pediatric Heart Surgery Program, Cites 'Inaccurate' Media Findings." *South Florida Sun Sentinel.* [https://www.sun-sentinel.com/local/palm-beach/fl-st-marys-heart-program-20150817-story.html]. Aug. 17, 2015.

Sherman, H., Castro, G., Fletcher, M., and others. "Towards an International Classification for Patient Safety: The Conceptual Framework." *International Journal of Quality in Health Care,* 2009, 21(1), 2-8.

Sievers, K. "Children's Hospital Lawsuit Highlights 'Own and Control' Issue." *Norfolk Daily News.* [http://norfolkdailynews.com/news/children-s-hospital-lawsuit-highlights-own-and-control-issue/article_8eae4e72-180e-11e9-8a15-cfc306063d3d.html]. Jan. 14, 2019.

Simpson, J., and Weiner, E. (eds). *Oxford English Dictionary.* London: Oxford University Press, 1989.

Singh, H., Thomas, E. J., Petersen, L. A., and Studdert, D. M. "Medical Errors Involving Trainees: A Study of Closed Malpractice Claims from 5 Insurers." *Archives of Internal Medicine,* 2007, 167(19), 2030-2036. doi: 10.1001/archinte.167.19.2030

Singh, H., Meyer, A. N., and Thomas, E. J. "The Frequency of Diagnostic Errors in Outpatient Care: Estimations from Three Large Observational Studies Involving US Adult Populations." *BMJ Quality & Safety,* 2014, 23(9), 727-731.

Small, S. D., and Barach, P. "Patient Safety and Health Policy: A History and Review." *Hematology/Oncology Clinics of North America,* 2002, 16, 1463-1482.

Solomon, M. Z., Gusmano, M. K., and Maschke, K. J. "The Ethical Imperative and Moral Challenges of Engaging Patients and the Public with Evidence." *Health Affairs (Millwood),* 2016, 35(4), 583-589.

Suliburk, J. W., Buck, Q. M., Pirko, C. J., and others. "Analysis of Human Performance Deficiencies Associated with Surgical Adverse Events." *JAMA Network Open,* 2019, 2(7), e198067. doi: 10.1001/jamanetworkopen.2019.8067

Sweet, M. P., and Bernat, J. L. "A Study of the Ethical Duty of Physicians to Disclose Errors." *Journal of Clinical Ethics,* 1997, 8(4), 341-348.

Tasker, R. C. "Training and Dealing with Errors or Mistakes in Medical Practical Procedures." *Archives of Disease in Childhood,* 2000, 83, 95-98.

Troxel, D. B. "Diagnostic Error in Medical Practice by Specialty." *The Doctor's Advocate.* [https://www.thedoctors.com/the-doctors-advocate/third-quarter-2014/diagnostic-error-in-medical-practice-by-specialty/]. 2014.

van Beuzekom, M., Boer, F., Akerboom, S., and Hudson, P. "Patient Safety: Latent Risk Factors." *British Journal of Anaesthesia,* 2010, 105(1), 52-59. doi: 10.1093/bja/aeq135

Weick, K. E., and Sutcliffe, K. M. *Managing the Unexpected: Assuring High Performance in an Age of Complexity.* San Francisco, CA: Jossey-Bass, 2001.

Werner, R., and Bradlow, E. "Public Reporting on Hospital Process Improvements Is Linked to Better Patient Outcomes." *Health Affairs (Millwood),* 2010, 29, 1319-1324.

Westrum, R. "Cultures With Requisite Imagination." In J. Wise, D. Hopkin, and P. Stager (eds.), *Verification and Validation of Complex Systems: Human Factors Issues.* New York, NY: Springer-Verlag, 1992, 401-416.

Wickens, C., Gordon, S., and Liu, Y. *An Introduction to Human Factors Engineering.* Reading, MA: Addison-Wesley, 1998.

World Health Organization. *Conceptual Framework for the International Classification for Patient Safety.* [http://www.who.int/patientsafety/taxonomy/icps_full_report.pdf]. 2009.

Wu, A. W., Folkman, S., McPhee, S. J., and Lo, B. "Do House Officers Learn from Their Mistakes?" *JAMA,* 1991, 265(16), 2089-2094.

Wu, A. W., Cavanaugh, T. A., McPhee, S. J., and others. "To tell the truth: Ethical and practical issues in disclosing medical mistakes to patients." *Journal of General Internal Medicine,* 1997, 12(12), 770-775. doi: 10.1046/j.1525-1497.1997.07163.x

Wu, A. W. "Handling Hospital Errors: Is Disclosure the Best Defense?" *Annals of Internal Medicine,* 1999, 131, 970-972.

Additional Resources

AHRQ Patient Safety Network, https://psnet.ahrq.gov/

AHRQ Patient Safety Tools and Resources, https://www.ahrq.gov/patient-safety/resources/pstools/

Centers for Disease Control (CDC), https://www.cdc.gov/

Division of Healthcare Quality Promotion (DHQP), https://www.cdc.gov/ncezid/dhqp/

National Center for Emerging and Zoonotic Infectious Diseases (NCEZID), https://www.cdc.gov/ncezid/

The Joint Commission National Patient Safety Goals, https://www.jointcommission.org/en/standards/national-patient-safety-goals/

Key Words/Terms

Active errors: A mistake that immediately injures a patient. Active errors result directly from the actions of healthcare professionals.

Catheter-Associated Urinary Tract Infection (CAUTI): A urinary tract infection (UTI) is an infection involving any part of the urinary system, including urethra, bladder, ureters, and kidney. UTIs are the most common type of healthcare-associated infection. Among UTIs acquired in the hospital, approximately 75 percent are associated with a urinary catheter, which is a tube inserted into the bladder through the urethra to drain urine. Between 15 and 25 percent of hospitalized patients receive urinary catheters during their hospital stay. The most important risk factor for developing a catheter-associated UTI (CAUTI) is the prolonged use of the urinary catheter. Therefore, catheters should only be used for appropriate indications and should be removed as soon as they are no longer needed (Source: CDC, NCEZID, DHQP).

Central Line-Associated Blood Stream Infection (CLABSI): A central line (also known as a central venous catheter) is a catheter (tube) placed in a large vein in the neck, chest, or groin to give medication or fluids or to collect blood for medical tests. A central line-associated bloodstream infection (CLABSI) is a serious infection that occurs when germs (usually bacteria or viruses) enter the bloodstream through the central line. Central line-associated bloodstream infections (CLABSIs) result in thousands of deaths each year and billions of dollars in added costs to the U.S. healthcare system (Source: CDC, NCEZID, DHQP).

Controlled Risk Insurance Company (CRICO): Founded more than 40 years ago, the CRICO insurance program includes all of the Harvard medical institutions and their affiliates, providing coverage to 32 hospitals, 15,500 physicians, more than 325 other healthcare organizations, and in excess of 100,000 other clinicians and employees.

Countermeasures: An action taken to counteract a danger or threat.

Diagnostic error: A diagnosis that is missed, wrong, or delayed, as detected by some subsequent definitive test or finding.

Haddon matrix: The most commonly used paradigm in the injury prevention field. Developed by William Haddon in 1970, the matrix looks at factors related to personal attributes, vector or agent attributes, and environmental attributes; before, during, and after an injury or death.

Hindsight bias: Refers to the common tendency for people to perceive events that have already occurred as having been more predictable than they actually were before the events took place.

Human factors: A science at the intersection of psychology and engineering – is dedicated to designing all aspects of a work system to support human performance and safety. Human factors, also known as ergonomics, uses scientific methods to improve system performance and prevent accidental harm. The goals of human factors in health care are twofold: (1) support the cognitive and physical work of healthcare professionals; and (2) promote high-quality, safe care for patients (Russ and others, 2013).

Latent factors: The systems approach focuses on working conditions rather than on errors of individuals, as the likelihood of specific errors increases with unfavorable conditions. Since the factors that promote errors are not directly visible in the working environment, they are described as latent risk factors (van Beuzekom and others, 2010).

Near miss: An unplanned event that has the potential to cause, but does not actually result in human injury, environmental or equipment damage, or an interruption to normal operation.

Psychological safety: Being able to show and employ one's self without fear of negative consequences of self-image, status, or career.

Public reporting: Data, publicly available or available to a broad audience free of charge or at a nominal cost, about a healthcare structure, process, or outcome at any provider level (individual clinician, group, organization).

Socio-technical: An approach to complex organizational work design that recognizes the interaction between people and technology in workplaces.

CHAPTER EIGHT

CREATING AN ACTIONABLE HEALTHCARE INFORMATION ENVIRONMENT TO INFORM INTELLIGENT ACTION

Brant J. Oliver, Eugene C. Nelson, John N. Mecchella, AnnMarie R. Hess, Marjorie M. Godfrey, Tina C. Foster, Julie K. Johnson

AIM

The aim of this chapter is to describe the fundamental importance of information and the information environment in micro- and mesosystems.

LEARNING OBJECTIVES

By the end of this chapter, the reader will be able to:

1. Discuss examples of actionable information environments at micro-, macro-, and mesosystem (*registry*) levels.
2. Make recommendations for creating rich information environments in specific situations.
3. Define principles that can be applied to develop powerful information environments.
4. Describe how measurement conceptualization approaches, design of information flow, and clinical *informatics* contribute to design of effective information environments.

Quality by Design: A Clinical Microsystems Approach, Second Edition. Edited by Marjorie M. Godfrey, Tina C. Foster, Julie K. Johnson, Eugene C. Nelson and Paul B. Batalden.

Introduction

This chapter discusses concepts and principles essential to developing, maintaining, and improving actionable information environments in microsystems, mesosystems, and macrosystems. We highlight features of rich information environments capable of producing actionable information for improvement. Features include feed forward/feedback data systems, *performance dashboards*, cascading measurement (*feed up/feed down* systems), and use of patient-reported outcomes and patient-facilitated networks (*feed in/feed out* systems). Rich information environments also educate and support all healthcare professionals in leveraging improvement measurement systems to inform improvement.

Rich Information Environments

A rich, actionable information environment supports the functioning of the smallest replicable unit of healthcare service delivery – the frontline clinical unit or clinical microsystem – that provides most health care to most people (Quinn, 1992; Nelson and others, 2002). Rich information environments also inform higher system levels, including mesosystems and macrosystems. Four case studies offer examples of how clinical microsystems, mesosystems, and macrosystems use data to create rich information environments, which can facilitate high-quality, cost-effective care and can lead to the development of *Learning Health Systems*:

1. Microsystem Level: The *Swedish Rheumatology Quality Register (SRQ)* case study provides an example of the robust development of an information environment within a clinical microsystem and discusses how that can be leveraged to create a Learning Health System.
2. Mesosystem Level: The *Cystic Fibrosis Foundation Dallas OneCF Center* case study provides a practical example of an improvement team's journey to develop a mesosystem-level data environment for improving the quality of care transitions.
3. Registries: The *Swedish National Diabetes Register (NDR)* and *Cystic Fibrosis Foundation (CFF)* registry examples illustrate the utilization of large-scale data registries for *benchmarking* and the application of cascading measurement from macrosystem to microsystem levels to inform improvement in collaboratives.
4. Clinical Informatics: An example from *MaineHealth* describes the critical and emerging role of the electronic medical record (EMR) in creating actionable information environments.

Case Study One: Evolution of the Learning Healthcare Microsystem: From Historic Beginnings in the Dartmouth Spine Center to National Adoption by the Swedish Rheumatology Quality Register (SRQ)

The Swedish Rheumatology Quality Register (SRQ) is an innovative, registry-enabled learning health system that includes over 60 rheumatology programs serving over 90 percent of Sweden's rheumatology patients. It was designed to efficiently improve care in busy medical practices and makes extensive use of patient-reported outcome measures (PROMs) along with clinical data to produce real-time "data dashboards," which are used by patients for self-management and used by healthcare providers for clinical *decision support* and outcomes measurement (Hvitfeldt and others, 2009). The SRQ, in addition to being used to improve care for individual patients, is also used for quality improvement, research, and public reporting on outcomes.

The Dartmouth Spine Center, launched in 1998, was the inspiration for the SRQ. It offered a new way of providing comprehensive and personalized care and a new outcome-tracking information environment to be used at the point of care, as well as for collaborative improvement, public reporting, and as a research platform (Weinstein and others, 2000). The Dartmouth Spine Center was founded by Dr. James Weinstein and featured its own data dashboards (Figure 8.1), which were based entirely on patient-reported outcomes (PROs). Dr. Staffan Lindblad, a prominent Swedish rheumatologist and founder of the Swedish Rheumatology Quality Register, made a visit to the Dartmouth Spine Center shortly after its opening. He was very impressed with the center's new information environment and the use of "feed-forward" dashboards, which brought the patient-reported outcomes and other patient-reported information to clinic providers ahead of the actual office visit. The information was then used to support shared decision-making in the Spine Center, to track individual patient outcomes over time, and to create a national spine registry, which was utilized for healthcare quality improvement and research purposes.

Use of SRQ Data to Improve Clinical Practice and National Outcomes

Dr. Sven Tegmark, a rheumatologist, was charged in 2008 with the coordination of rheumatology services in four hospitals in the county of Gävle, Sweden, about 100 miles north of Stockholm. Dr. Tegmark championed clinical integration of the SRQ computerized modules into the clinical workflows of physicians as they were seeing rheumatology patients and the use of patient-friendly dashboards between

FIGURE 8.1 DARTMOUTH SPINE CENTER DASHBOARD.

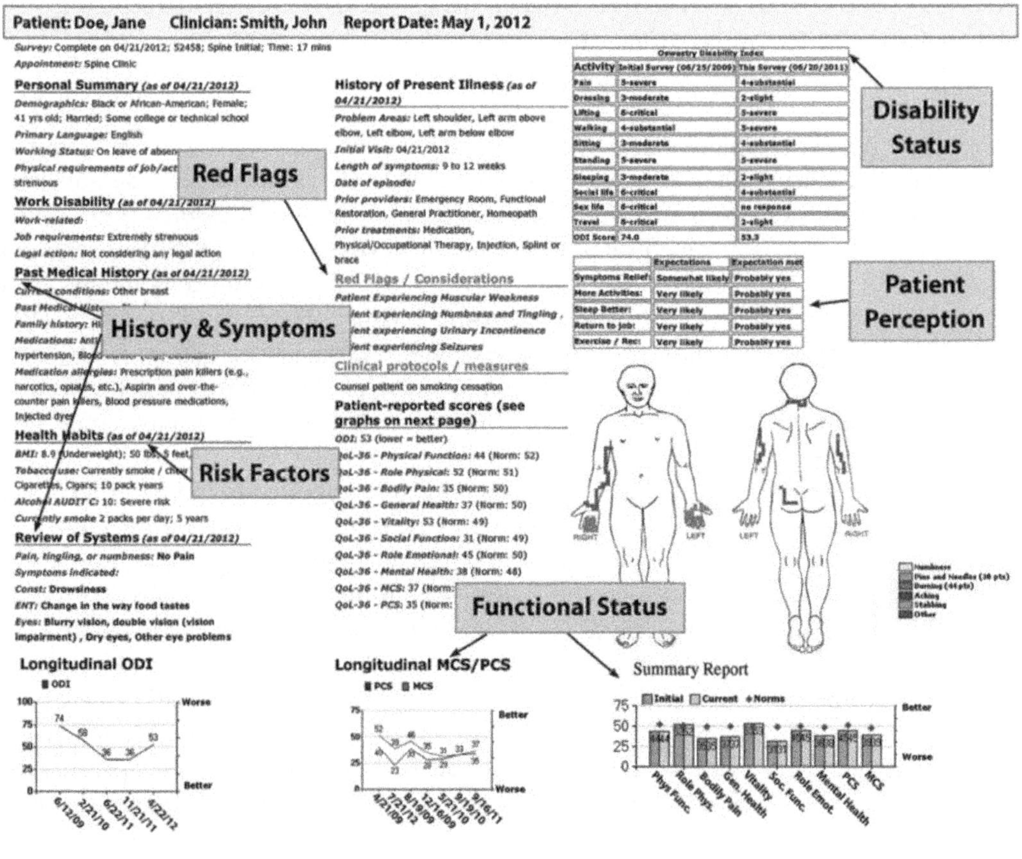

Source: Adapted from Nelson, E. C., and others, 2007, p. 181. Used with permission.

visits by patients for self-management and disease monitoring. In just one year, the four clinics became national exemplars by making significant improvements in both clinical processes and outcomes.

Patients reported information relevant to their disease (for example, health assessment, pain, self-examination of swollen and tender joints, and smoking) in the patient self-registration module, which allowed PROMs to be fed forward to the care delivery system and summarized before the clinical encounter, as was first demonstrated at the Dartmouth Spine Center. The healthcare provider then added clinical examination findings (joint counts) and laboratory results (C-reactive protein) and then used the clinical module to produce a dashboard (Figure 8.2) to visualize

FIGURE 8.2 SRQ DASHBOARD FOR A RHEUMATOID ARTHRITIS PATIENT.

År	2010	2010	2010	2010	2010	2010
Dag Månad	05-Jan	23-Feb	28-Mar	03-Jun	05-Sep	08-Dec
Årskontroll						
Månads-Kontroll	0	2	3	5	8	11
MK-grupp	1	3	3	6	9	12
Arbetsförmåga	/	/	/	/	/	/
Allmän hälsa	75	75	71	35	35	36
SR	54	63	48	25	15	5
Läkarbedömning	Hög	Hög	Hög	Måttlig	Låg	Låg
EQ5D	-0.045		-0.045		0.808	0.931
CRP	35	35	20	8	2	1
Spond.artrit, Ank.spond.						
BASFI						
Svullna leder (66)						
Ömma leder (68)						
Daktylit						
Entesit						
Funktionsneds. - HAQ	1,75	1,75	1,63	0,88	0,88	0
Smärta	81	80	75	40	30	27
Svullna leder (28)	12	12	11	2	0	1
Ömma leder (28)	12	12	11	3	1	2
TIRA						
Trombocyter						
DAS28	6.75	6.86	6.49	4.11	2.95	2.7
BASDAI						
DAS28CRP	6.21	6.21	5.84	3.61	2.41	2.79
NSAID	COX1	COX1	COX1	COX1	COX1	COX1
KORT	PRE	PRE	PRE	PRE	PRE	PRE
KORT dos	10/1d	15/1d	10/1d	10/1d	10/1d	10/1d
DMARD 1	MTX	MTX	MTX	MTX	MTX	MTX
DMARD 1 dos	20/1v	20/1v	20/1v	20/1v	20/1v	20/1v
DMARD 2	SAL	SAL				
DMARD 2 dos	2000/1d	2000/1d				
DMARD 3						
DMARD 3 dos						
DMARD 4						
DMARD 4 dos						
Uppföljd månad			0	0	3	6
Uppföljd läkemedel			ENB	REM	REM	REM
Läkemedelsdos			50/1v	200/8v	200/8v	200/8v

longitudinal changes in the treatment regimen regarding changes in disease activity and outcomes, thereby enabling well-informed decisions for future treatment.

The clinical integration of the SRQ modules led to clinical process improvements. Rather than simply scheduling routine follow-up visits, which rarely coincided with disease flare-ups, patients now had the knowledge and the patient module to track their disease activity from home and request a follow-up when needed. This type of scheduling is called "Open" Clinic. Follow-up visits that are scheduled frequently to optimize treatments when needed based on disease activity are called "Tight" Visits. This patient-driven scheduling, called "Open-Tight Clinics," frees up providers so that they meet only with patients who need them and allows any patient requesting an appointment to be seen within two weeks. These clinical process changes enabled outstanding outcome improvements. Over the last 10 years, inflammatory activity among patients with rheumatoid arthritis (measured by the mean value of serum C-reactive protein) has been reduced by half nationally, but in Gävle county (approximately three percent of the Swedish population) the results are even better with a stable mean that has remained well below the national average since 2009 (Figure 8.3).

FIGURE 8.3 LONGITUDINAL OUTCOMES FOR RHEUMATOID ARTHRITIS PATIENTS IN SWEDEN.

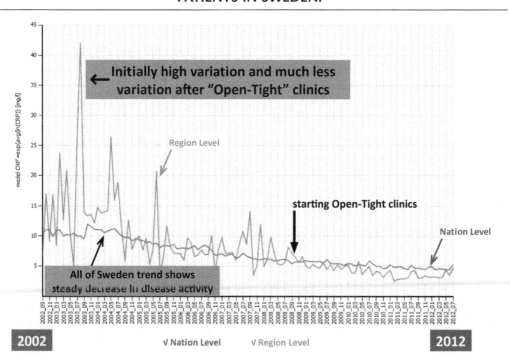

The Learning Health System

The Institute of Medicine (IOM; 2001) has popularized the idea of the learning health system, but there are not many models for connecting the learning health system idea with frontline clinical microsystems (Nelson, Fisher, and Weinstein, 2011a). The development of the SRQ provides a pathway toward building a learning health system based on a special type of data registry that is used to support better care and coproduction for individuals, quality improvement at the microsystem level, and research at the national level (Forsberg and others, 2015; Nelson and others, 2015). In the United States, the Inflammatory Bowel Disease Quorus Learning Health System is another exemplar (Johnson and others, 2017). The learning health system is designed to enable learning at three levels. First, learning occurs at the level of the individual patient about what treatments work best to provide personalized, evidence-based care. Second, learning occurs at the level of the clinical microsystem about how to apply evidence-based processes and how to track the impact on outcomes on the patient population served to improve quality and outcomes for individuals and populations. Third, learning occurs at the national and international levels to form a platform for treatment research and to enable people with disparate conditions to build new evidence on what treatments work best. The Dartmouth Spine Center and SRQ approaches are examples of how individual clinical microsystems can be part of dynamic national and international learning health systems.

Case Study Two: Using Data from Multiple Microsystems to Create a Mesosystem-Level Information Environment: The *Dallas OneCF Center* Pediatric to Adult CF Care Mesosystem Measurement Journey

Over the past few decades, cystic fibrosis (CF) care has improved dramatically due to significant biomedical advances and a substantive investment in healthcare quality improvement, resulting in significantly increased life expectancy in the CF population and improvements in CF research, quality of care, and quality of life (Berlinski and others, 2014; Marshall and Nelson, 2014; Mogayzel and others, 2014; Savant and others, 2014; Stevens and Marshall, 2014; Zanni and others, 2014). This has effectively created a new challenge for the CF community. With more people with CF living into adulthood, pediatric and adult CF centers now have to learn how to collaborate more effectively to care for people with CF who are transitioning into adult CF care. The *OneCF* Learning and Leadership Collaborative (*OneCF* LLC) utilized an improvement collaborative and team coaching approach (Godfrey and

Oliver, 2014) to focus on the pediatric to adult CF care transition. Participating CF centers in the *OneCF* LLC consisted of pediatric and adult CF clinics that combined to form *OneCF* centers or a CF mesosystem. The *Dallas OneCF Center* improvement team volunteered to develop a mesosystem-level data dashboard that could measure the quality of the pediatric to adult CF care transition and could serve as an exemplar for other *OneCF* centers participating in the *OneCF* LLC.

Conceptualizing Transition Quality Using a Modified Clinical Value Compass Balanced Scorecard Approach

The Dallas improvement team wanted a "living measurement system" that could get to the heart of the transition process and how it was experienced by people with CF and their families. They began by conceptualizing what transition quality meant and what factors would need to be measured to assess it. Utilizing a modification of the clinical value compass (CVC) as originally developed by Nelson and others (1996) and the *balanced scorecard* model (Kaplan and Norton, 1992), they developed a *OneCF* Center modified CVC/scorecard with population, process, outcome, and experience-of-care domains that reflected the quality of the transition process (Figure 8.4). Similar to the traditional CVC's focus on the individual level, the *OneCF* mesosystem CVC/scorecard utilized a person-level focus and included clinical and patient-experience domains. It also included mesosystem-level foci on population readiness for transfer and transfer process performance.

FIGURE 8.4 DALLAS ONECF CENTER MODIFIED SCORECARD.

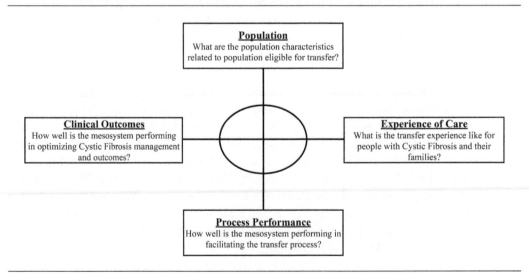

Developing Population, Process, and Outcome Measures

Building upon their mesosystem CVC/dashboard model, the Dallas team next worked to identify elements within each domain that could be operationalized, quantified, and measured to guide care design and delivery. These elements included how well people with CF respiratory function and nutritional status were maintained during the care transition process, how efficiently people with CF were transitioned, how well prepared they were for transition, and how they experienced the transition. They organized candidate "measurement grids" in three categories: (1) population demographics; (2) process measures; and (3) outcome measures (including clinical, functional health, and experience of care). Each "measurement grid" contained a listing of candidate measures, their operational definitions, and options for data display (Tables 8.1–8.3).

TABLE 8.1 DALLAS ONECF CENTER POPULATION MEASURES.

Domain	Measures	How can I measure it?	What kind of display can I use?
Age	Age distribution of the clinic population	% in each age category	Bar chart or Pie chart
Gender	Gender distribution	% in each gender category	Pie chart
Eligible for transfer	People with CF eligible for transfer	% of total clinic population eligible for transfer in 90 and 180 days	Bar chart
Planned transfers	When you are planning to transfer people with CF	Frequency counts by season or quarter	Bar chart
Comorbidities	What other conditions are present besides CF?	% of people with CF with each co-morbidity	Bar chart or Pareto chart

TABLE 8.2 DALLAS ONECF CENTER OUTCOME MEASURES.

Domain	Measures	How can I measure it?	What kind of display can I use?
Clinical	FEV1 (respiratory status)	% at goal	p Chart
		Average FEV1	XmR chart or run chart
Clinical	BMI (nutritional status)	% at goal	p Chart
		Average BMI	XmR chart or run chart
Clinical	Exacerbations ("CF flare frequency")	% with no flares	p Chart
		Average # flares	XmR chart or run chart
Experience	Satisfaction with transfer experience	Average summary score by quarter (Questionnaire)	Bar chart, XmR chart, or run chart

TABLE 8.3 DALLAS ONECF CENTER PROCESS MEASURES.

Domain	Measures	How can I measure it?	What kind of display can I use?
Efficiency	Time to transfer	% transferred in 90 days	p Chart
		Average transfer time	XmR chart or run chart
Readiness	1st adult visit appointment	% with 1st adult visit scheduled at last pedi appointment	p Chart
Readiness	Readiness assessment completed	% with assessment completed at time of last pedi visit	p Chart
Problems	Categories of most common problems	Frequency counts of problems by category	Pareto chart or bar chart
Utilization	Categories of service utilization	Frequency counts of utilization by category, for example, ED, office visits	Pareto chart or bar chart

Starting Simple

Like many engaged in innovation and improvement work, the Dallas center did not have the time or resources to create a full clinical informatics infrastructure when first developing the *OneCF* mesosystem performance dashboard; they had to rely on basic methods. This meant narrowing the full list of candidate measures to develop a parsimonious display containing two population measures, one clinical measure, one experience-of-care measure, and two process measures that could display the most important and actionable information for pediatric to adult transition. They utilized a simple *dummy display* to visually organize the dashboard (Figure 8.5) and then populated it with visual displays of priority measures (Figure 8.6).

Developing a Robust and Parsimonious Information Environment for the Dallas *OneCF* Mesosystem

The Dallas improvement team built upon the basic performance dashboard and progressively refined and expanded the mesosystem performance dashboard based on ongoing work to improve transition performance. Throughout this process, they maintained the measurement domains that they had established in the original measurement development process using the CVC domains and the three measurement categories (population, process, and outcome). They then expanded the reach of these by adding further measurement capability and changing the focus of the measures for better effectiveness. The result of this journey was the development of an interactive, Excel-format performance dashboard, which provided a

FIGURE 8.5 DUMMY DASHBOARD STRUCTURE.

POPULATION MEASURE #1	POPULATION MEASURE #2
CLINICAL OUTCOME MEASURE	EXPERIENCE OUTCOME MEASURE
PROCESS MEASURE #1	PROCESS MEASURE #2

well-articulated and actionable information environment (Figure 8.7) that could be used to monitor and improve the pediatric to adult CF care transition process within a *OneCF* Center mesosystem (Microsoft® Excel, 2019). The template they developed, as well as the measurement development process they created, was shared with the *OneCF* LLC collaborative. The *Dallas method* is now being utilized by many *OneCF* centers to start their mesosystem measurement journey.

Over time, the Dallas group further developed their dashboard through successive iterations informed by ongoing improvement work. They aimed to simplify the dashboard and to capture the most important performance measures while optimizing fidelity and efficiency of data collection. Ultimately, they utilized *statistical process control* (SPC) methods (Benneyan, Lloyd, and Plsek, 2003) to create a more focused, parsimonious, and analytic real-time performance dashboard capable of real-time monitoring and better detection (Figure 8.8).

Key Aspects of the Dallas *OneCF* Mesosystem Measurement Journey

The Dallas *OneCF* example highlights a number of key factors for developing effective information environments for mesosystems. First, they started with an understanding of the microsystems (the pediatric and adult CF clinic) that

FIGURE 8.6 DALLAS ONECF CENTER POPULATED DUMMY DASHBOARD.

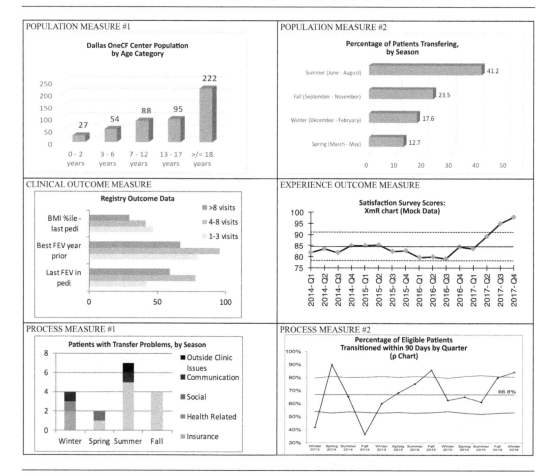

comprised the mesosystem, the population they served (people with CF transitioning from pediatric to adult CF care), and the pathway linking the two microsystems that was of priority interest (pediatric to adult transition). Second, they applied methods that are effective in conceptualizing and developing measurement approaches for clinical microsystems, such as the CVC and balanced scorecard. Third, they did not allow innovation to be impeded by lack of a robust informatics infrastructure to support the initial work. Instead, they created parsimonious, but actionable, simple displays as a foundation for later expansion, which eventually could be incorporated into a larger clinical informatics strategy. Finally, they kept measurement linked and responsive to the ongoing improvement work in a mutually beneficial way. Just as the performance dashboard

FIGURE 8.7 DALLAS ONECF CENTER INITIAL DASHBOARD.

Cystic Fibrosis Healthcare Quality Improvement
Dallas OneCF Cystic Fibrosis Center: Pediatric to Adult Care Transition

Population and Performance Characteristics	Narrative Summary	Performance Measures

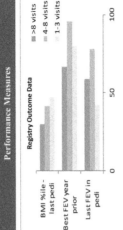

Dallas OneCF Center Population by Age Category

Age Category	Count
0 - 2 years	27
3 - 6 years	54
7 - 12 years	88
13 - 17 years	95
>/= 18 years	222

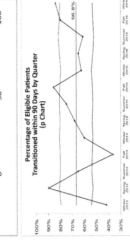

Percentage of Patients Transfering, by Season

Season	%
Summer (June - August)	41.2
Fall (September - November)	23.5
Winter (December - February)	17.6
Spring (March - May)	12.7

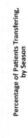

Patients with Transfer Problems, by Season

■ Outside Clinic Issues
■ Communication
■ Social
■ Health Related
■ Insurance

(Winter, Spring, Summer, Fall)

Narrative Summary

- OneCF Center project is focused on the handoff from the pediatric center to the adult center at the point of transfer.
- Goals include improving communication between medical teams and improving follow-up care and overall health following transition to adult care.
- Criteria for beginning transition include being 17 or senior in high school, whichever is later.
- Patients with developmental impairments may benefit from delayed transfer.
- Time of year for transfer will be a joint decision with family but recommended based on post-graduation plans.
- Medical handoff communication tool was created and implemented for use.
- Current focus is on refinement and measure of both process and medical outcomes.

Performance Outcomes for 2014 (Year 3):

- 58.8% transferring patients are meeting CFF goals for FEV_1, greater than 80% predicted.
- 41.2% transferring patients are meeting CFF goals for BMI percentile, greater than 50%.
- 70.6% transferring patients are meeting CFF goals for completing 4 visits to the clinic per calendar year.
- 35.3% transferring patients met criteria for a CF exacerbation at their last pediatric visit.

Performance Measures to be implemented:

- Patient and Parent Satisfaction Survey will be completed following first adult clinic visit, except for year one, which will receive it ASAP.
- Analysis of BMI and FEV_1 patterns for 2 years prior to and following transfer.

Performance Measures

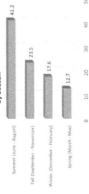

Registry Outcome Data

■ >8 visits
■ 4 -8 visits
■ 1-3 visits

- BMI %ile - last pedi
- Best FEV year prior
- Last FEV in pedi

(0, 50, 100)

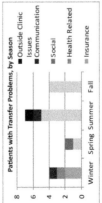

Percentage of Eligible Patients Transitioned within 90 Days by Quarter (p Chart)

66.8%

(30%, 40%, 50%, 60%, 70%, 80%, 90%, 100%)

Satisfaction Survey Scores: XmR chart (Mock Data)

(75, 80, 85, 90, 95, 100)

(2014-Q1 … 2017-Q4)

FIGURE 8.8 DALLAS ONECF CENTER SPC DASHBOARD

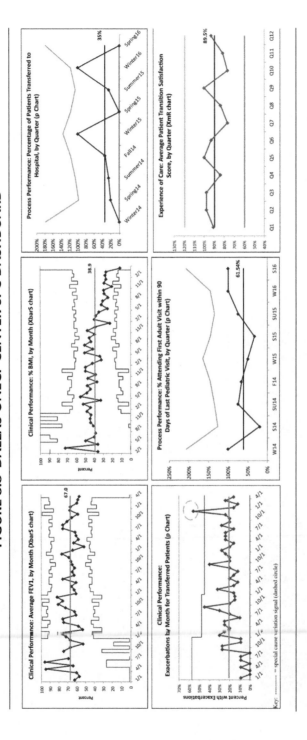

informed the improvement work, so did the improvement work inform the iterative modifications and redesign of the information environment. This mutual synergy of improvement and measurement exemplifies the potential of rich information environments in action.

Case Study Three: Cascading Data from the Macrosystem Level to Inform Performance and Improvement: Examples of Data Registry Applications from Sweden and the United States

The first two case studies focused on the creation of rich information environments in microsystems and mesosystems. Case Study 1 described an application of feedforward data design that can contribute to a Learning Health System. Building upon this foundation, Case Study 3 introduces the concept of cascading data from the microsystem level to higher system levels including macrosystems and population data registries (Figure 8.9). Two brief case studies illustrate the concept of *cascading measures* and the use of registries in two major applications: (1) benchmarking for improvement; and (2) facilitating and evaluating the effects of large-scale improvement initiatives on outcomes.

FIGURE 8.9 CASCADING MEASURES.

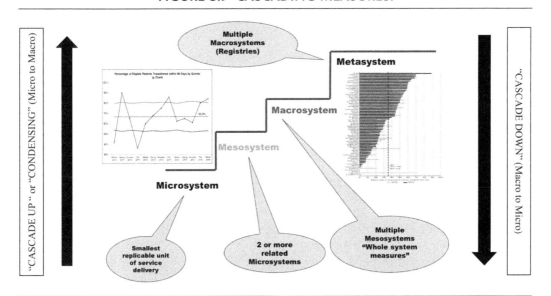

Using Registries for Benchmarking: The Cystic Fibrosis Foundation Benchmarking Project

Benchmarking involves the comparison of the performance of multiple entities on similar measures (Griffith, Alexander, and Jelinek, 2002; Johnson and others, 2007). Benchmarking is often associated with accountability and can therefore carry a negative connotation within healthcare teams who seek to avoid punishment for underperformance versus comparators. However, benchmarking can be used to identify high performers who can be studied and emulated to influence improvement. Benchmarking can be done within a single macrosystem to compare the performance of different service lines (mesosystems), or the performance of different clinical units within service lines (microsystems), or at scale as in a national improvement collaborative composed of multiple participating centers.

The Cystic Fibrosis Foundation has utilized a national registry over the past two decades to monitor and study CF population health, quality of care processes, and outcome measures. This has supported the study of regional variation in performance across CF centers. The registry, generated and sustained by data contributions from individual CF center microsystems and mesosystems, has the capability of providing center-level reports back to contributing CF centers. The use of aggregate benchmarking data in a registry gave CFF improvement collaboratives the ability to identify priority improvement needs and areas of high variation in performance (Boyle and others, 2014), and also identified exemplar centers that could serve as benchmarking site visits for the rest of the improvement collaborative to learn from. A hallmark of the CFF Learning and Leadership Collaborative model is the inclusion of site visits to high-performing centers for this purpose (Godfrey and Oliver, 2014). The registry also allowed the CFF collaborative to evaluate the impact of improvement interventions on population health outcomes (Mogayzel and others, 2014).

Using Registries for Improvement: The Swedish National Diabetes Register Improvement Collaborative

Population health data registries can also be utilized to drive large-scale, coordinated improvement efforts. Peterson and colleagues (2015) describe a 20-month improvement initiative conducted from 2008 to 2009 utilizing the National Diabetes Register (NDR) to drive a national-level improvement initiative across Sweden. A total of 23 teams participated and contributed clinical outcomes data for people with diabetes in their populations, including serum hemoglobin A1c (HgbA1c), low-density lipoprotein levels (LDL), and systolic blood pressure (SBP). The total sample size for the collaborative was just below 8,000 adults with diabetes. The NDR collaborative was a collaborative learning model and utilized the registry to track individual center and total collaborative outcomes. Individual teams focused on improving performance on processes linked to improving HgbA1c, SBP, or LDL. The processes the teams included smoking cessation counseling, use of the NDR patient profile to inform patients of their diabetes status at clinic visits, and clinical service bundles to improve diabetes comprehensive care provision. These process measures were actionable at the microsystem level and were assumed to be related to improved outcomes. The collaborative realized greater improvement in SBP and LDL control compared to the general Swedish population but did not realize comparative improvements in HgbA1c. This highlights a key role that population-level registries can play in determining the association between improvement interventions and outcomes. Here, the NDR enabled the Swedish diabetes collaborative to determine an effect on outcomes compared to the general Swedish population, which, in turn, allowed them to make some basic determinations concerning the effects of the improvement collaborative on priority outcomes.

Case Study Four: The Role of Clinical Informatics: Using Data from an Electronic Health Record (EHR) to Improve Health Maintenance Outcomes in the MaineHealth System

An EHR has been the source of monthly quality reporting for primary care practices across the MaineHealth system. MaineHealth is an integrated, not-for-profit care network of 1,500 providers and 12 member organizations serving Maine and northern New Hampshire (https://mainehealth.org). The clinical measures produced from EHR data extraction provide data for analysis from the MaineHealth system level down to the region, practice, team, provider, and individual patient level. Historically, regional-level data has been used for comparison purposes (Table 8.4) and to identify outliers. Most providers will argue that the aggregate results that demonstrate regional performance are not "actionable" as they likely represent a provider other than themselves.

Data Capture Challenges

Provider-level data such as colorectal cancer screening rates (Figure 8.10) can be used to challenge assumptions about what is driving performance. However, data discussions at this level can be challenging as the discussions often focus on how "the data are wrong." The data are not actionable because they are not

TABLE 8.4 PERCENTAGE OF HEALTH MAINTENANCE ACTIVITIES COMPLETED (FEBRUARY 2016).

Measure	Falls Screening	Depression Screening	Colorectal Cancer Screening	Adult BMI	HbA1c >9%	HTN Control	DM Eye Exam	Tobacco	Peds BMI
Target	60.90%	64.00%	64.00%	88.00%	18.20%	71.00%	60.00%	94.00%	88.00%
Region A	87.85%	46.57%	65.29%	81.25%	19.61%	64.25%	54.13%	96.39%	85.54%
Region B	84.44%	76.67%	51.13%	94.93%	16.55%	57.82%	54.65%	72.45%	48.15%
Region C	83.85%	53.81%	51.59%	84.66%	21.24%	67.77%	42.42%	95.69%	76.39%
Region D	68.98%	70.82%	57.08%	86.73%	19.53%	67.63%	51.30%	97.03%	72.52%
Region E	78.13%	56.28%	57.99%	88.85%	19.15%	65.05%	53.46%	95.59%	80.54%

* Shading indicates below performance target/goal

FIGURE 8.10 COLORECTAL SCREENING STRATIFIED BAR CHART.

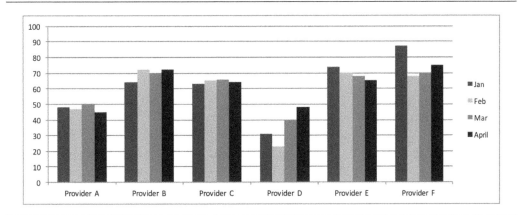

trusted. In 2012 clinical teams at MaineHealth became increasingly frustrated with their patterns of performance that showed trends consistently below targets at all levels of reporting. They blamed the system for not capturing clinical information that they were reportedly documenting. Analysts provided documentation and found that multiple fields in the electronic record that accepted data entry were not mapped to any reporting workflows, which validated the providers' concerns.

The discovery of errors in the documentation process validated provider distrust of the electronic record. In another example, the documentation of depression screening was entered in a flowsheet row that did not communicate with a health maintenance reporting function. Therefore, teams were not getting credit for completed screenings. Recognizing that distrust in the data and variation in documentation were barriers to improving outcomes, a clinical informatics workgroup was organized to systematically research all documentation and technical workflows for key performance indicators. The aim was to eliminate all technical barriers to accurate reporting of clinical outcomes. The workgroup included a process for generating operational definitions for key measures, mapping technical workflows and reminder mechanisms, eliminating multiple documentation pathways, and improving data-reporting queries to reflect the measure definition. The workgroup postulated that with improved trust in the data, the regular reporting could be actionable and focus resources to improve care.

One small primary care practice used its team data to close gaps in care management using a documentation guide as the "source of truth" for accurate data capture and reporting (Table 8.5). In addition to accurate documentation, new decision supports were built to alert clinicians when best practice guidelines were not

TABLE 8.5 PERCENTAGE OF HEALTH MAINTENANCE ACTIVITIES COMPLETED (IMPROVEMENT PHASE).

Measure	Target	Jan	Feb	Mar	Apr	May	Jun	Jul	Aug	Sep	Oct	Nov	Dec
Falls Screening	61%	90%	89%	94%	92%	90%	90%	93%	92%	90%	93%	94%	95%
Depression Screening	64%	46%	46%	48%	52%	56%	60%	62%	72%	78%	78%	77%	79%
Colectal Cancer Screening	64%	45%	45%	45%	46%	46%	46%	46%	47%	46%	46%	46%	46%
Adult BMI	88%	82%	82%	81%	81%	81%	82%	82%	96%	96%	97%	97%	97%
HbA1c >9%	18%	20%	20%	20%	20%	18%	19%	19%	17%	17%	16%	15%	15%
HTN Control	71%	63%	63%	62%	62%	63%	63%	63%	62%	60%	59%	57%	58%
DM Eye Exam	60%	55%	54%	54%	54%	54%	54%	53%	55%	55%	55%	55%	55%
Tobacco	94%	96%	96%	96%	97%	97%	96%	96%	96%	96%	97%	96%	96%
Peds BMI 5210	88%	86%	86%	86%	86%	85%	85%	86%	85%	86%	86%	86%	86%

Shading indicates performance measures targeted by improvement efforts.

FIGURE 8.11 DEPRESSION SCREENING RUN CHART.

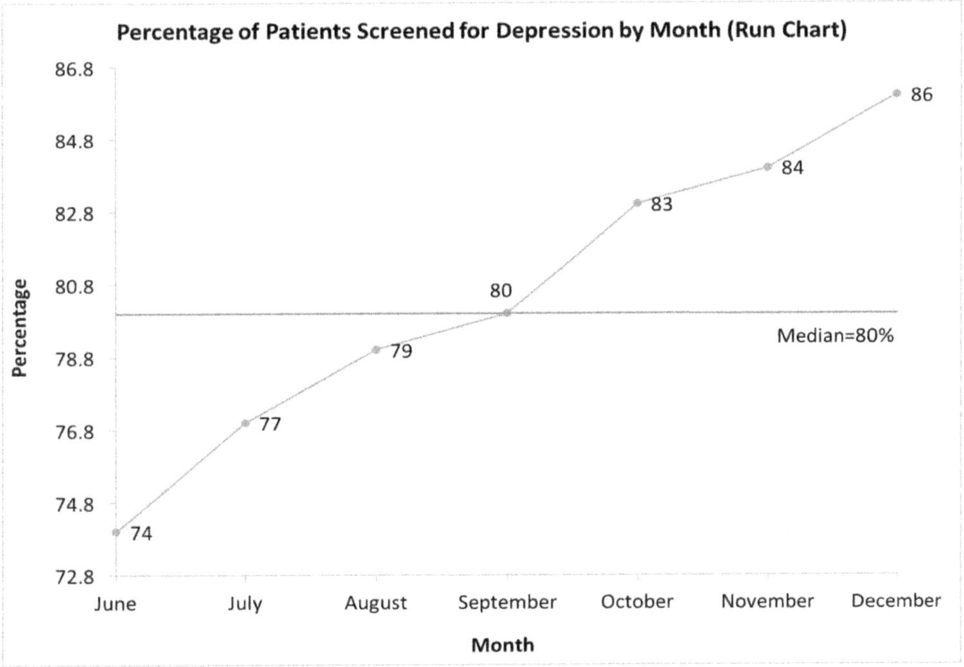

Percentage of Patients Screened for Depression by Month (Run Chart)

followed. Patients also received reminders through the *patient portals* when health maintenance activity was due and overdue. With these interventions, the results for completion of depression screening, adult body mass index (BMI) documentation, and patients with HbA1c >9 improved significantly.

Clinical teams can also use an EHR to create longitudinal monitoring charts to monitor progress over time. *Run charts* (Figure 8.11) can be used for this purpose and are capable of describing median performance and variation patterns, such as common cause and special cause variation (Perla, Provost, and Murray, 2011). Teams can also "drill down" into the data to the patient lists to close care gaps through targeted outreach or through an office visit. The implementation of electronic reminder systems that alert both clinical teams and patients when depression and other screenings are due has improved outcomes. Ensuring the systems are built for accurate, efficient, and valid data collection and providing teams with a documentation "source of truth" has resulted in providers becoming more trusting of the reports they use on a daily, weekly, and monthly basis to improve care for patients and families.

Creating a Rich Information Environment

A rich information environment does not just happen. It must be designed and improved over time. It begins with engineering an information environment that can support an organization's ability to deliver high-quality services to patients and families within a clinical microsystem and propagates across system levels up to the macrosystem level. The case studies highlight three key factors that are important for designing, developing, and sustaining a rich and actionable information environment:

- Conceptualizing measures
- Designing information flow
- Leveraging clinical informatics.

Conceptualizing Measures: The Value Compass, Balanced Scorecard, and Inverted Triangle Approaches

The patient value compass, also called the CVC, can be used to determine whether the microsystem is providing care and services that meet the needs of patients and families and whether the healthcare delivery system is producing high-quality and high-value care (Nelson and others, 1996). The CVC is designed to provide a balanced view of outcomes – health status, patient satisfaction, and patient care costs – for an individual patient or a defined population of patients. Like a compass used for navigation, the CVC has four cardinal points that can be pursued in exploring answers to critical questions:

- West: What are the biological and clinical outcomes?
- North: What are the functional status and risk status outcomes?
- East: How do patients experience and participate in health care? What is their level of satisfaction with services and perceived health benefit?
- South: What costs are incurred in the process of delivering care? What direct and indirect costs do patients and families incur?

The CVC can be adapted to virtually any population of patients – such as outpatients, inpatients, home health clients, and community residents (see Figure 8.12; Nelson and others, 1996). It assumes that patient outcomes – health status, satisfaction, and costs – evolve over time and through wellness and illness episodes. For example, a person may be in generally good health at 32 years of age and then suffer a herniated disc, undergo short-term treatment for the disc problem, and regain full health. Then, at age 35, he may reinjure his back, suffer from prolonged chronic back pain, lose his job, and become clinically depressed. At each point in the

FIGURE 8.12 CLINICAL VALUE COMPASS.

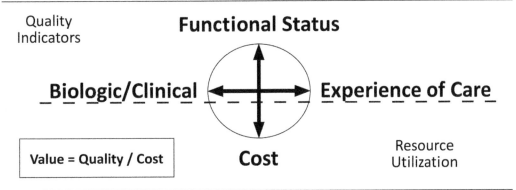

Source: Adapted from Nelson, E. C., and others, 1996, p. 252. Used with Permission.

patient's illness journey, it is possible, through data collection, to explore that individual patient's CVC for that point in time and compare it to his CVC at earlier points in time. CVC data can be collected and analyzed to answer the question, "Is this patient improving or declining with respect to health status and satisfaction and in relation to his need for care, and at what cost?" Finally, the CVC has applicability to the coproduction model, which calls for measurement that reflects process and outcomes that are coproduced rather than produced by a system and delivered to those receiving care (Batalden and others, 2016).

Organizational and Strategic Perspective. The Balanced Scorecard. The balanced scorecard approach (Kaplan and Norton, 1993, 2000, 2004) can be used to answer the question, "Is the microsystem making progress in areas that contribute to operating excellence and strategic progress?" It is a powerful approach that has gained popularity (Oliveira, 2001; Griffith, Alexander, and Jelinek, 2002). In contrast to the CVC, which uses the patient as the unit of analysis, the balanced scorecard examines the organization or a smaller operational unit (microsystem) within the organization. Just as the CVC can work at multiple levels – the individual patient or a discrete subpopulation – the balanced scorecard can work at the level of the clinical microsystem, the mesosystem, or the macrosystem.

The balanced scorecard is designed to provide a well-rounded view, specifying and assessing an organization's strategic progress from four critical perspectives – learning and growth, core processes, customer viewpoint, and financial results. It can be used to answer fundamental questions such as:

- Are we learning and growing in business-critical areas?
- How are our core processes performing?

FIGURE 8.13 BALANCED SCORECARD.

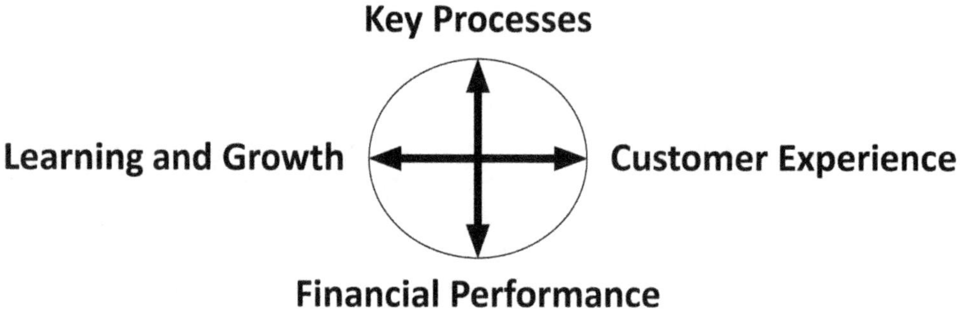

Key Processes

Learning and Growth   **Customer Experience**

Financial Performance

Source: Adapted from Nelson, E. C., and others, 2007, p. 193. Used with permission.

- How do we look in the eyes of our customers (patients, families, specific populations)?
- How are we doing at managing costs?

The balanced scorecard approach can be adapted to virtually any type of organization – a manufacturing plant, a service enterprise, or a healthcare delivery system (see Figure 8.13; Nelson and others, 2007, p. 193). Balanced scorecards offer a simple, yet elegant, way to link strategy and vision with the following:

- Objectives for strategic progress
- Measures of objectives
- Target values for measures
- Initiatives to improve and innovate.

Other positive features of the balanced scorecard framework are its capacity to align different parts of a system toward common goals, deploy high-level themes to ground-level operating units that directly serve the patient or customer, and establish a succinct method for communicating results and for holding operating units accountable for generating essential results.

Linking Aims, Change Ideas, and Measures for Improvement: The "Inverted Triangle" Approach. Continuous improvement is a core activity of clinical microsystems and affects all system levels. Regardless of the level of system involved (microsystem, mesosystem, or macrosystem), engaging in improvement activities requires a strong focus on three critical aspects: (1) aims that are derived from organization and strategic priorities; (2) change ideas (interventions) that are designed to achieve

FIGURE 8.14 BASIC IMPROVEMENT MEASUREMENT PROCESS.

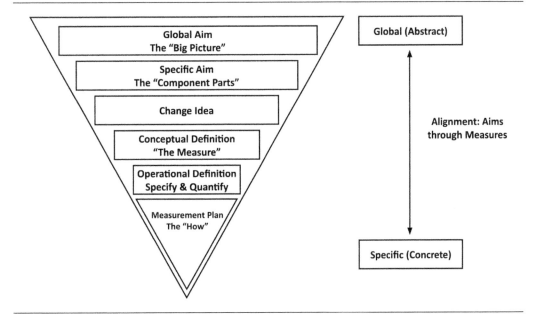

those aims; and (3) measures that can assess whether the change ideas, when put into action, are achieving those aims. These aspects can be visualized as an inverted triangle with the wide top representing the most abstract and global ideas, and the narrow point at the bottom representing the most concrete, specified, and quantified aspects. Each aspect of the inverted triangle can be populated with the global aim, associated specific aims, change ideas, and finally, operationally defined measures that are most feasible to collect and most effective to assess performance (Figure 8.14). This simple design can be further expanded to include the use of driver diagrams, which can organize these linkages for multiple improvement efforts simultaneously and delve deeper into factor relationships that affect aims and outcomes (Bennett and Provost, 2015).

As one moves down the inverted triangle, the broadly-based global aim must be specified by one or more specific aims, and each specific aim must then be linked to a defined change idea (intervention). Each intervention in turn must be linked to at least one operationally defined measure. Conversely, as one moves up the triangle, a clear linkage must exist from each operationally defined measure to its associated change ideas and aims. If a deviation of alignment is detected, it may indicate a poor match between measures, aims, and change ideas, which if left unmediated, could result in inefficient or ineffective measurement, or information that does not inform improvement. Unmediated deviations can create excess waste and confusion in the information environment.

The inverted triangle approach can be linked to the CVC or Balanced Scorecard approach. Case Study 2 (*Dallas OneCF Center*) illustrates the use of a modified CVC/Scorecard (Figure 8.4) to develop performance dashboards (Figures 8.6–8.8). A brief application of the inverted triangle approach for the Dallas example is given below:

- Global aim: Improve the overall quality of the pediatric to adult care transition process for persons with CF.
- Specific aim: Improve the percentage of people with CF who are transitioned from pediatric to adult CF care within 90 days of final pediatric CF visit to 80 percent by spring 2016, with a stretch goal of 100 percent.
- Change ideas: Utilize a transition checklist and modified transition care process including case management and real-time measurement of mesosystem performance to identify eligible persons for transfer and follow them through the transition process.
- Measures: (from Performance Dashboard, see Figure 8.8).
- Primary: Percentage of people eligible for transfer attending first adult CF clinic appointment within 90 days of final pediatric visit (process measure).
- Secondary: Experience of transition survey (outcome measure).

Note that this process can be used to validate alignment of the performance dashboard measures with the aims (priorities) for improvement and includes foci on system performance and experience of care. Patient and family experience of care measures could reflect a measure of quality that aligns with the concepts of coproduction and the learning healthcare system model (Sabadosa and others, 2014; Batalden and others, 2016; Johnson and others, 2017).

Failure to maintain focus and alignment of aims, change ideas, and measures can lead to inefficient and ineffective improvement efforts, and disorganized and duplicative information pathways supporting them, leading to "death by a thousand measures." Concerns about the unintended consequences of unbridled measurement and unrestrained informatics have been voiced by many as both areas grow in application in health care (Meyer and others, 2012; Rosenbaum, 2015; Watcher, 2016). Conversely, maintaining a focus on alignment can lead to parsimony in measurement, an emphasis on reducing measurement complexity to prioritize the use of the most important measures, and the standardization and simplification of informatics measurement. Data-collection structures can aid rather than disrupt the performance and improvement trajectory of the system.

Designing Information Flow to Support Systems: *Feed Forward/ Feedback, Feed Up/Feed Down,* and *Feed In/Feed Out* Approaches

High-performing systems use *feed-forward* data to engineer timely data collection and interpretation into the microsystem, which enables the healthcare delivery system to anticipate the needs of patients and families and to prepare to "do the right thing at the right time." In addition, the same information can be displayed as *feedback* (such as graphical data displays; SPC charts; data walls; and weekly, monthly, quarterly, and annual reports) to *aggregate up* performance measures and use the resulting information to manage and improve performance. Both feed-forward and feedback methods are commonly used in care delivery. For example, many healthcare practices caring for patients with hypertension have a nurse or medical assistant measure the patient's blood pressure level and feed this information forward to the healthcare provider, who then uses it to guide decision-making concerning the treatment and the need for adjustments to the regimen. Likewise, many primary care practices show the level of control of hypertension by the panel of hypertensive patients under the care of each physician in the practice and will feed these comparative data back to the providers to identify the degree of success and to identify improvement opportunities.

Cascading Measures from Micro- to Macrosystem Levels: A *Feed up/Feed down* Approach

Case Studies 1, 2, and 3 describe the use of rich information environments at different system levels (microsystem, mesosystem, and registry/macrosystem levels) to measure and improve performance. Building upon this, now imagine an information environment that is capable of linking information across system levels, "cascading upstream (or condensing)" from micro- to meso- to macro- to population levels, or "cascading downstream" from a large data registry to inform lower system levels. At the simplest level, measurement cascades can be viewed as linkages between short- and long-term measures or between measures from smaller systems and measures aggregated at higher system levels, such as whole system measures (Meyer and others, 2012).

Starting Simple: Linking Short-Term Process and Long-Term Outcome Measures. A common application of cascading measures involves the linkage of short-term process measures at the microsystem level with longitudinal outcome measures at the macrosystem or population (registry) level. An example can be derived from Case Study 2 (*Dallas OneCF Center* mesosystem). Figure 8.15 includes a mixture of short-term process measures (for example, percent of patients transferred within 90 days)

FIGURE 8.15 LINKING SHORT- AND LONG-TERM MEASURES.

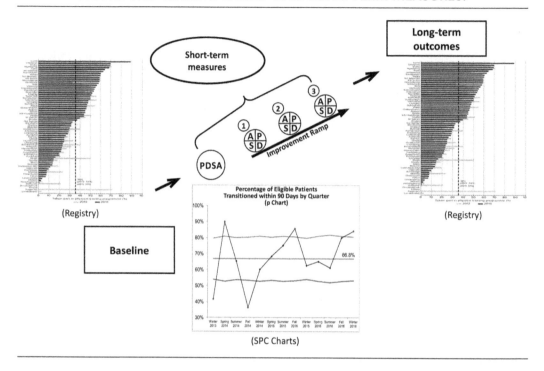

and longitudinal outcome measures (FEV1 and BMI). If a number of *OneCF* mesosystems contributed this data to a population registry, as exists within the Cystic Fibrosis Foundation, then the impact of multiple mesosystems on adult to pediatric care transition on population level FEV1 and BMI outcomes can be assessed. Conceptualizing and linking measures in this way creates a method by which improvement work can be focused at the frontline on improving performance on short-term process measures that are actionable at the microsystem level and can improve outcomes at higher system levels.

Facilitating the Cascade: Following Measures Upstream and Downstream. The concept of measurement cascades builds upon the basic "short-term/long-term" measurement linkage concept and assumes a pathway by which frontline data from clinical microsystems can be aggregated at successively higher levels, creating a population data registry (Figure 8.16). Similarly, aggregate data at the registry level should "disaggregate" down to lower system levels or be connected to measures at those levels. As described in Case Studies 1 (*SRQ*) and 3 (*CFF and Sweden Diabetes Improvement*), aggregated data in registries can be used for benchmarking to identify priorities for improvement, to identify actions needed to create the conditions for success for

FIGURE 8.16 CASCADING MEASURES ACROSS SYSTEM LEVELS.

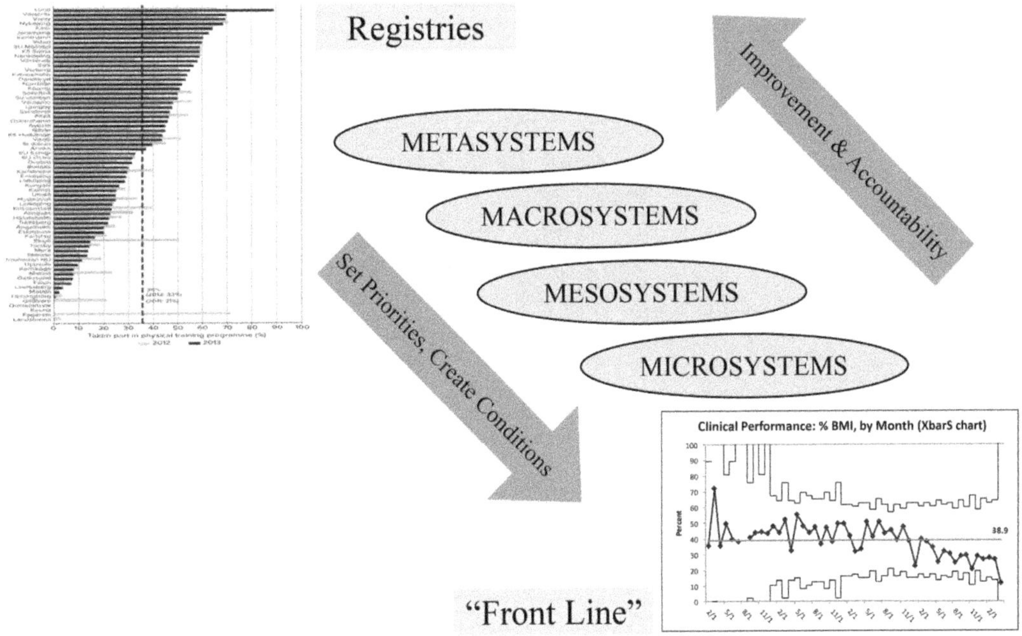

frontline improvement, and to demonstrate the effects of frontline improvement on macrosystem and population health outcomes. A critical assumption of measurement cascades is that measures linked across system levels are actually correlated. For this reason, empirically and statistically testing the associations between linked measures is recommended when designing a cascading measurement pathway.

Creating a Coproduced Learning Healthcare System: A Feed in/Feed out *Approach.* The IOM has popularized the learning healthcare system concept and describes it as a system that generates and applies the best evidence for the collaborative healthcare choices of each patient and provider and drives the process of discovery as a natural outgrowth of patient care (IOM, 2001). In fact, the groundbreaking work done by the Spine Center at Dartmouth and the Swedish Rheumatology Quality Registry (SRQ) actually contributed to this powerful concept and gives form and function to the idea of a learning healthcare system (Nelson, Fisher, and Weinstein, 2011a). Patient-generated information and clinical information *feed in* to contribute to a dashboard that shows changes in outcomes over time as well as treatments. This enriched information environment is then used at the point of care to coproduce judgments about the effectiveness of prior treatments and to make new, shared

FIGURE 8.17 INFORMATION FLOW SYSTEMS ("FEED SYSTEMS").

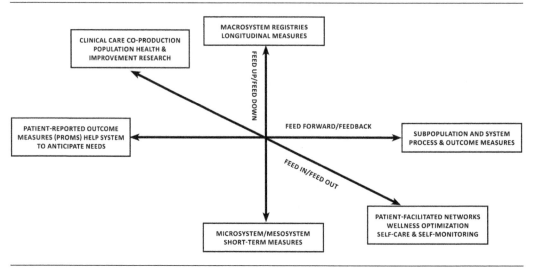

decisions about next steps in the treatment plan that is informed by the evidence base, as well as the patient's treatment history and preferences. Then, key process and outcome data can be *fed out* into a data registry that can be used for research and new scientific knowledge about treatment effectiveness, which can then be used for future patients to answer the question about what treatments or interventions work best for what kinds of people under what conditions. In addition, the *feed in* patient-reported and clinical data can be used for learning about how to improve a practice (for quality improvement learning) as well as to *feed out* to patient-facilitated networks, which patients and families can access to learn about what is already known and what is being learned from peers, experts, and the literature (see Figure 8.17). Patient-facilitated networks can be facilitated by a robust, clinical informatics infrastructure and enable the creation of an environment that is capable of coproducing health care using information that is optimally shared between the people engaged in the healthcare experience (Sabadosa and others, 2014; Batalden and others, 2016).

Leveraging Clinical Informatics to Optimize the Information Environment

Clinical (biomedical) informatics can be defined as "the interdisciplinary field that studies and pursues the effective uses of biomedical data, information, and knowledge for scientific inquiry, problem solving, and decision making, motivated by efforts to improve human health" (Kulikowski and others, 2012, p. 931). The explosive growth of the EHR has provided unprecedented opportunities for healthcare quality improvement initiatives. The ability to leverage the data captured within the EHR allows for the quantification of measures on a large scale for data of interest that was not easily accessible in narrative notes.

In the recent past, most clinical information was documented in narrative form within progress notes. Measurement of process and outcome required extensive, individual-patient chart review that was labor-intensive and often resulted in small samples, the results of which were extrapolated. Given the lack of readily accessible data, billing or claims data was often used as a surrogate for clinical data. This approach is often problematic given the lack of billing specificity and the time lag to obtaining the data. These limitations made QI initiatives difficult and measurement time consuming, particularly on a large scale. However, in the new world of EHRs, with vast quantities of clinical data being captured electronically, we are now able to leverage various tools to allow for the integrated collection of specific data points in field-defined ways. This allows for the near-real-time measurement of thousands of variables and the capability to use that information to improve care while scientifically studying it (Nelson and others, 2016).

Workflow Considerations

While the EHR can be used to generate a rich data environment, careful consideration of clinical workflows is required for the successful collection and measurement of valuable data. As we learned in Case Study 4 (MaineHealth), if there are multiple ways in which the data are documented and collected, the reporting structure has to take that into account. Either the documentation should be standardized to reduce variation, or the reporting structure must take into account such variation. Creating field-defined locations for data capture is only a small portion of the work. If the data capture is not seamlessly integrated within the workflow, it has a low chance of adoption by members of the clinical team. However, if important data element capture is incorporated into the clinical workflow in an efficient, standardized way, the downstream possibilities for using data for improvement are improved.

The choice of measures and stratification of targets should be carefully considered. If outcomes for improvement are trusted by providers and influence the clinical care of the patient, improvement teams are likely to have a high rate of provider adoption. Setting targets for measures can affect team engagement. If the goal is at an unrealistic level, team members may be less engaged. The MaineHealth case study also highlights the importance of data validation. In the case study, providers did not trust the data and found examples where the reporting failed. Therefore, it is imperative to validate the data prior to sharing reports with clinical team members. If incorrect data is shared, trust in the data may be lost within the improvement team.

Data Display Considerations

Once measures are chosen and baseline data are obtained and validated, data display aspects should be considered. Often the EHR can display some patient-level data over time (for example, weight, lab results) and some summary data (for example, total patients in clinic with a given clinical condition). However, it is often necessary to use other methods outside of the EMR to create appropriate data display to help tell the story. A stratified bar chart (Figure 8.18) shows the starting and ending frequency of a given measure by team but tells little of the improvement story that led to better results. By tracking data over time, as in the chart below (Figure 8.19), we can see Team A had dramatic improvement in May 2015, which then generally leveled off. Team C began to improve during July and continued to improve over time. Lastly, Team B demonstrated no substantive improvement.

Another option is the "stop light" display, which combines the use of color-coded tables (see Table 8.4) with data tables to demonstrate if performance is at target levels across different sites. In this example, we see that Region A was above target for falls screening but well below target for depression screening and nearing target for diabetic eye exams (DM Eye Exam). Similarly, Region D performed at or above target for fall, diabetes, and tobacco screening, but had a higher percentage of

FIGURE 8.18 STRATIFIED BAR CHART.

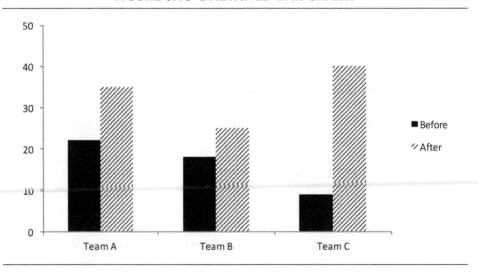

FIGURE 8.19 STRATIFIED TIME PLOT.

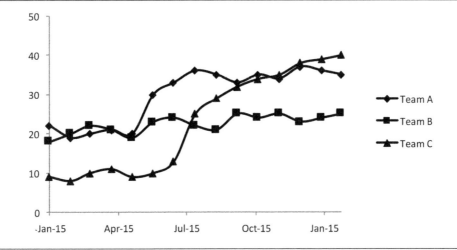

patients with HbA1c levels >9 percent (above target) and was nearing target performance on the remaining measures.

Finally, more advanced approaches for real-time visualization and longitudinal analytic data displays, such as run charts (Figure 8.11) and SPC methods (Figure 8.8), can provide displays that are able to both describe performance and analyze patterns of performance variation over time.

Clinical Decision Support and Shared Decision-Making

Clinical decision support (CDS) can assist clinicians by applying patient-specific recommendations to reduce the cognitive burden and improve adherence to evidence-based practices. The CDS tools strive to get the right information to the right healthcare team member at the appropriate time to improve outcomes. While alerts within the EHR constitute one mode of CDS, there are many additional formats of CDS. Tools such as templated notes, order sets, and corollary orders represent the various modalities of decision support. When designing such CDS tools, we recommend considering the five "rights" (Sirajuddin and others, 2009):

1. Is the right information being presented?
2. Is the right person being presented the information?
3. Is the decision support in the right format?
4. Is the CDS displayed in the right mode (channel)?
5. Is the CDS being presented at the right time within the workflow?

CDS targeted to providers should not simply be "accepted" but should be used to inform conversations around shared decision-making. While clinical decision support has historically been targeted to the care team, it can (and should) be directed toward patients to facilitate the coproduction of health. The EHR has the potential to leverage large volumes of data to help present the right information, at the right time, to the right person to improve the quality of care and improve the health of the population. The right information can facilitate more effective and efficient shared decision-making processes in the healthcare experience and can also contribute to quality improvement (Ruland, 2004; Deegan and Drake, 2006; Lee and Emanuel, 2013).

The Future Potential of Clinical Informatics: Coproduction and the Learning Healthcare System

Clinical informatics, the study of information technology and how it can be applied to health care, remains in its relative infancy. With appropriate systems to analyze patient-reported measures, clinical variables, and care team assessments, the potential to develop a learning healthcare system is within our reach (Johnson and others, 2017). CDS and improved visual displays of patient-reported data and clinical data can ensure personalized, evidence-based care delivered to the right patient at the right time. Data aggregation (often in the form of registries) can support the cascading performance measurement as discussed previously. Registries can and should be studied to track quality of care and outcomes at various system levels and for population health (Nelson and others, 2016). Ultimately, aggregated microsystem data should feed national and international collaborations to determine best practices and drive improvement and implementation efforts to optimize population health outcomes of healthcare delivery systems. Similarly, optimized informatics systems should effectively link and cascade data down to the front line to enable clinical microsystems to engage fully in the coproduction and continuous improvement of health care.

Tips and Principles to Foster an Actionable Information Environment

Without actionable information, healthcare delivery systems operate blindly, unable to monitor and improve performance, and unable to fully engage in the coproduction of health care with patients and families to generate optimal population health outcomes. System-level performance measurement must be employed effectively and efficiently to create rich information environments, which can facilitate continuous improvement in health care. Each of the case studies highlights specific tips for creating effective information environments in different applications (Table 8.6), including microsystems, mesosystems, use of registries, and clinical informatics.

These tips for success can be categorized into five general principles that facilitate actionable information environments in healthcare systems:

- Principle 1: Design It!
- Principle 2: Link It!
- Principle 3: Use It!
- Principle 4: Teach It!
- Principle 5: Cascade It!

Principle 1: Design It – Provide Access to a Rich Information Environment

This is the primary principle. Information guides intelligent action. Lack of information precludes the ability to take intelligent action. Actions that support Principle 1 include:

- Design an information system that transforms data into parsimonious, actionable, and important information that is critical to the work and to optimizing performance.
- Design the information environment to support and inform daily work, and to promote core competencies and core processes essential for care delivery.
- Establish multiple formal and informal communication channels to keep all players – patients, families, and staff – informed at the right time with the right type and amount of information needed.
- Design ease of access and use to optimize the access to and utilization of information using effective informatics design.

Principle 2: Link It – Connect People with Priorities and Enable Productive Work

Success at all system levels is contingent on the interactions between the key players – patients, families, professionals (clinical staff, administrators, support staff), and ultimately, populations. The players must be connected for positive and productive interactions to take place and for the right things to be done in the right way at the right time. Additionally, the information environment must be linked to priority goals for patients and families, to organizational priorities, and to focused improvement initiatives. Leveraging clinical informatics to connect patients, families, and

TABLE 8.6 TIPS FOR DEVELOPING AND SUSTAINING AN ACTIONABLE RICH INFORMATION ENVIRONMENT.

Case Study	Tips
Case Study 1: Swedish SRQ Rheumatology Microsystem	• Fit convenient collection and instant display of process and outcome information into flow of care for patients and clinicians. • Use "dashboards" to put key information together all in one view to avoid "hunting and gathering" of needed information stored in different locations. • Co-design the feed forward information with end users—patients, clinicians, improvement experts, researchers—to be accurate, easy to understand, and easy to use. • Design the information system to capture the data once and then to use it for multiple purposes such as personalizing patient care, clinical decision support, outcomes tracking, quality improvement, public reporting and research.
Case Study 2: Cystic Fibrosis Foundation Dallas OneCF Mesosystem	• Start with a defined subpopulation and priority outcome of interest. • Define the component microsystems that comprise the mesosystem environment. • Build a conceptual model of how quality is conceptualized in the mesosystem environment for that subpopulation and priority outcome. • Operationally define process and outcomes measures and select data displays—organize this using data definition tables. • Create simple displays (data dashboards) using priority measures. • Use the data dashboard to inform ongoing frontline improvement work in the mesosystem and use the improvement work to iteratively improve and further develop the data dashboard. • Move from simple to more complex technological applications.
Case Study 3: Registries (Cascading Measures)	• Utilize registries to identify improvement priorities at the macrosystem or metasystem level. • In improvement collaboratives, registries can enable benchmarking to identify regional variation in performance and best practices, which can then be shared for accelerated improvement. • Link registry measures to frontline microsystem and mesosystem improvement efforts using a cascading measurement approach. • People working at different system levels can utilize registry measures for leadership, coaching, or frontline improvement purposes. • Test the linkage between measures at system levels to assure that the measurement cascade is aligned with the aims and priorities of the organization and continuous improvement work.

TABLE 8.6 (*Continued*)

Case Study	Tips
Case Study 4: Electronic Medical Record (Informatics)	• Standardize the technical workflows for data capture and reporting based on well-defined operational definitions and accurate documentation. • Develop real-time measurement systems accessible to clinical teams for improving care day to day. • Build decision support mechanisms to remind clinical teams and patients when prevention plans are due. • Build best practice alerts that are the right type, to the right provider, and at the right time in a clinical workflow. • Implement a clinical information system review process for interpreting quality measures, developing documentation standards, and building technical solutions for accurate data collection.

providers with actionable information can facilitate linking the information environment to goals at all levels.

Actions that contribute to Principle 2 include:

- Conceptualize measures that connect to priorities for patients and families, the organization, and improvement goals.
- Give people the right information at the right time to do the best work possible.
- Invest in software, hardware, and expert staff to develop an effective informatics infrastructure and take full advantage of information technology to support healthcare delivery.
- Provide multiple channels for people to interact within a system, and to contribute to and receive information from the system (for example, written materials, telephone calls, email, web-based information, shared medical appointments).
- Use the information environment to inform practice and improvement and use the experience of the system to inform the continued development and improvement of the information environment.

Principle 3: Use It – Use Effective Data Analytics and Data Displays to Empower Performance and Facilitate Improvement

To improve performance or to maintain performance in a desired range of excellence, it is important to set goals that are aligned with critical values, competencies, and processes, and to measure goal attainment over time. Information being gathered must provide insight to all the key players involved in the system, instigate actions to improve or innovate, and use information streams to assess the impact of system process and design changes. To achieve this, information must be organized and displayed effectively so that it can be consistently utilized to monitor and improve performance.

Actions that promote Principle 3 include:

- Work with teams to set goals and link rewards and incentives to measured results.
- Use measures to gauge performance, ideally in real time, using information flow pathways (for example, feed forward/feedback).
- Build data collection into the daily work of clinical and support staff and into the clinical informatics infrastructure.
- Turn the primary customer – the patient/person engaged in care – into an active information source so that his or her interactions with care systems produce critical data elements in a standard and systematic manner.
- Design work processes and supporting technology to automatically generate real-time data displays, such as data walls and performance dashboards. Include the use of run charts and SPC methods that demonstrate how well the system is performing over time.
- Design informatics structures capable of generating information that can contribute to a learning healthcare system, including information for clinical care; for patients, families, and specific populations; and for improvement and outcomes research.
- Use registries and benchmarking to identify priorities for improvement and best practices.

Principle 4: Teach It – Develop Capacity for Systems to Utilize Basic Measurement Skills

Professional development is one of three critical activities required to create, develop, and sustain continuous healthcare improvement (Batalden and Davidoff, 2007). It follows that people engaged in the business of healthcare delivery and improvement cannot be expected to develop, utilize, and sustain rich information environments without being given basic knowledge and skills to do so. People engaged in day-to-day practice need to understand how and why information produced by the system is used, and people engaged in improvement work need to understand how to develop and utilize improvement measurement to inform that work.

Practical and basic education using experiential learning, simulation, and application to improvement work supported by improvement coaching and improvement collaboratives can be effective in developing frontline capability. Basic skills include measurement for assessment, defining measures and linking them to aims and change ideas, developing and pilot testing an effective data collection plan, and use of real-time, system-level analytic approaches such as run charts and SPC to assess performance and variation in systems (Table 8.7). In the Cystic Fibrosis

TABLE 8.7 FUNDAMENTAL AND INTERMEDIATE IMPROVEMENT MEASUREMENT SKILLS EDUCATION IN DARTMOUTH MICROSYSTEM ACADEMY PROGRAMS.

Module	Core Skills	Learning Activities
Fundamental Skills	Creating Data Displays	• Create basic descriptive data displays (pie charts, bar charts, and time plots) using basic Excel functions.
	Using Measurement for Assessment	• Create a data display containing key measures describing important characteristics and performance aspects of a selected microsystem or mesosystem.
	Using the Clinical Value Compass	• Use the clinical value compass to conceptualize measures.
	Denning Improvement Measures and Linking to Aims	• Use the inverted triangle approach to define measures and link to improvement aims and change ideas.
	Creating a Basic Data Collection Plan	• Create and pilot test a basic data collection plan that facilitates consistent fidelity of data capture.
	Using Modified Driver Diagrams	• If engaged in multiple improvement efforts in parallel, use modified driver diagrams to link specific aims, change ideas, and measures to the global improvement aim.
Intermediate Skills	Understanding Variation	• Education on system-level performance variation, including variation types (common cause and special cause).
	Short-term and Long-term Measures	• Articulate linkages between short-term and long-term measures for improvement.
	Using Run Charts	• Create run charts manually and using software programs to measure and analyze performance variation in a selected system.
	Using Basic Statistical Process Control (SPC): XmR and p Charts	• Using software, create and interpret basic SPC charts for continuous data (XmR charts) and proportions data (p Charts) for a selected microsystem or mesosystem.
	Creating Basic Performance Dashboard	• PDSA simulation exercises using a linked cascading measures registry.
		• Create a basic data dashboard using Excel or other platform to monitor the performance of a selected microsystem or mesosystem (See Case Study 2: OneCF mesosystem).

Learning and Leadership Collaborative, the use of a diversified teaching team including an improvement measurement expert, an experienced improvement coach with measurement experience, and a registry and informatics analyst was particularly effective in balancing the competing needs for rigor and practicality in developing and facilitating the learning experience (Godfrey and Oliver, 2014).

Actions that promote Principle 4 include:

- Provide basic measurement skills and knowledge for frontline teams.
- Create experiential learning activities including simulation and application to frontline work that reinforce basic skills.
- Promote coaching and improvement collaboratives that can provide support, guidance, and structure.
- Focus on core skills, including using data displays, defining measures, creating a data collection plan, using run charts and basic SPC, and developing basic data dashboards.
- Build basic measurement education into the usual and customary work of improvement.

Principle 5: Cascade It – Link Levels of Data to Help Leaders Create Conditions for Success, Coaches to Support Leaders and Teams, and Frontline Teams to Engage in Improvement Work

A focus on clinical microsystems is critical to optimizing healthcare delivery performance, but the influence of microsystems can only be realized if the information environment enables a linkage between system levels using cascading measures from microsystem to macrosystem. Figure 8.9 shows how measures can cascade up from the microsystem to the macrosystem level, and conversely, how they can cascade down from the macrosystem to microsystem level. Cascading measures can help an organization link longitudinal organizational performance metrics to short-term, micro-, and mesosystem-level performance and improvement measures. Organizational performance metrics can create the ability to measure the impact of system performance on population health outcomes and the capability to conduct benchmarking for improvement (Griffith, Alexander, and Jelinek, 2002; Johnson and others, 2007).

Data registries can be utilized, as described in the CFF registry case study, to help leaders identify priorities for improvement, predict resource and system needs, and create conditions necessary to facilitate optimal frontline performance and improvement at the microsystem and mesosystem levels (Boyle and others, 2014). People working in different roles will focus on different aspects of the measurement cascade. Improvement coaches can use cascading measures to inform, develop, and bridge leaders and frontline teams to optimize collaboration, communication, improvement, and effectiveness. Frontline teams can use cascading measures to find meaning in macrosystem-level metrics, to connect them with their microsystem work environment, and to ultimately understand how the microsystem can influence organizational and population health outcomes in the long term.

Actions that promote Principle 5 include:

- Focus bidirectionally from microsystem upstream (cascade up) and from macrosystem downstream (cascade down) emphasizing the measurement connections between different system levels.
- Link short-term microsystem measures to longitudinal macrosystem measures.
- Utilize clinical informatics structures to facilitate measurement cascades across system levels.
- Involve leaders, coaches, and frontline teams in creating a "shared language" of cascading measures, allowing leaders to create conditions for success and frontline teams to engage in improvement and "manage up."

Conclusion

In the new age of accountable and value-based health care, the clinical microsystem remains the cornerstone of value generation for healthcare organizations and for population health. Effective information environments are critical for continuously improving microsystem performance and communicating effectively and efficiently across system levels; between patients and healthcare systems; and between patients and families, the healthcare delivery system, and research. In this chapter, four case examples described the development of intelligent information environments in a microsystem, a mesosystem, using registries, and using clinical informatics. Tips and principles from these case studies can guide the development of actionable information environments, which can inform and facilitate optimal health system performance. Actionable information environments can provide methods for conceptualizing effective and parsimonious measures aligned with, and informed by, organizational priorities and improvement efforts. Actionable information environments can design effective information flows that link people, systems, and processes, and leverage clinical informatics to facilitate data collection, data display, decision support, data registries, and shared decision-making.

Care must be taken to avoid potential pitfalls, such as a loss of parsimony and alignment of measurement with the work of health care (Meyer and others, 2012; Watcher, 2016); the potential for the burgeoning machine of informatics to disrupt rather than facilitate more efficient and effective care (Rosenbaum, 2015); and the potential for an overreliance on system productivity and population health metrics that do not incorporate the voice of patients and families or allow for inclusion of a coproduction perspective (Sabadosa and others, 2014; Batalden and others, 2016). Following guidance from this chapter, healthcare professionals and healthcare systems can intelligently design rich information environments that are efficient, effective, and actionable, which can facilitate (rather than disrupt) innovation, improvement, and research to optimize system performance and population health outcomes.

Mesosystem Considerations

The second case study (*OneCF Center*) is an example of a mesosystem application of the concepts described in this chapter. In a mesosystem setting, two or more microsystems are engaged in the care of a specified population in a specified context – in the case of the *OneCF Center* example, the mesosystem included a pediatric CF center and an adult CF center working together to maintain continuity of care for people with CF who were transitioning from pediatric to adult CF care. In a mesosystem situation, care must be taken to design and facilitate the measurement plan to treat the mesosystem as a whole rather than a sum of its constituent parts, and with a central focus on the journey of the patient through the mesosystem. The result is an approach that can inform monitoring and improvement efforts not only within each microsystem but also within the mesosystem as a whole. Concept-forward design approaches are strongly recommended in mesosystem situations. It is important to design the measurement approach beginning with mesosystem-specific needs and aims in mind, rather than trying to fit separate measurement approaches currently used in the participating microsystems. As was the case in the *OneCF Center* situation, many mesosystems are newly formed or do not yet have an accompanying informatics infrastructure allowing for immediate "high-tech" development. Starting simple and iteratively developing beginning with a "low-tech" prototype can help the mesosystem learn about itself while developing an optimal measurement approach and simultaneously informing the informatics build of the final dashboard version.

Summary

A key message of this chapter is the important role of the mesosystem in harmonizing measurement across microsystems and between the macro- and microsystems. It also highlights the importance of information and information technology in the day-to-day work of most health systems and the implications for measurement at micro- and mesosystem levels, as seen in the discussion of cascading measures. At the microsystem level, tick and tally and other methods to collect data by hand, while doing the work, are powerful and often underutilized resources that should not be overlooked. The mesosystem will often be more dependent on data from the EHR or other existing reporting mechanisms. As shown in the CF example, the conversations between microsystems within a mesosystem are vitally important to ensure that the data collected is meaningful and seen as important by all involved, including patients and families. Mesosystem support for transparency and sharing of data is also needed, and the material in this chapter on considerations for data display is worth studying. Finally, the concept of parsimony is especially relevant at the mesosystem level where sometimes it feels as though the data are overwhelming. Creating ownership of a small number of important data points will help guide the mesosystem through the sometimes-baffling landscape of multiple metrics.

Review Questions

1. What is a registry? Provide at least three examples of registries currently in use.
2. Differentiate the concepts of feedback/feed forward, feed in/feed out, and feed up/feed down as described in this chapter.
3. Provide an example of cascading measures.
4. Describe an example of Clinical Decision Support (CDS) and how it might improve safety and/or quality.
5. What are some differences between a "rich" information environment and an "actionable" information environment?

Discussion Questions

1. What are the mechanisms by which the SRQ might have achieved its outstanding results? What might you need to consider if you wanted to introduce this approach to another health condition?
2. A number of clinicians in the MaineHealth case distrusted the data they were shown. What are the factors that contributed to that distrust? How could a trustworthy data system be created?

Additional Activities

1. Pick a patient population (for example, people with diabetes or adolescents). Develop a clinical value compass for that population.

2. Pick a health system you know or have heard of. What measures do they report themselves? What can you learn from a website such as www.medicare.gov/hospitalcompare? What micro- and mesosystems might be involved in creating those results? How helpful are they for you as a patient or family member?

3. Look at some data displays on the Internet – from health systems, from other businesses, whatever you can find. Compare how you respond to them and how easy they are to interpret.

References

Batalden, M., Batalden, P. B., Margolis, P., and others. "Coproduction of Healthcare Service." *BMJ Quality & Safety*, 2016, 25(7), 509-517. doi: 10.1136/bmjqs-2015-004315

Batalden, P. B., and Davidoff, F. "What Is 'Quality Improvement' and How Can It Transform Healthcare?" *Quality & Safety in Health Care*, 2007, 16(1), 2-3. doi: 10.1136/qshc.2006.022046

Bennett, B., and Provost, L. "What's Your Theory? Driver Diagram Serves as a Tool for Building and Testing Theories for Improvement." *Quality Progress*, 2015, 36-43.

Benneyan, J. C., Lloyd, R. C., and Plsek, P. E. "Statistical Process Control as a Tool for Research and Healthcare Quality Improvement." *Quality & Safety in Health Care*, 2003, 12(6), 458–464. doi:10.1136/qhc.12.6.458

Berlinski, A., Chambers, M. J., Willis, L., and others. "Redesigning Care to Meet National Recommendation of Four or More Yearly Clinic Visits in Patients with Cystic Fibrosis." *BMJ Quality & Safety*, 2014, 23, i42-i49. doi: 10.1136/bmjqs-2013-002345

Boyle, M. P., Sabadosa, K. A., Quinton, H. B., and others. "Key Findings of the US Cystic Fibrosis Foundation's Clinical Practice Benchmarking Project." *BMJ Quality & Safety*, 2014, 23, i15-i22. doi: 10.1136/bmjqs-2013-002369

Deegan, P. E., and Drake, R. E. "Shared Decision Making and Medication Management in the Recovery Process." *Psychiatric Services*, 2006, 57(11), 1636-1639.

Forsberg, H. H., Nelson, E. C., Reid, R., and others. "Using Patient-Reported Outcomes in Routine Practice: Three Novel Use Cases and Implications." *Journal of Ambulatory Care Management*, 2015, 38(2), 188-195. doi: 10.1097/JAC.0000000000000052

Godfrey, M. M., and Oliver, B. J. "Accelerating Improvement in Cystic Fibrosis Care: The Learning and Leadership Collaborative Model." *BMJ Quality & Safety*, 2014, 23, 123-132. doi: 10.1136/bmjqs-2014-002804

Griffith, J. R., Alexander, J. A., and Jelinek, R. C. "Measuring Comparative Hospital Performance." *Journal of Healthcare Management*, 2002, 47(1), 41-57.

Hvitfeldt, H., Carli, C., Nelson, E. C., and others. "Feed Forward Systems for Patient Participation and Provider Support: Adoption Results from the Original US Context to Sweden And Beyond." *Quality Management in Health Care*, 2009, 18(4), 247-256.

Institute of Medicine (U.S.), Committee on Quality of Health Care in America. *Crossing the Quality Chasm: A New Health System for the 21st Century.* Washington, DC: National Academies Press, 2001. doi: 10.17226/10027

Johnson, J. K., Mahoney, C. C., Nelson, E. C., and others. "Learning From the Best: Clinical Benchmarking for Best Patient Care." In E. C. Nelson, P. B. Batalden, and J. S. Lazar (eds.), *Practice-Based Learning and Improvement: A Clinical Improvement Action Guide,* 2nd edition. Oakbrook Terrace, IL: Joint Commission Resources, 2007, 65-80.

Johnson, L. C., Melmed, G. Y., Nelson, E. C., and others. "Fostering Collaboration Through Creation of an IBD Learning Health System." *American Journal of Gastroenterology,* 2017, 112, 406-408. doi: 10.1038/ajg.2017.9

Kaplan, R. S., and Norton, D. P. "The Balanced Scorecard: Measures That Drive Performance." *Harvard Business Review,* 1992, 71-79.

Kaplan, R. S., and Norton, D. P. "Putting the Balanced Scorecard to Work." *Harvard Business Review,* 1993, 71(5), 134-147.

Kaplan, R. S., and Norton, D. P. *The Strategy Focused Organization: How Balanced Scorecard Companies Thrive in the New Business Environment.* Boston, MA: Harvard Business Review Press, 2000.

Kaplan, R. S., and Norton, D. P. *Strategy Maps: Converting Intangible Assets Into Tangible Outcomes.* Boston, MA: Harvard Business School Press, 2004.

Kulikowski, C. A., Shortliffe, E. H., Currie, L. M., and others. "AMIA Board White Paper: Definition of Biomedical Informatics and Specification of Core Competencies for Graduate Education in the Discipline." *JAMIA,* 2012, 19(6), 931-938. doi: 10.1136/amiajnl-2012-00105

Lee, E. O., and Emanuel, E. J. "Shared Decision Making to Improve Care and Reduce Costs." *New England Journal of Medicine,* 2013, 368, 6-8. doi: 10.1056/NEJMp1209500

Marshall, B. C., and Nelson, E. C. "Accelerating Implementation of Biomedical Research Advances: Critical Elements of a Successful 10 Year Cystic Fibrosis Foundation Healthcare Delivery Improvement Initiative." *BMJ Quality & Safety,* 2014, 23, i95-i103. doi: 10.1136/bmjqs-2013-002790

Meyer, G. S., Nelson, E. C., Pryor, D. B., and others. "More Quality Measures Versus Measuring What Matters: A Call for Balance and Parsimony." *BMJ Quality & Safety,* 2012, 21(11), 964-968. doi: 10.1136/bmjqs-2012-001081

Mogayzel, P. J., Dunitz, J., Marrow, L. C., and others. "Improving Chronic Care Delivery and Outcomes: The Impact of the Cystic Fibrosis Care Center Network." *BMJ Quality & Safety,* 2014, 23, i3-i8. doi: 10.1136/bmjqs-2013-002363

Nelson, E. C., Mohr, J. J., Batalden, P. B., and Plume, S. K. "Improving Health Care, Part 1: The Clinical Value Compass." *Joint Commission Journal on Quality Improvement,* 1996, 22(4), 243-258.

Nelson, E. C., Batalden, P. B., Huber, T. P., and others. "Microsystems in Health Care: Part 1. Learning from High-Performing Front-Line Clinical Units." *Joint Commission Journal on Quality Improvement,* 2002, 28(9), 472-493.

Nelson, E. C., Fisher, E. S., and Weinstein, J. N. (eds). "A Perspective on Patient-Centric, Feed-Forward. Collaboratories.'" In *Engineering a Learning Healthcare System: A Look at the Future,* Workshop Summary, IOM (Institute of Medicine). Washington, DC: The National Academies Press, 2011, *149-170.* Available online: http://nap.edu/12213.

Nelson, E. C., Lazar, J. S., Godfrey, M. M., and Batalden, P. B. "Partnering With Patients to Design and Improve Care." In E. C. Nelson, P. B. Batalden, M. M. Godfrey, and J. S. Lazar (eds.),

Value by Design: Developing Clinical Microsystems to Achieve Organizational Excellence. San Francisco, CA: Jossey-Bass, 2011, 77.

Nelson, E. C., Eftimovska, E., Lind, C., and others. "Patient Reported Outcome Measures in Practice." *BMJ*, 2015, 350, g7818. doi: 10.1136/bmj.g7818

Nelson, E. C., Dixon-Woods, M., Batalden, P. B., and others. "Patient-Focused Registries Can Improve Health, Care, and Science." *BMJ*, 2016, 354, i3319. doi: 10.1136/bmj.i3319

Oliveira, J. "The Balanced Scorecard: An Integrative Approach to Performance Evaluation." *Healthcare Financial Management*, 2001, 55(5), 42-46.

Perla, R. J., Provost, L. P., and Murray, S. K. "The Run Chart: A Simple Analytic Tool for Learning from Variation in Healthcare Processes." *BMJ Quality & Safety*, 2011, 20, 46-51. doi: 10.1136/bmjqs.2009.037895

Peterson, A., Gudbjörnsdottir, S., Löfgren, U. B., and others. "Collaboratively Improving Diabetes Care in Sweden Using a National Quality Register: Successes and Challenges – a Case Study." *Quality Management in Health Care*, 2015, 24(4), 212-221. doi: 10.1097/qmh.0000000000000068

Quinn, J. B. *Intelligent Enterprise: A Knowledge and Service Based Paradigm for Industry.* New York, NY: Free Press, 1992.

Rosenbaum, L. "Transitional Chaos or Enduring Harm? The EHR and the Disruption of Medicine." *New England Journal of Medicine*, 2015, 373(17), 1585-1588. doi: 10.1056/NEJMp1509961

Ruland, C. M. "Improving Patient Safety Through Informatics Tools for Shared Decision Making and Risk Communication." *International Journal of Medical Informatics*, 2004, 73, 551-557. doi: 10.1016/j.ijmedinf.2004.05.003

Sabadosa, K. A., and Batalden, P. B. "The Interdependent Roles of Patients, Families and Professionals in Cystic Fibrosis: A System for the Coproduction of Healthcare and Its Improvement." *BMJ Quality & Safety*, 2014, 23, i90-i94. doi: 10.1136/bmjqs-2013-002782

Savant, A. P., Britton, L. J., Petren, K., and others. "Sustained Improvement in Nutritional Outcomes at Two Paediatric Cystic Fibrosis Centres After Quality Improvement Collaboratives." *BMJ Quality & Safety*, 2014, 23, i81-i89. doi: 10.1136/bmjqs-2013-002314

Sirajuddin, A. M., Osheroff, J. A., Sittig D. F., and others. "Implementation Pearls from a New Guidebook on Improving Medication Use and Outcomes with Clinical Decision Support: Effective CDS Is Essential for Addressing Healthcare Performance Improvement Imperatives." *Journal of Healthcare Information Management*, 2009, 23(4), 38-45.

Stevens, D. P., and Marshall, B. C. (eds). "Ten Years of Improvement Innovation in Cystic Fibrosis Care." *BMJ Quality & Safety*, 2014, 23.

Van Citters, A. D., Gifford, A. H., Brady, C., and others. "Formative Evaluation of a Dashboard to Support Coproduction of Healthcare Services in Cystic Fibrosis." *Journal of Cystic Fibrosis*, 2020, 3(9), 14-26. doi: 10.1016j.jcf.2020.03.009

Watcher, R. M. "How Measurement Fails Doctors and Teachers." *The New York Times*, Jan. 16, 2016. Available online: http://nyti.ms/1NdiQIV.

Weinstein, J. N., Brown, P. W., Hanscom, B,, and others. "Designing an Ambulatory Clinical Practice for Outcomes Improvement: From Vision to Reality – the Spine Center at Dartmouth-Hitchcock, Year One." *Quality Management in Health Care*, 2000, 8(2), 1-20.

Zanni, R. L., Sembrano, E. U., Du, D. T., and others. "The Impact of Re-Education of Airway Clearance Techniques (REACT) on Adherence and Pulmonary Function in Patients with Cystic Fibrosis." *BMJ Quality & Safety*, 2014, 23, i50-i55. doi: 10.1136/bmjqs-2013-002352

Additional Resources

MaineHealth, https://mainehealth.org

Key Words/Terms

Balanced scorecard: A strategy performance management tool – a semi-standard structured report that can be used by managers to keep track of the execution of activities by the staff within their control and to monitor the consequences arising from these actions.

Benchmarking: A systematic process of searching to identify best practices.

Cascading measures: A method that allows for simultaneous and linked analysis and visualization of data at increasing levels of aggregation, including individual, system, and population levels.

Clinical decision support (CDS): Timely information, usually at the point of care, to help inform decisions about a patient's care. CDS tools and systems help clinical teams by taking over some routine tasks, warning of potential problems, or providing suggestions for the clinical team and patient to consider.

Data dashboard: A visual display that features the most important information needed to achieve specific goals captured on a single screen. Effective dashboards should be designed as monitoring tools that are understood at a glance. Dashboards are useful tools because they can leverage visual perception to communicate dense amounts of data clearly and concisely.

Decision support: A decision support system is an information system that supports decision-making activities.

Dummy display: A make-believe figure or table showing the results you might get. Helps you find relationships between data, discover what variables you will need to answer your questions, and decide how you will analyze data and display results (Nelson and others, 2011b, p. 77).

Feed forward/feedback: Describes the use of clinical and patient-reported data in learning health systems: (1) *feed-forward* refers to the use of data to predict needs of patients ahead of clinical visits or to inform clinical encounters at the point of care; (2) *feed-back* refers to the transmission of data to health systems describing the outcomes of care for use in monitoring and improving system performance, healthcare outcomes, and related research.

Feed in/feed out: Refers to data flow pathways used in learning health systems that use patient reported data to inform coproduction, comparative effectiveness research, and/or predictive analytics. Patient-generated clinical data can be *fed in* to health systems to inform care coproduction, including decision support, shared decision-making, self-monitoring, and patient facilitated networks. Data can also be *fed out* to registries that can be used to inform research about effectiveness and can be used to inform predictive analytics and precision healthcare approaches.

Feed up/feed down: Refers to the application of cascading measurement in multi-center learning health system or collaborative improvement contexts in which short-term measures are used at micro- and mesosystem levels to inform frontline improvement efforts and aggregated into or linked to longitudinal outcome measures used at the macrosystem or population level to inform collaborative improvement efforts and research.

Informatics: The science of processing data for storage and retrieval; information science.

Learning health system: Healthcare systems in which knowledge generation processes are embedded in daily practice to produce continual improvement in care.

Patient portals: A secure online website that gives patients convenient, 24-hour access to personal health information from anywhere with an Internet connection. By using a secure username and password, patients can view health information.

Patient-reported outcome (PRO): A health outcome directly reported by the patient who experienced it. It stands in contrast to an outcome reported by someone else, such as a physician-reported outcome, a nurse-reported outcome, and so on.

Performance dashboard: Provides consolidated, real-time displays of patient- and clinician-generated information, including well-being, needs, goals, and interventions. The impact of using dashboards to improve knowledge, health, and care delivery has been demonstrated: outcomes are optimized when patients, families, and clinicians have information they need at a point-of-care, over time, and in a supportive delivery system capable of making and sustaining improvements (VanCitters and others, 2020).

Registry: An organized data repository that houses data gathered for use in research and improvement for a specified population or clinical condition, such as the SRQ registry for adults with rheumatoid arthritis in Sweden.

Run chart: A time plot (line graph) of data plotted over time, which also includes a measure of central tendency (usually the median). By collecting and charting data over time, you can find trends or patterns in the process. Because they do not include control limits, run charts are not as sophisticated as SPC charts. However, run charts are very simple and easy to use, can be constructed manually, and can accurately detect common signals of non-random (special cause) variation, including shifts and trends.

Statistical process control (SPC): Refers to a body of measurement, analytical, and statistical approaches focusing on the study of performance variation. SPC is commonly used in quality control and quality improvement to monitor, analyze, improve, and control process performance.

CHAPTER NINE

INTERPROFESSIONAL EDUCATION AND THE CLINICAL MICROSYSTEM

Tina C. Foster, Paul N. Uhlig, Brant J. Oliver, Gay L. Landstrom, Julie K. Johnson, Marjorie M. Godfrey

AIM

The aim of this chapter is to explore the clinical microsystem's unique opportunities for interprofessional learning by both students and working professionals and to describe the use of microsystem thinking to design *educational microsystems*.

LEARNING OBJECTIVES

By the end of this chapter the reader will be able to:

1. Discover recent trends in health professional education.
2. Describe the importance of the clinical microsystem in contemporary *interprofessional education*.
3. Understand how microsystem thinking can be applied in educational design.
4. Become familiar with the concept of social fields and how they relate to work and learning in clinical microsystems.

Quality by Design: A Clinical Microsystems Approach, Second Edition. Edited by Marjorie M. Godfrey, Tina C. Foster, Julie K. Johnson, Eugene C. Nelson and Paul B. Batalden.
© 2025 John Wiley & Sons, Inc. Published 2025 by John Wiley & Sons, Inc.

Introduction

In this chapter, we explore education, professional formation, and the microsystem as a learning environment. We introduce and describe "educational microsystem" and "social field" concepts that can help microsystems become rich sites for both personal professional learning and collective organizational learning. At the foundation of both is recognition that learning in microsystems is a highly social activity with deep structural roots. Careful attention must be devoted to intentionally shaping the underlying organizing structures, learning routines, and social patterns that guide learning interactions.

Central to these concepts is a shift of emphasis from individual knowledge to collective knowledge as the focus of learning and improvement in microsystems. Additionally, acknowledging the importance of collective tacit knowledge, more than the individual explicit knowledge, is the primary source of reliability and resilience in microsystems. Shifting from learning that generates explicit knowledge in individual learners to learning that generates a blend of explicit and tacit knowledge in the care environment as a whole is the primary source of reliability and resilience in clinical microsystems. This shift of emphasis is necessarily accompanied by increased awareness of the care setting as a system, including its interdependencies and interactions.

Education in Clinical Microsystems

We begin with the premise that education in clinical microsystems includes not only formally designated learners, but also all of the professionals, patients, and families interacting within the microsystem; and that it involves all of the processes by which the accumulating knowledge and abilities carried within the microsystem are codeveloped and coproduced. We view the microsystem as a living entity – a constantly renewing ecosystem – whose functions and vitality are built and sustained by ongoing learning, improvement, and transformation.

When considering the role of the clinical microsystem in health professions education, two major trends are important – a focus on *competency-based education* and the recognition of the interprofessional nature of health care. The Institute of Medicine report (2003) on health professions education identified five core competencies for all health clinicians: provide patient-centered care, utilize informatics, employ evidence-based practice, apply quality improvement, and work in interprofessional teams. The Accreditation Council for Graduate Medical Education (2019) and the American Board of Medical Specialties (1999) endorsed six competencies for physicians in 1999. The Quality and Safety Education for Nursing (2020) competencies have also been widely accepted for use in education (http://qsen.org/competencies/pre-licensure-ksas/). With a move to competencies, the learning trajectory of novice to expert (Dreyfus and Dreyfus, 1980; Benner, 1982; Dreyfus, 2004) has been applied widely in health professional education. More recently and importantly for understanding education in the clinical microsystem, the idea of *team competencies* has come into focus (Mitchell and others, 2012; Nancarrow and others, 2013).

The 2011 Interprofessional Education Collaborative (IPEC) Expert Panel report describes four competency domains for interprofessional collaborative practice:

- Values/ethics
- Roles/responsibilities
- Interprofessional communication
- Teams and teamwork.

Interprofessionality has been defined by D'Amour and Oandasan (2005, p. 9) as "the process by which professionals reflect on and develop ways of practicing that provides an integrated and cohesive answer to the needs of the client/family/population." The "interdependence between health professional education and interprofessional practice" is captured in the IPEC report, which calls attention to the importance of the clinical microsystem as an essential learning site for health professional education. To maintain vitality, microsystems must tend to outcomes, system improvement, and professional development of those new to their discipline as well as seasoned professionals (Batalden and Foster, 2012). To develop and maintain engagement of patients and families, clinical microsystems must become sites of continuous sharing and learning where the unique needs and gifts of everyone present are exchanged and care is coproduced. Without attention to personal and professional education and growth, those working in the microsystem risk exhaustion and burnout (Bodenheimer and Sinsky, 2014), and the microsystem itself does not reach its full potential. Meaningful engagement in mutual education of self and others creates a sense of pride and joy in work and enables the microsystem to remain relevant and effective.

As we consider the microsystem as a learning environment, the connections to the future of health care become increasingly important. How can we prepare today's teachers to help students learn what will be needed in tomorrow's microsystems? How can we prepare today's students for their future work of creating and staffing those microsystems? This focus on the future means that we will need to continuously develop our understanding of the work of the microsystem and create new support structures especially as it relates to the collective (across staff, patients, and families) nature of that work. Equally important is the fact that in the microsystem the social nature of learning is brought into stark relief.

New Opportunities for Learners in Microsystems

Earlier chapters in this book have described the centrality of the clinical microsystem as the place where safety, value, and patient and family experiences are created. Microsystems are not only the setting for the clinical component of training for most health professionals, but also where much professional formation occurs.

The microsystem is the first place many health professions students have real clinical interactions with other members of the healthcare team and experience the complex dynamics of *team-based care*. It is often the first place where learners experience multiple nested systems of care and can appreciate the function (or dysfunction) that working within, between, and around microsystems can produce. The clinical microsystem may also be the first place that learners experience the emotional and physical challenges of real-world care and teamwork.

Those who teach using interprofessional simulation know the electricity that can be generated during simulations when medical, nursing, and other health professions students work together for the first time and begin to explore the fascinating experience of collaboration. Because they have nothing to unlearn, students quickly adapt to collaborative practice. Unfortunately, that same energy may not always be present in non-simulated, established clinical settings where established, professionally siloed patterns run deep and the benefits and accompanying joy of learning as a team may be harder to access and explore.

Traditionally, clinical education in medicine focuses on multiple individual patient-care experiences and the development of individual clinical skills and knowledge. Opportunities to connect those patient-care experiences to the structure, processes, and outcomes of the microsystem may provide a chance to develop a deeper appreciation for the work and habits of inquiry of different disciplines. In many traditional education models, individual patient experiences may be discussed, but the roles of patients and families in the microsystem often are not. All too often there is little formal time for collaborative reflection or opportunity to discuss the sometimes-harsh realities that learners and staff face. The discipline of learning about the 5Ps (purpose, patients, professionals, processes, and patterns) of the microsystem provides a tangible opportunity for learners and staff to work together to understand the nature of the microsystem. The transient nature of many learners who are likely to move between many microsystems offers multiple opportunities to consider similarities, differences, and experiences with change. Many medical and nursing students rotate at a variety of institutions. How often do we convene them to discuss what they noticed in the different places they worked? What made one place feel different from another? Who was on the teams they worked with? How were learners engaged? What were the apparent attitudes toward safety, collaboration, and diversity? The opportunity to discuss these differences can help learners create a mental model of where they would like to work in the future or what further training they would like to pursue. The discussions can also provide windows for faculty to learn about the actual experiences of trainees.

Tierra Byrd, a wise medical student, noted that "socialization negates education" (Byrd, 2017). This comment highlights the importance of the hidden curriculum. The hidden curriculum (Hafferty, 1998) has been described as "what is implicitly taught by example, day to day" (Mahood, 2011). Hidden learning occurs outside academic institutions and in the absence of people formally designated as "students." It occurs in the "real-life" setting where care is delivered: the clinical microsystem. Just as the hidden curriculum is omnipresent in the microsystem, so are the teaching and learning habits of health professionals. Hidden learning is happening all the time, often unrecognized, and it could happen even better if the myriad opportunities for connections between microsystems and the learning process in health care were made explicit and intentionally optimized.

Case Studies – New Models for Enhancing Interprofessional Education and Practice in Microsystems

Through three case studies we discuss the educational benefits offered by microsystems and describe how incorporating a learning orientation in microsystems translates into enhanced learning opportunities for all. The following case studies consider application of clinical microsystem theory to inform nursing education and the implications of a re-orientation of the work of the microsystem for the education of students and others who populate it.

We begin with a case study highlighting how microsystem principles can be applied to the educational process by creating "educational microsystems" in a nursing curriculum innovation program. We then offer a discussion of how shared knowledge arises and becomes useful in groups that learn together, developing this into a conceptual model for understanding care and education in microsystems called the Social Field Model of Collaborative Care. We then use this model to consider strategies and methods for implementing collaborative care and strengthening interprofessional education in clinical microsystems. A second case study illustrates how social, field-based interventions can be used to intentionally reconfigure microsystems to support interprofessional education and team learning. We end with a case study that explores the development of nurse leaders and the synergistic opportunities of combining practice and education in that clinical environment. Throughout, we emphasize the foundational importance of education in collaborative microsystems for co-creating health care of high value, and how microsystem approaches to education and practice can help generate exceptional care that is deeply responsive to the expertise, needs, and perspectives of practitioners, patients, and families alike.

Case Study One: Using "Educational Microsystems" to Develop a "Clinician-Leader-Improver" Curriculum

The *IOM Nurse of the Future* report (IOM, 2010) envisions nurses as "clinician-leader-improvers" who are able to diagnose and improve systems of care delivery just as readily as they are able to assess and care for patients. Nursing education faces a number of key challenges in meeting this call (Table 9.1).

Headrick and colleagues (2012) discuss key challenges in early efforts to integrate improvement science into medical and nursing education programs. These challenges include lack of faculty appropriately trained in improvement science, structural and financial constraints, a culture focused on traditional clinical and research education models, and the early developmental stage of healthcare improvement science as an academic discipline. Many nursing faculties presented with the daunting task of integrating new content into standard curriculum already filled to bursting bristle at being asked to add "one more thing."

Nursing has made substantive progress in developing structure, competencies, and resources but most is in the form of national organizations, specialized master's degree programs and advanced fellowships such as Quality and Safety Education for Nurses (QSEN), Institute for Healthcare Improvement Open School, *Clinical Nurse Leader* (CNL), and Veterans Administration Quality Scholar (VAQS).

All of these resources have moved the field forward but represent small pockets of opportunity or large compendiums of resources that are not optimally utilized or are only superficially applied. Unfortunately, they are not accessible to a majority of nursing faculty and students and are not scalable to create the "critical mass" of trained professionals in improvement science who are needed to "mainstream" quality and safety into health professions education (Headrick and others, 2012). What is needed now is a way to bring these resources to bear in a meaningful and

TABLE 9.1 KEY CONSTRAINTS CREATING BARRIERS TO QUALITY AND SAFETY INTEGRATION.

Key Constraints

- Cost
- Credit burden
- Packed student schedules
- Lack of faculty with expertise in quality and safety
- Competing demands
- Lack of experiential learning opportunities

non-superficial way by actively embedding them within the everyday life, work, and culture of health professions education and practice. This case study describes an innovative approach taken by a school of nursing to get past the barriers and move culture and practice towards full integration of quality and safety.

Context for This Work

The MGH Institute of Health Professions (MGH Institute) is a non-profit, interprofessional, health professions education institution that is part of a large academic healthcare system and offers undergraduate, graduate, and doctoral degree programs in nursing, physical therapy, occupational therapy, speech language pathology, and physician assistant studies. The School of Nursing at the MGH Institute offers generalist (Registered Nurse), graduate (Nurse Practitioner), and doctoral (Doctor of Nursing Practice) nursing programs. Nursing students participate in the interprofessional IMPACT, a one-year overarching approach program to incorporate the principles of interprofessional learning, setting the stage for interprofessional collaborative practice for entry-level students from across all MGH Institute programs.

Like many health professions programs, the MGH Institute School of Nursing (SON) faced many of the key constraints previously discussed, including lack of trained faculty and lack of capacity to expand credit hours without substantively impacting cost. However, there was significant positive tension for change driven by an upcoming re-accreditation process, visionary leadership at the SON that prioritized quality and safety and created conditions for effective change, and the growing need for health professionals who are ready to function as "clinician-leader-improvers" when they enter the workforce. These conditions created an environment that demanded creative, cost-effective, innovative approaches to move quality and safety into the usual and customary work of nursing education and role socialization across the School of Nursing programs.

The Concept of "Educational Microsystems"

The MGH Institute School of Nursing based its approach on a belief that health professions education could adapt perspective and methods from clinical microsystems theory and related methods to create an educational microsystems approach to health professional education. An educational microsystem (EM) can be defined as a group of people who work together in a specified educational setting on a regular basis to provide educational services to members of a discrete subpopulation of students, faculty, and/or administrators. It has educational, administrative, and business aims; linked processes; a shared information environment; and produces services that can be measured as process and outcomes performance.

It was assumed that this new "EM perspective" would not only empower nursing faculty to effectively integrate quality and safety into courses and programs, but would also view health professions education as a process and system that can be continuously improved by the students, faculty, and/or administrators in the educational microsystem. The EM perspective approach utilized the foundational work on critical success characteristics of clinical microsystems (Nelson and others, 2002) to structure a four-part strategy aimed at directing the SON faculty to create and own a new culture of educational improvement. The approach included four main steps:

1. Developing a strong frontline focus capable of building capacity and driving rapid innovation.
2. Engaging the SON faculty in applied experiential learning within EMs.
3. Formalizing and coproducing EM-based improvement.
4. Linking the work to scholarship.

Using Modified Improvement Coaching to Build Capacity and Drive Rapid Curriculum Innovation

The first step was to build faculty capacity while generating successive, consistent progress in quality and safety curriculum integration and innovation over time. A modification of the team coaching approach (Godfrey and others, 2014b), which is often used to build capacity and accelerate improvement in health care (Godfrey and Oliver, 2014a) was utilized to create a situation in which early faculty adopters with interest in quality and safety innovation could be coached by faculty "coach-consultants" with training and expertise in improvement methods. Together they would design, integrate, and evaluate new quality and safety learning activities.

Conceptualizing each course as an educational microsystem helped the faculty to better recognize the structures, processes, and patterns inherent in the courses they were redesigning. Through that knowledge, they were able to creatively redesign and navigate around barriers that had previously thwarted their efforts. Working within this structure, the "coach-consultant" helped course faculty assess their EM courses and build knowledge and skills "as they needed it." There were two key facilitators discovered across EMs during this work: (1) quality and safety learning experiences could be integrated with standard clinical didactic and applied education without substantively changing course objectives or creating more work for faculty or students; and (2) attempting multiple "small curriculum integration tests" instead of large-scale curriculum redesign and implementation efforts could allow for iterative, consistent, and cost-effective curriculum integration over time (similar to the way that plan–do–study–act cycles are utilized in healthcare improvement). A continuous improvement approach was utilized to iteratively evaluate and improve learning

FIGURE 9.1 PERCEIVED KNOWLEDGE OUTCOMES AND STUDENT EXPERIENCE OUTCOMES FROM A SCHOOL OF NURSING COURSE IN WHICH STUDENTS USED THE MICROSYSTEMS ASSESSMENT TOOL (MAT).

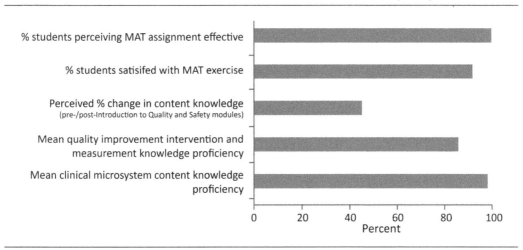

experiences over time utilizing an outcomes measurement system that was integrated with the student online learning environment. This enabled real-time assessment of performance and outcomes during curriculum integration work. An example of an embedded data display is given in Figures 9.1 and 9.2.

Over a two-year period participating in the EM approach, 10 faculty members teaching six courses spanning all three program levels integrated quality and safety into their courses one semester at a time (Oliver and others, 2017). Together, the faculty members created a curriculum thread spanning a developmental trajectory aligning with the *AACN Essentials* for nursing education and subsequently linking to post-graduate residency education (academic-clinical partnerships) and advanced fellowships (Figure 9.3).

Engaging Experiential Learning and Culture Change: The QI Task Force Initiative

The second step aimed to engage a majority of the nursing faculty in experiential learning. Essential in this effort were context-specific factors of leadership prioritization and support of the work, which created the conditions for conducting the work, and the identification of five areas for improvement through benchmarking against comparator schools of nursing using a benchmarking process similar to that utilized in health care (National Higher Education Benchmarking Institute, 2019).

FIGURE 9.2 KNOWLEDGE OUTCOMES FROM A SCHOOL OF NURSING COURSE EMBEDDED WITHIN AN ONLINE LEARNING ENVIRONMENT.

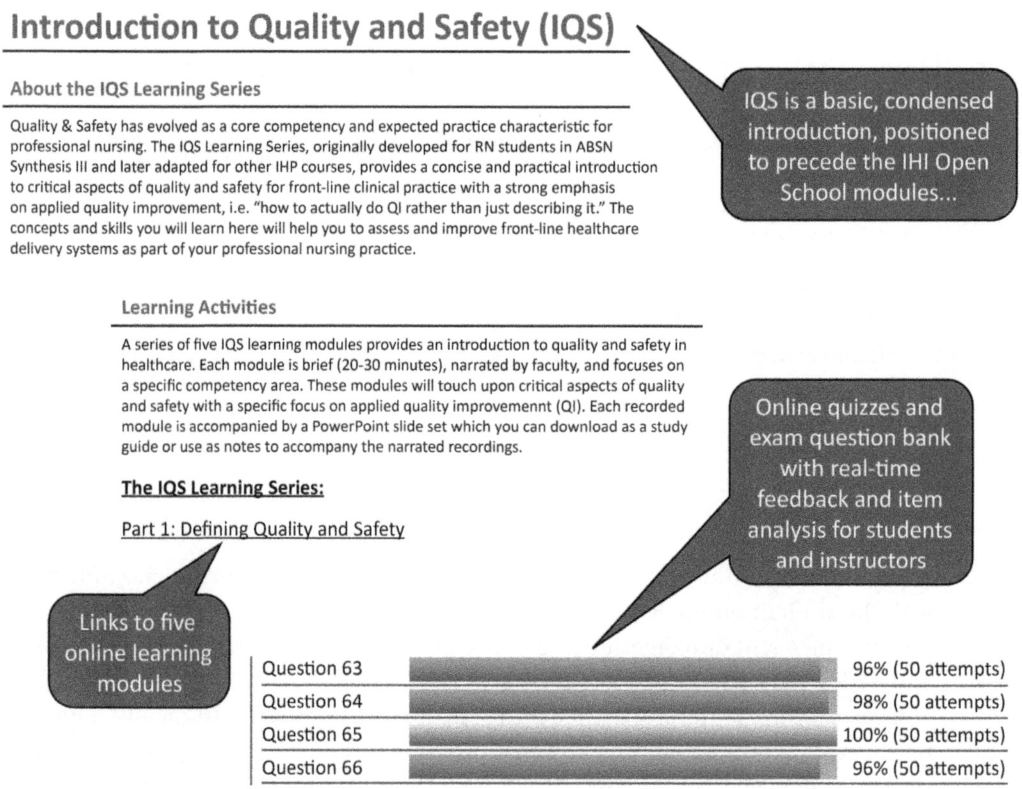

Introduction to Quality and Safety (IQS)

About the IQS Learning Series

Quality & Safety has evolved as a core competency and expected practice characteristic for professional nursing. The IQS Learning Series, originally developed for RN students in ABSN Synthesis III and later adapted for other IHP courses, provides a concise and practical introduction to critical aspects of quality and safety for front-line clinical practice with a strong emphasis on applied quality improvement, i.e. "how to actually do QI rather than just describing it." The concepts and skills you will learn here will help you to assess and improve front-line healthcare delivery systems as part of your professional nursing practice.

IQS is a basic, condensed introduction, positioned to precede the IHI Open School modules...

Learning Activities

A series of five IQS learning modules provides an introduction to quality and safety in healthcare. Each module is brief (20-30 minutes), narrated by faculty, and focuses on a specific competency area. These modules will touch upon critical aspects of quality and safety with a specific focus on applied quality improvemennt (QI). Each recorded module is accompanied by a PowerPoint slide set which you can download as a study guide or use as notes to accompany the narrated recordings.

Online quizzes and exam question bank with real-time feedback and item analysis for students and instructors

The IQS Learning Series:

Part 1: Defining Quality and Safety

Links to five online learning modules

Question 63		96% (50 attempts)
Question 64		98% (50 attempts)
Question 65		100% (50 attempts)
Question 66		96% (50 attempts)

Source: Adapted from Oliver, B. J., and colleagues at the MGH Institute of Health Professions School of Nursing. Used with permission.

EM improvement teams consisting of eight faculty members and one coach-consultant were created, and each team was tasked with improving performance in one improvement area. In sum, these teams represented approximately 75 percent of the total full-time SON faculty. The teams were organized into an EM improvement collaborative designed to share experiences, compare results, and accelerate improvement in a way similar to that employed in successful healthcare improvement collaboratives, such as the Cystic Fibrosis Foundation Learning and Leadership Collaborative (Godfrey and others, 2014b). Teams completed a series of improvement skills training sessions focused on basic clinical microsystems theory (adapted to EMs), rapid cycle improvement Institute for Healthcare Improvement – IHI improvement model (Langley and others, 2009), and basic improvement measurement methods. Coach-

FIGURE 9.3 SCHOOL OF NURSING CURRICULUM THREAD FOR QUALITY AND SAFETY INTEGRATION ACROSS PROGRAMS.

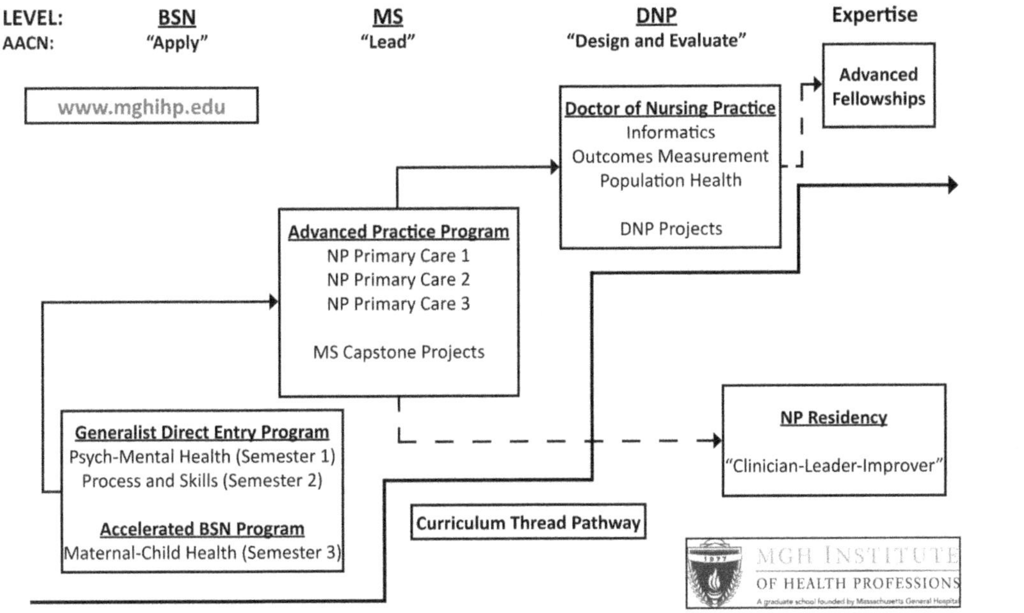

consultants guided and developed improvement teams that worked over a one-year period and completed multiple PDSA cycles (Table 9.2).

Like many engaged in early-stage improvement work, the teams struggled with assessment, proper execution of PDSA cycles, and measurement; and teams varied in productivity during the work period. Improvement teams were invited to report on their progress during SON faculty meetings; progress and results were shared in a web-based environment that could be accessed by all teams for shared learning. This resulted in an experiential learning experience similar to a healthcare improvement collaborative (Godfrey and others, 2014b) but in an educational setting and created an experiential learning exposure for a majority of the School of Nursing faculty over a one-year period.

Formalizing, Deepening, and Coproducing: The QI Action Committee Improvement Journey to Improve First-Time Board Examination Pass Rates

The second step in the MGH Institute plan created significant awareness and engagement by the SON faculty and empowered them to utilize basic improvement

TABLE 9.2 SUMMARY OF SCHOOL OF NURSING QUALITY IMPROVEMENT TASK FORCES AND PDSA CYCLES.

	PDSA 1	PDSA 2	PDSA 3	PDSA 4	PDSA 5	PDSA 6
Organization	Unified online calendar	Syllabus posted one week prior to start of semester	Coordinate exam and assignment dates across courses	Revised coordinated exam and assignment schedule linked to online calendar system		
Technology	Needs assessment (no intervention)	Implemented monthly faculty "Quick Tech Tips."	IT Focus group session (no intervention)	Increased integration of instructional designers	Second IT focus group (no intervention)	Revised "Tech Tips" resource on faculty website
Advising	Assessment survey (no intervention)	"Online tools guide" for online advisor resources implemented	Online calendar tool developed to remind advising faculty of key dates	Explore use of validated advising quality questionnaire	Explore changes to existing advising guide to better assist advisors	
Responsiveness	Increase use of faculty "away messaging" during vacations and time off	Student expectations and needs survey (no intervention)	Communication expectations tool developed for faculty to use with students			
Inclusiveness	Inclusiveness awareness survey and pilot continuing education session	ABSN program faculty training session (clinical instructors)				

Source: Adapted from Oliver, B. J., and colleagues at the MGH Institute of Health Professions School of Nursing. Used with permission.

methods adapted from health care to improve educational service quality. It started a shift in the general culture toward the active recognition and inclusion of quality and safety throughout the School of Nursing. However, more work was needed to further develop and formalize the presence of improvement within the School of Nursing and to continue a developmental trajectory.

In the third step, again with the benefit of committed leadership support, a formal improvement committee (the QI Action Committee) was formed and tasked with the further development of a core group of "faculty improvers" organized into an EM improvement team capable of tackling priority improvement need areas identified by the School of Nursing. Topics included faculty responsiveness to student concerns, academic advising, technology, inclusiveness, and organization of administrative processes. The QI Action Committee was comprised of faculty and students from each of the School of Nursing programs and a faculty coach-consultant. The committee utilized a shared online information environment for the organization of data, measures, and ongoing learning and development activities. Notable in this stage of development in the EM journey is the addition of students to the improvement team, an element with a clear parallel to the addition of patients to highly successful healthcare improvement teams, which has been documented (Nelson and others, 2002; Godfrey and others, 2014b; Sabadosa and Batalden, 2014).

The QI Action Committee was tasked to improve RN licensure examination pass rates for first-time takers after a change in testing format at the national level had adversely impacted test performance across many regional schools of nursing. The committee collaborated with faculty and students from two key courses in the undergraduate nursing program, treating each as a separate EM, and worked to improve educational service delivery quality in each. Process performance (learning activities) and longitudinal outcomes (licensure exam first-time pass rates) were measured and used to guide improvement work (Figures 9.4 and 9.5). Over a one-year period, process performance and pass rates improved significantly (Oliver and others, 2018).

The Academy for Improvement Science

The final step in the School of Nursing EM journey was the creation of a sustainable environment to study the improvement journey and generate scholarship related to this new application of EM improvement to educational microsystems performance. Faculty from all three previous stages, again assisted by coach-consultant faculty, were gathered into a writing, scholarship, and continuing education collaborative (the Academy for Improvement Science) and engaged in telling the story of their three-year improvement journey. This practice has been utilized by successful improvement collaboratives (Nelson and others, 2002) and improvement residency and

FIGURE 9.4 SHORT-TERM PROCESS AND OUTCOMES PERFORMANCE RESULTS.

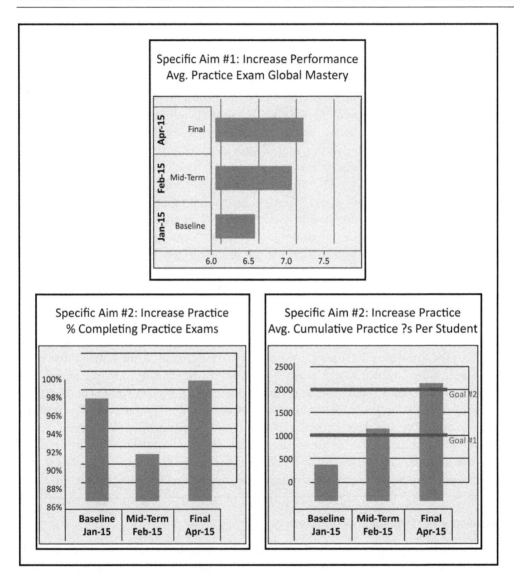

fellowship programs to develop improvement scholarship skills and to further develop and disseminate the science of improvement. The School of Nursing Academy of Improvement Science utilizes a shared online information environment and monthly meeting structure to create a supportive collegial scholarship

FIGURE 9.5 STATISTICAL PROCESS CONTROL (SPC) CHART OF PASS RATE PERFORMANCE OUTCOMES (P CHART).

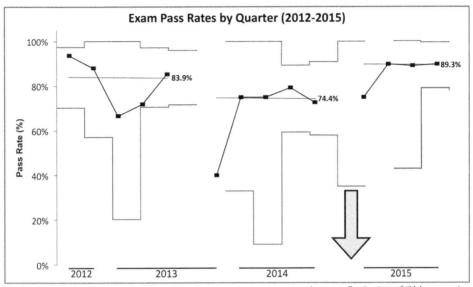

Arrow = Beginning of QI Intervention

Source: Adapted from Oliver, B. J., and others, 2018. Used with permission.

environment, develop faculty improvement scholars, and disseminate results using the *SQUIRE* framework (Standards for QUality Improvement Reporting Excellence) for improvement scholarship (Ogrinc and others, 2015).

Discussion

The MGH Institute School of Nursing Education microsystems journey is an example of how education can utilize improvement frameworks and methods that have been successful in health care, such as the clinical microsystems framework, and adapt them for application in educational contexts similar to the way healthcare improvement frameworks and methods were initially derived from business, industry, and military contexts. The derivation of the educational microsystems concept and the use of PDSA cycles, modified improvement coaching, and improvement collaborative structure and organization of improvement work according to factors known to optimize microsystem performance (such as a focus on students, using a shared information environment, and an emphasis on staff and the front line) were all helpful in moving the SON culture forward into a new "improvement culture" that included everyone in the work and where quality and safety is a part of the usual and everyday work of nursing education. A successive, consistent, incremental change approach (mirroring PDSA cycles), improvement coaching, the support of leadership, the involvement of students in the work, and connection of the work to scholarship were strong contributors to generating and sustaining improvement and culture change. The experiential learning fashion of the journey also created opportunities to develop and embed knowledge and skills over time and to develop increased faculty capacity that will reach the critical mass needed to enable sustainable improvement education in the health professions settings (Headrick and others, 2012). The involvement of students in educational improvement work, which parallels the involvement of patients and families in healthcare improvement work, accelerates and informs improvement work, and aligns with the modern concept of coproduction (Batalden and others, 2016). Coproduction of care that includes patients and families can be adapted to health professions education and include faculty, students, and administration. Finally, the MGH Institute SON educational microsystem experience suggests a way past the constraints that have historically hampered progress in educational services innovation and improvement. Adapted clinical microsystems framework and use of basic improvement methods applied to educational services can help produce better outcomes for faculty and students one educational microsystem at a time.

Case Study Two: The Social Field Model of Collaborative Care

Despite efforts to transform educational structures, habits, and roles within the microsystem, true collaborative care is still an aspiration in many health systems. Reaching this goal in both outpatient and inpatient settings may require a deeper look at the underlying assumptions and structures at work in our current care system and accompanying redesign efforts.

The *Social Field Model of Collaborative Care* was developed by Paul N. Uhlig and Ellen Raboin with colleagues Jeff Brown, Cindy Dominguez, Olga Gurevich, and Lorri Zipperer as a way of synthesizing more than 15 years of research implementing collaborative care and studying exceptional healthcare teamwork in diverse clinical settings (Dominguez and others, 2005; Gurevich, 2005). Rather than focusing on individual teamwork behaviors, the approach underpinning this model focuses on the collective abilities of care teams situated in their environments, and how those abilities are socially constructed (or not) through ongoing shared interactions and team learning over time. The Social Field Model is about learning at a collective level, with special emphasis on the preconditions that make collective team learning likely, and on the emergence of certain team-level resources that characterize highly reliable and resilient care.

Relationship to Microsystem Theory

The Social Field Model is closely related to microsystem theory but places more emphasis on structural and relational aspects of frontline microsystems, with special attention on the local development of collective tacit knowledge through ongoing team learning. A generalized understanding of system monitoring and improvement is emphasized through curiosity, outcomes awareness, shared reflection, collective learning, and ongoing system refinement, with exact methods for doing this left open for development and use by each individual team in its own way.

The Social Field Model emphasizes the importance of social structures and relationships, intentionally optimizing structural and social preconditions in the care environment with the intent of setting the stage for the emergence of collaborative interactions and enabling local team learning.

What Is a Social Field?

A social field is the *living collective intelligence* of a care team in its local environment. It is built through shared learning as a team accumulates experiences, memories, and connections that arise and grow among members of the team who are able to work together regularly, reflect together about their interactions, and learn together in ongoing cycles of action and reflection.

The experiences and connections that develop in a care environment become familiar to the people who create them. The collective capabilities of the team develop and become available to the team in its daily interactions, making the work of the team easier and giving it special meaning. A team with a well-developed social field can draw upon these connections and shared abilities in its work together. The following section from the *Field Guide to Collaborative Care – Implementing the Future of Health Care* describes the growth of a social field. "At first, as people are just starting to work together and getting to know one another, their social field is not very well developed. As people are able to work together consistently and come to know one another better, a reservoir of shared history develops, and it becomes easier to work together. People learn what to expect by doing things together and carry with them what they have learned. Their social field is developing" (Uhlig and Raboin, 2015, p. 227).

Figure 9.6 illustrates the growth of a social field from early "transactional" interactions to a richly developed social field.

The people represented on the right side of the figure have worked together before, know one another, and have an accumulated history of shared experiences, collective knowledge, and mutual insights from their previous interactions together. This accumulated knowledge of what to expect and do is represented by the multicolored space that surrounds them – their social field.

FIGURE 9.6 BEFORE AND AFTER THE DEVELOPMENT OF A SOCIAL FIELD.

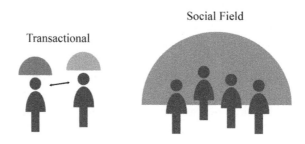

Source: Uhlig and Raboin, 2015, p. 228. Used with permission.

In contrast, the people represented on the left side of the figure do not have a well-developed social field. They have individual professional role knowledge and expertise represented by the colored space over each person. However, individual expertise is all they are able to contribute. They do not have prior shared experiences in their work together that they can draw from. Their interactions must be coordinated in transactional ways because team members haven't developed shared collective knowledge.

Our research suggests that many dimensions of the "goodness" of exceptional care teams – including reliability and resilience as well as human dimensions of compassion and caring – depend a lot on the development of rich social fields. The social field of a care team is made up of experiences and patterns of interaction that the team can draw upon based on their shared history together – resources for connecting, coordinating, learning, making decisions, managing differences – and many other things they need to do as a team that they have "made" together in prior interactions. A care team in a well-developed social field can do much of this without words, often without conscious thought.

Learning is Central to the Development of Social Fields

Social fields are built from collective learning that occurs for all in the care environment, including patients, family members, care team members, and anyone who is in the social field long enough to impact and be impacted by it. The social field of a care environment is continually enriched and changed by new experiences, questions, ideas, and insights sparked by patients, families, students, and new care team members as they flow through the care environment and participate in shaping its social field and the resources it carries.

One of the most important insights about social fields is they are constantly in active formation, renewal, and reformation. Social fields are constantly being formed and reformed through the actions of the people who build and inhabit them. As such, they can be intentionally modified and reshaped by changing the conditions under which the people who co-create them interact and learn together.

What Preconditions Give Rise to Rich Social Fields?

The foundational preconditions for rich social fields set the stage for people to be able to work consistently together, feel safe and supported, actively engage patients and families, reflect and learn together, improve care, and collectively remember and apply what they have learned.

These preconditions are under the control of people in the care environment and can be purposefully modified and intentionally implemented. This is not always easy to do but can be done.

Preconditions

1. Organization for consistency and continuity (based on "natural work clusters" of roles/resources).
2. Leadership that models and encourages respect, dignity, inclusion, and collaboration.
3. Regular opportunities for team-level reflection (weekly system meetings).
4. Familiar processes for daily interprofessional collaborative care (daily collaborative rounds).
5. Active engagement of patients and families (always "nothing about me without me").
6. Ways of monitoring and staying intentionally aware of care outcomes.
7. Ways of monitoring and improving systems and processes of care.
8. Thoughtfully maintained alignment and connections at micro-, meso-, and macrosystem levels.

What Resources Develop in Rich Social Fields?

The development of collective tacit knowledge in rich social fields creates resources that the care team can utilize in its work together, enabling reliability and resilience. These team-level resources include:

1. Knowledge of what to do and expect.
2. Ability to invite and welcome.
3. Web of monitoring.
4. Alertness, responsiveness, and patience.
5. Ability to actively engage patients and families.
6. Commitment to learning and change.

7. Emergence of new ideas.

8. Aliveness of the human spirit.

A more complete description of the preconditions and resources is available on the Collaborative Care Alliance website at https://www.createbettercare.org/.

New Approaches to Care Transformation

The Social Field Model points to new ways of conceptualizing care transformation that emphasize culture, relationships, meaning, and social construction of local resources. This approach stands in contrast to the more typical belief that best practices can be brought from one environment to another with predictable results. The theoretical approaches underpinning the Social Field Model are less deterministic, and more co-creative and local. The Social Field Model looks upstream for sites of action, to preconditions that set the stage for socially constructed local transformation, rather than to teamwork training, individual behaviors, and generalizable best practices. These differences are summarized in Figure 9.7.

FIGURE 9.7 DIFFERENCES BETWEEN TRADITIONAL AND SOCIAL FIELD APPROACH TO CARE TRANSFORMATION.

Individual ⟶		**Social Field**	
Traditional approach:		Alternative approach:	
Study:	attributes of teamwork	Study:	how culture works
Identify:	best practices and teamwork behaviors	Identify:	optimum preconditions and underlying social processes
"Roll out:"	policies and procedures teamwork training hold accountable	Implement:	structural changes in context opportunities for new dialog invitations to participate
Expect:	improved results (because of new techniques)	Expect:	improved results (through cultural transformation)
Nature:	mechanistic/cause-effect	Nature;	organic/evolutionary
Requires:	adherence	Requires:	voluntary engagement
Valued most:	generalizable knowledge	Valued most:	local meaning

Source: Uhlig and Raboin. Used with Permission.

FIGURE 9.8 GROWTH OF RELIABILITY AND RESILIENCE IN CARE TEAMS.

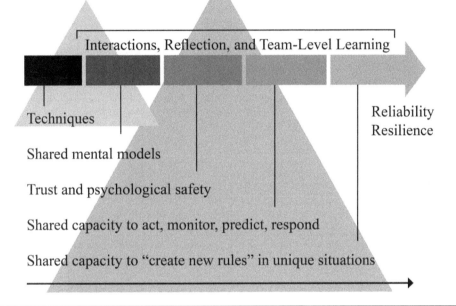

Source: Uhlig and Raboin, 2015, p. 186. Used with permission.

Figure 9.8 illustrates the growth of reliability and resilience in care teams from the perspective of the Social Field Model. The initial steps can be taken with team training at an individual level. However, the Social Field Model assumes that reliability and resilience depend on higher-level collective abilities that arise and develop in the social field through team interactions, reflection, and team-level learning.

There are observable differences between traditional and collaborative care. These differences are summarized in Figure 9.9 (Uhlig and others, 2018).

There are also differences in the perceptions about experiences of care between traditional and collaborative care. Some of these differences in reported emotions are summarized in Table 9.3.

The Social Field Model approach has been used to implement and study collaborative care in diverse settings across different kinds of inpatient and outpatient care. In several of these settings, careful assessments of care outcomes have been made. The initial implementation was at Concord Hospital in Concord,

FIGURE 9.9 OBSERVABLE DIFFERENCES BETWEEN TRADITIONAL AND COLLABORATIVE CARE.

Traditional Care	Collaborative Care
Physicians direct	Physicians participate
Disciplines report	Professions confer
Patient and family informed	Patient and family actively engaged
Patient progress updated	Care progress mutually assessed
Orders given through hierarchy	Care plan jointly developed in real time
Come "knowing everything"	Come "prepared but incomplete"
Patients talked "about"	Patients talked "with"
Begins with synopsis, physiologic update	Begins with introductions, goals, questions, concerns
Focus on disease/treatment/problems	Focus on people/needs/goals/suggestions
Third person ("he" "she" "they")	First person ("you" "we" "I")
Medical language/acronyms	Ordinary language or immediate translation
Bullet points	Conversational
Frequent side/silo conversations	Inclusive conversation together
"Who will do what" unspoken/assumed	"Who will do what" clarified/agreed upon
Uniprofessional teaching and learning	Collaborative teaching and learning
Patients and families as recipients of knowledge	Patients and families as co-teachers and co-learners
Care and education "delivered/provided"	Care and education "co-created" – generative

Source: Uhlig, P. N., and others, *Academic Medicine,* 2018, p. 1442. Used with permission.

New Hampshire. Notable improvements in mortality, complications, patient satisfaction, and provider satisfaction occurred during the implementation. This work was recognized with the Eisenberg Patient Safety Award in System Innovation by the Joint Commission and National Quality Forum.

A second implementation was accomplished over three years in a cardiac surgery program at Wesley Medical Center in Wichita, Kansas. Notable improvements were seen in care outcomes as reflected in markedly improved reliability of care and marked improvement in Society of Thoracic Surgeons Database composite quality scores. Examples of these shifts in outcomes are illustrated in Figure 9.10 (Uhlig and others, 2002; 2010).

Everyone Teaches, Everyone Learns – But There Are Surprises!

In the well-developed social field of a highly evolved collaborative care environment, teaching and learning are natural and every encounter is filled with reciprocal learning. Patient and family members participate, contribute, and learn; students from multiple health professions participate, contribute, and learn; established

TABLE 9.3 SUMMARY OF PATIENT AND TEAM SELF-PERCEPTION.

Emotions Reported			
Collaborative approach		Heirarchical approach	
Patients	Treatment team	Patients	Treatment team
Safe to ask questions	Safe to express opinions	Scared, unsafe at times	Insecure, at risk
Appreciative	More compassionate	Angry	Angry
Confident	Confident	Confused	Confused at times
Empowered	Empowered	Disempowered	Disempowered
Pleasurable	Pleasurable	Frustrated	Frustrated
Energized	Energized		Exhausted
Comforted	Calm	Stressed	Stressed, agitated
Supported	Supported by team members	Helpless at times	Helpless at times, lacking support from team
Satisfied	Satisfied	Less satisfied	Unsatisfied
Hopeful		Less hopeful	
Responsible	Responsible	Not responsible	Not responsible
Engaged	Engaged	Disconnected, uninvolved	Isolated
Valued, respected	Appreciated		Unappreciated
	Interested, eager to learn	Unable to comprehend	Meaningless at times
In control	In control	Not in control	Not in control
	Growing		Regressing, stuck

Source: Data from Gurevich. Used with permission.

practitioners participate, contribute, and learn; and the care environment is being reshaped with every new interaction and insight.

However, this state is not easily reached at first, because there is so much to unlearn. Patterns that are deeply ingrained in traditional health professions education, for example, the time-honored ritual of "presenting the patient," which is expected of every medical student and resident, must be unlearned.

Imagine a room full of health professionals including nurses, therapists, pharmacists, care coordinators, and others, as well as the patient and family, who are actively engaged in a warm, human conversation of what matters to everyone as people. The patient is telling about her new grandchild, family members are nodding in agreement, the professional members of the care team are taking delight in understanding the importance of this special child within this family circle, there is frequent laughter and warm smiles all around – and now imagine, at this moment, we ask the

FIGURE 9.10 EXAMPLES OF CARE OUTCOME IMPROVEMENTS – SOCIAL FIELD MODEL OF COLLABORATIVE CARE.

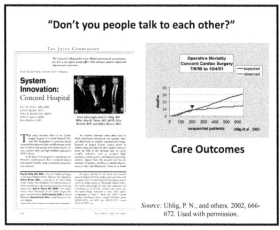

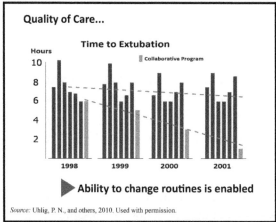

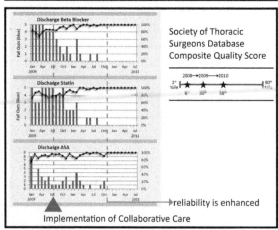

medical student to "present the patient" in a traditional way in this very human, warmth-filled, collaborative care context.

She begins, "Mrs. Garcia is a 67-year-old Latino female who presented with. . ." The student continues, "She denies constipation, hematochezia, melena. . ." "CT scan of the abdomen reveals a six-centimeter mass in the head of the pancreas with dilated. . ." It doesn't fit, and it doesn't work. The nurses become restless, the RT is sighing, the pharmacist is looking at her iPad, the care coordinator is taking a call, the parents are tending to their children, and the patient is lost in another world.

In the simulation lab, with the patient and family acting their roles and a care team composed only of students, things can be very different. The interprofessional students are unburdened by deeply held patterns of how rounds need to happen and how learning encounters should be structured. There are some simple ground rules: sit down, have everyone introduce themselves including the patient and family members, direct all conversation to the patient, and actively engage the patient and family. Use ordinary language or immediately translate medical concepts, find ways so that everyone can bring each other up to speed on what is happening, and invite everyone into jointly planning next steps. Run the simulation for a few minutes, stop, debrief, try again, and debrief again. Then try it again with another scenario. And then another. With each scenario, ramp up the complexity and acuity of the simulation (see Figure 9.11).

What happens? In less than an hour and a half, the interprofessional student team will be functioning at the highest level of collaboration with active patient and family engagement. The students, together with the patients and family members they are caring for, will have invented entirely new patterns for communicating with each other, sharing information, supporting each other, and making plans together. There will be laughter, possibly tears, new respect, new bonds of friendship, and a

FIGURE 9.11 UNIVERSITY HOSPITALIST TEACHING SERVICE PREPARING TO IMPLEMENT COLLABORATIVE CARE.

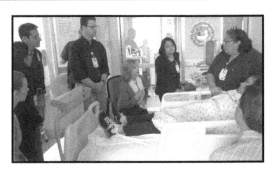 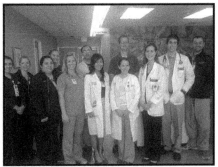

Source: Uhlig, 2015. Used with permission.

striking sense of shared excitement and optimism about the future of their work together in health care.

When students, patients, and families are asked to say a few words about what they just experienced, their comments express a deep appreciation for each other and for each other's roles. Student nurses will say, "The medical students were so nice. They weren't mean to us. I felt included." The student physicians will say, "The nurses were so knowledgeable. I was so grateful they were here. I was terrified but we did it, together." The patients and family members will say, "Everyone was so caring. She held my hand. They listened to me. I felt seen and heard." Others will say, "It was eye opening." "It was so real." "It was scary but we did it!" "We need to do more of this." "We need to do this all the time."

Case Study Three: The Clinical Nurse Leader Role – Two Stories of Clinical Microsystem Transformation

The role of clinical nurse leader (CNL) was created to provide a change leader focused on improving the quality of patient outcomes at the center of the clinical microsystem. The American Association of Colleges of Nursing (AACN) introduced the CNL in 2004 (Hix, McKeon, and Walters, 2009) and it is the first new role in nursing since the nurse practitioner was introduced more than 40 years ago. Nursing, similar to medicine, had become more specialized, increasingly high-tech, and required strong partnering and intersecting with other disciplines to create the integrated actions and responses to patient needs. Also, healthcare organizations had been dependent on nurses to compensate for poor structure, inadequate processes, and organizational barriers (Porter-O'Grady, Clark, and Wiggins, 2010). Waste and inefficiencies impeded the ability of the healthcare team to provide the patient care required to achieve the best patient outcomes. AACN recognized the need for an advanced nurse generalist educated at the master's level to facilitate high-quality and safe nursing care in a complex healthcare environment, mentor novice and advanced beginner nurses to design complex plans of patient care, and provide integration of care services and evidence-based strategies to improve team performance within the clinical microsystem. The CNL curriculum includes advanced coursework in leadership, teamwork, quality, informatics, and data analysis designed to help the CNL meet these challenges (Murphy, 2014).

The CNLs develop integration skills in their academic program through educational experiences unique in nursing education. During the graduate program, the CNL student spends time with individuals from other clinical disciplines (for example, pharmacy, respiratory therapy, physical therapy, and medicine) and with other structures and processes within the healthcare system (for example, quality specialists, patient experience/satisfaction specialists, and environmental sustainability leaders). Through these experiences, the student develops an appreciation of how other disciplines contribute to the care of patients and families with complex conditions and understands the complex interplay of the various components of the healthcare system. CNL students are then taught the organizational and interactional determinants of interprofessional integration (Bender, Connelly, and Brown, 2013). Organizational determinants include the institution's mission, values, management structures, level of administrative and clinical leadership, and the resources that can be dedicated to support interdisciplinary collaboration. Interactional determinants are the cultural and individual skill elements brought into the collaborative team, including a willingness to collaborate, mutual trust, common goals, respect for members of the team, and personal communication skills.

Reported outcomes of the implementation of the CNL role include the institution of consistent processes that result in early extubation of ICU patients (Bartley, 2015), reduced surgery cancellations in ambulatory surgery units (Hix, McKeon, and Walters, 2009), reduced blood transfusions after total knee replacements (Hix, McKeon, and Walters, 2009), reduced length of stay and lowered cost of care (Murphy, 2014), and improved levels of patient, staff, and physician satisfaction (Bender and others, 2012; Murphy, 2014).

Trinity Health Story

Trinity Health, a large, Catholic-integrated healthcare system distributed across 21 states within the United States, needed a mechanism to help facilitate significant care transformation in its acute care facilities. The organization was focused on meeting desired quality outcomes and patient satisfaction results. While these metrics were slowly improving, a number of the system's hospitals were interested in finding a mechanism to help accelerate this desired improvement. In 2007, after investigating the early outcomes of CNL implementation across the United States, the Trinity system made the decision to invest in the development of 40 CNLs. Candidates were selected from the best nurses within the system. Trinity Health formed a partnership with the University of Detroit Mercy, developing the curriculum for the master's program using the AACN guidelines for the program. Knowing that the transformational skills of the CNLs would be crucial to the achievement of the system's goals for the program, the curricular elements focused on process improvement skills were amplified and all application projects were aligned with significant goals set by Trinity's hospitals. CNL students were able to select from a number of potential projects and practice their newly acquired skills while helping the organization achieve desired goals.

Graduate CNLs were deployed into three of Trinity's medium-sized hospitals and the care model was redesigned to optimize the impact of the CNL on the interprofessional care team. Leadership focused effort not only on engaging representatives from various disciplines in the redesign of the care model, but also equally focused on the communication of that new model, the new connections, and the new ways for the team to interact to facilitate patient outcomes. The CNLs were advocates of the CNL model, explaining the purpose of their role and using relationships to help facilitate change. Physicians, care managers, and other members of the healthcare team learned to listen to the CNL and enjoy the improved cohesiveness and communication between members of the team.

Only a brief five years after implementing the CNL team model, the system leadership applauded and highlighted the transformative power of the CNL role and the outcomes that could be obtained. Outcomes achieved in the three CNL implementation sites were consistent with outcomes reported in the literature, resulting in the desired actual return on the organization's investment.

Dartmouth-Hitchcock Story

Leaders within Dartmouth-Hitchcock's (D-H) academic medical center in Lebanon, New Hampshire, also recognized that the acute care systems were in need of transformation. Patients repeatedly spoke about the need for someone in the healthcare team to really know their full story. Nurses working 12-hour shifts typically worked one to two days and then were scheduled off. The patient and family often would never see the same nurse twice during their hospital stay. While hand-offs were a standard procedure, the patients frequently noted that their caregivers did not seem to have all the information they needed to provide individualized care. Residents rotated to a patient unit for a limited period of time and would often rotate off service during the middle of a patient's stay, creating discontinuity in medical direction for the team. Someone needed to carry the patient's story, ensure that the patient's preferences were incorporated into all plans of care, and facilitate the integration of all members of the healthcare team.

Typical of academic medical centers that frequently attract new nursing graduates, Dartmouth-Hitchcock's nursing staff included many registered nurses with less than three years of clinical experience. With an organizational case mix index of 2.1, the second highest in New England, the care required by the inpatient populations was complex. The younger nurses needed mentors not only to develop their critical thinking skills, but also to help them develop the complex plans of care required to help patients recover and successfully transition to their next site of care following an acute care episode. Nurse educators and clinical nurse specialists provided some of the required mentoring but only as a byproduct of other work rather than as a core role expectation.

Dartmouth-Hitchcock evaluated the CNL role and determined that this newer nursing role had the potential to be the catalyst needed to transform the inpatient structure and processes, yielding improved outcomes. D-H partnered with a local college to develop that academic institution's first master's-level nursing program. With the launch of the program in the fall of 2017, D-H funded 12 RNs to earn their CNL master's degree and be part of the implementation of the new role within the academic health system.

Conclusion: A New Future Waiting

The clinical microsystem is a rich learning environment for both students and practicing professionals. It provides real and meaningful opportunities for interprofessional learning and teaching, and it serves as the place where competence is developed and demonstrated. Both formal and informal learning occur around the clock. As shown in case study one (*Using "Educational Microsystems" to Develop a "Clinician-Leader-Improver" Curriculum*), the microsystem concept can also be used in a purely educational setting to understand the purpose, people, processes, and patterns of courses. Case study two (*The Social Field Model of Collaborative Care*) hints at what the future can bring: new models of care in restructured physical and social environments, new ways of teaching and learning that are embedded and essential for the optimized microsystems that are their new home, and new patterns that move away from time-honored education and practice traditions to new ways of interacting, which produce even better results. Case study three (*The Clinical Nurse Leader Role – Two Stories of Clinical Microsystem Transformation*) describes the intersection of practice and learning, and the role of leader as learner.

These new approaches weave teaching and learning into every aspect of care and practice. They actively engage patients and families in the respectful co-creation of care that emerges from rich human connections rather than being "delivered" to people. They are more about meaning and life wholeness and involve healthcare science in supportive ways rather than as a central focus. They move from care that is delivered and consumed, to care that is a sustainable, renewable resource.

The steps to that new future are slow, uncertain, and difficult but remarkably rewarding. As authors of this chapter, we challenge you to imagine and take a step, any step that will allow you and others in your care environment to begin to experience and explore the integration of education and care transformation through interprofessional approaches in your microsystem. From our own experiences, we believe you will be thankful you did, and that you will never want to go back.

Mesosystem Considerations

This chapter once again illustrates the important role of the mesosystem in facilitating and communicating the work of the microsystems it includes. The first case study discusses the educational microsystem, as well as the educational mesosystem that was needed to support and spread the concept. In the second case study, the mesosystem played an important role in facilitating and enabling the interprofessional work. Finally, the third case study clearly shows how the CNL is at the intersection of meso- and microsystems and plays a crucial role in connecting the two. As health professions students move from microsystem to microsystem, they must also be prepared to see functional and mutually supportive relationships between mesosystem and microsystem. All too often, students are visible to the microsystem but invisible to the mesosystem. Including learners in the routine activities of both micro- and mesosystem will develop professionals who have a more complete and nuanced understanding of how small systems in healthcare function, what is needed to optimize that function, and an enhanced understanding of the multiple roles and (sometimes conflicting) priorities of any clinical setting.

Summary

Education of both students and professionals is an important function of the clinical microsystem. As the place where teamwork skills are honed, where clinical competency is developed and assessed, and where the explicit and hidden curricula are juxtaposed, the microsystem provides rich opportunities for learning and reflection. Microsystem principles can also be exported to purely education settings. Finally, the social field model of collaborative care points to future models for high-performing microsystems.

Review Questions

1. Name and describe two recent trends in health professional education.
2. What is the hidden curriculum?

3. What are the principles of social field theory?
4. Describe the role of the clinical nurse leader. If you are not a nurse, what might be a similar role in your profession?

Discussion Questions

1. What is your experience with interprofessional education? What has worked well? What could be improved?
2. What are some of the defined competencies for your profession? How are you assessed on your attainment of those competencies?
3. Describe your class as an "educational microsystem."
4. Have you seen elements of the social field in your own work or education? If so, describe them. How did they contribute to your learning?
5. Imagine you are a student in the clinical microsystem of the future. How will you work and learn?

Additional Activities

1. Describe in words and images an educational microsystem you are or have been a part of. (This is best done as a group with learners, faculty, staff, and others.) Consider the 5Ps of your educational microsystem. What are the important measures of the success of the microsystem; consider the perspectives of learners, faculty, patients, and accreditors.
2. Review the material in this chapter on Social Fields and the Collaborative Care Model. Working with other members of the microsystem, describe what steps might be taken to implement collaborative care and learning.
3. Explore resources related to interprofessional education and team competencies. Compare these to current curricula and assessments in programs you are a part of. Prepare a presentation on how that program is doing, including suggested first steps to address gaps.

References

Accreditation Council for Graduate Medical Education website. [http://www.acgme.org/]. 2019.
American Board of Medical Specialties. "A Trusted Credential." [http://www.abms.org/board-certification/a-trusted-credential/]. 1999.

Bartley, M. "Clinical Nurse Leader: Achieving Improved Outcomes Through Teams." Nursing Grand Rounds, Dartmouth-Hitchcock Medical Center, Lebanon, NH, Apr. 23, 2015.

Batalden, M., Batalden, P., Margolis, P., and others. "Coproduction of Healthcare Service." *BMJ Quality & Safety*, 2016, 25(7), 509-517. doi: 10.1136/bmjqs-2015-004315

Batalden, P., and Foster, T. *Sustainably Improving Health Care: Creatively Linking Care Outcomes, System Performance and Professional Development.* London: Radcliffe Publishing, 2012.

Bender, M., Connelly, C. D., and Brown, C. "Interdisciplinary Collaboration: The Role of the Clinical Nurse Leader." *Journal of Nursing Management*, 2013, 21, 165-174.

Bender, M., Connelly, C. D., Glaser, D., and Brown, C. "Clinical Nurse Leader Impact on Microsystem Care Quality." *Nursing Research*, 2012, 61(5), 326-332.

Benner, P. "From Novice to Expert," *American Journal of Nursing*, 1982, 402-407.

Bodenheimer, T., and Sinsky, C. "From Triple to Quadruple Aim: Care of the Patient Requires Care of the Provider." *Annals of Family Medicine*, 2014, 12(6), 573-576. doi: 10.1370/afm.1713

Byrd, T. Personal conversation with Tina C. Foster, Jul. 20, 2017.

D'Amour, D., and Oandasan, I. "Interprofessionality as the Field of Interprofessional Practice and Interprofessional Education: An Emerging Concept." *Journal of Interprofessional Care*, 2005, Suppl 1, 8-20. doi: 10.1080/13561820500081604

Dominguez, C., Uhlig, P., Brown, J., and others. "Studying and Supporting Collaborative Care Processes." Paper presented at the Human Factors and Ergonomics Society Annual Meeting, Orlando, Sep. 2005.

Dreyfus, S. E., and Dreyfus, H. L. *A Five-Stage Model of the Mental Activities Involved in Directed Skill Acquisition.* (Under contract F49620-C-0063) Berkeley, CA: United States Air Force Office of Scientific Research. [http://www.dtic.mil/dtic/tr/fulltext/u2/a084551.pdf]. 1980.

Dreyfus, S. E. "The Five-Stage Model of Adult Skill Acquisition." *Bulletin of Science, Technology & Society*, 2004, 24(3), 177-181.

Gilbert, J. H. V., Yan, J., and Hoffman, S. J. "A WHO Report: Framework for Action on Interprofessional Education and Collaborative Practice." *Journal of Allied Health*, 2010, 39(3 pt 2), 196-197.

Godfrey, M. M., and Oliver, B. J. "Accelerating the Rate of Improvement in Cystic Fibrosis Care: Contributions and Insights of the Learning and Leadership Collaborative." *BMJ Quality & Safety*, 2014a, 23(s1), i23-i32. doi: 10.1136/bmjqs-2014-002804

Godfrey, M. M., Andersson-Gare, B., Nelson, E. C., and others. "Coaching Interprofessional Health Care Improvement Teams: The Coachee, the Coach and the Leader Perspectives." *Journal of Nursing Management*, 2014b, 22(4), 452-464. doi: 10.1111/jonm.12068

Gruppen, L. D., Mangrulkar, R. S., and Kolars, J. C. "The Promise of Competency-Based Education in the Health Professions for Improving Global Health." *Human Resources for Health*, 2012, 10, 43.

Gurevich, O. Personal conversation with Paul N. Uhlig, 2005.

Hafferty, F. W. "Beyond Curriculum Reform: Confronting Medicine's Hidden Curriculum," *Academic Medicine*, 1998, 73(4), 403-107. doi: 10.1097/00001888-199804000-00013

Headrick, L. A., Barton, A. J., Ogrinc, G., and others. "Results of an Effort to Integrate Quality and Safety into Medical and Nursing School Curricula and Foster Joint Learning." *Health Affairs*, 2012, 31(12), 2669-2680. doi: 10.1377/hlthaff.2011.0121

Hix, C., McKeon, L., and Walters, S. "Clinical Nurse Leader Impact on Clinical Microsystems Outcomes." *Journal of Nursing Administration*, 2009, 39(2), 71-76.

Institute of Medicine (US) Committee on the Health Professions Education Summit. In Greiner, A. C. and Knebel, E. (eds.), *Health Professions Education: A Bridge to Quality*. Washington, DC: National Academies Press, 2003. [https://www.ncbi.nlm.nih.gov/books/NBK221528/]

Institute of Medicine (US) Committee on the Robert Wood Johnson Foundation Initiative on the Future of Nursing. *The Future of Nursing: Leading Change, Advancing Health*. Washington, DC: National Academies Press, 2010. [http://www.nationalacademies.org/hmd/Reports/2010/The-Future-of-Nursing-Leading-Change-Advancing-Health.aspx]

Langley, G. L., Moen, R., Nolan, K. M., and others. *The Improvement Guide: A Practical Approach to Enhancing Organizational Performance* 2nd edition. San Francisco, CA: Jossey-Bass, 2009.

Mahood, S. C. "Medical Education: Beware the Hidden Curriculum." *Canadian Family Physician*, 2011, 57(9), 983-985.

Mitchell, P., Wynia, M., Golden, R., and others. *Core Principles & Values of Effective Team-Based Health Care*. Discussion Paper, Institute of Medicine. Washington, DC: National Academies Press, 2012. [https://nam.edu/wp-content/uploads/2015/06/VSRT-Team-Based-Care-Principles-Values.pdf]

Murphy, E. A. "Healthcare Reform – A New Role for Changing Times: Embracing the Clinical Nurse Leader Role – a Strategic Partnership to Drive Outcomes." *Nurse Leader*, 2014, 12(4), 53-57. doi: 10.1016/j.mnl.2014.05.010

Nancarrow, S. A., Booth, A., Ariss, S., and others. "Ten Principles of Good Interdisciplinary Team Work." *Human Resources for Health*, 2013, 11, 19. doi: 10.1186/1478-4491-11-19.

National Higher Education Benchmarking Institute. [https://benchmarkinginstitute.org/], 2019.

Nelson, E. C., Batalden, P. B., Huber, T. P., and others. "Microsystems in Health Care: Part 1. Learning from High-Performing Front-Line Clinical Units." *The Joint Commission Journal on Quality Improvement*, 2002, 28(9), 472-493. doi: 10.1016/s1070-3241(02)28051-7

Oliver, B. J., Potter, M., Pomerleau, M., and others. "Rapid Health Care Improvement Science Curriculum Integration Across Program in a School of Nursing." *Nurse Educator*, 2017, 42(5S), S38-43. doi: 10.1097/NNE.0000000000000428

Ogrinc, G., Davies, L., Goodman, D., and others. "SQUIRE 2.0 (Standards for Quality Improvement Reporting Excellence): Revised Publication Guidelines from a Detailed Consensus Process." *The Permanente Journal*, 2015, 19(4), 65-70. doi: 10.7812/tpp/15-141 Also available online: www.squire-statement.org.

Oliver, B. J., Potter, M., Pomerleau, M., and others. "Rapid Health Care Improvement Science Curriculum Integration Across Program in a School of Nursing." *Nurse Educator*, 2017, 42(5s), s38-s43. doi: 10.1097/NNE.0000000000000428

Oliver, B. J., Pomerleau, M., Potter, M., and others. "Optimizing NCLEX-RN Pass Rate Performance Using an Educational Microsystems Improvement Approach." *Journal of Nursing Education*, 2018, 57(5), 265-274. doi: 10.3928/01484834-20180420-03

Porter-O'Grady, T., Clark, J. S., and Wiggins, M. S. "The Case for Clinical Nurse Leaders: Guiding Nursing Practice into the 21st Century." *Nurse Leader*, 2010, 8(1), 37-41. doi: 10.1016/j.mnl.2009.11.002

Quality and Safety Education for Nurses. "QSEN competencies." [http://qsen.org/competencies/pre-licensure-ksas/].

Sabadosa, K. A., and Batalden, P. B. "The Interdependent Roles of Patients. Families and Professionals in Cystic Fibrosis: A System for the Coproduction of Healthcare and its Improvement." *BMJ Quality & Safety*, 2014, 23, i90-i94. doi: 10.1136/bmjqs-2013-002782

Uhlig, P. N., Brown, J., Nason, A., and others. "The John M. Eisenberg Patient Safety Awards. System Innovation: Concord Hospital." *Joint Commission Journal on Quality Improvement,* 2002, 28(12), 666-672.

Uhlig, P. N., Berry, W. R., Raboin, E. W., and others. "Preventing Complications: New Frontiers of Safety Science in Cardiothoracic Surgery." In A. G. Little and W. H. Merrill (eds.), *Complications in Cardiothoracic Surgery: Avoidance and Treatment,* 2nd edition. West Sussex, UK: Blackwell Publishing, 2010.

Uhlig, P. N., and Raboin, W. E. *Field Guide to Collaborative Care: Implementing the Future of Health Care.* Overland Park, KS: Oak Prairie Health Press, 2015, 227. (ISBN 978-0-99141-129-0)

Uhlig, P. N., Doll, J., Brandon, K., and others. "Interprofessional Practice and Education in Clinical Learning Environments: Frontlines Perspective." *Academic Medicine,* 2018, 93(10), 1441-1444. doi: 10.1097/ACM.0000000000002371

Additional Resources

American Board of Medical Specialties, http://www.abms.org/
board-certification/a-trusted-credential/based-on-core-competencies/

Center for Interprofessional Education, University of Toronto, http://www.ipe
.utoronto.ca/

Centre for Advancement of Interprofessional Education, https://www.caipe.org

Collaborative Care Alliance, https://www.createbettercare.org/

Interprofessional Education Collaborative, https://www.ipecollaborative.org/

National Center for Interprofessional Practice and Education, https://nexusipe.org/

National Higher Education Benchmarking Institute, https://benchmarkinginstitute.org/

Key Words/Terms

Clinical nurse leader (CNL): A graduate-level nursing role that was developed in the United States to prepare registered nurses focused on the improvement and leadership of quality and safety outcomes for patients or patient populations.

Competency-based education: Competency-based education refers to systems of instruction, assessment, grading, and academic reporting that are based on students demonstrating that they have learned the knowledge and skills they are expected to learn as they progress through their education (Gruppen, Mangrulkar, and Kolars, 2012).

Interprofessional education: Refers to occasions when students from two or more professions in health and social care learn together during all or part of their professional training with the object of cultivating collaborative practice for providing client- or patient-centered health care (Gilbert, Yan, and Hoffman, 2010).

SQUIRE (Standards for QUality Improvement Reporting Excellence): Guidelines that provide a framework for reporting new knowledge about how to improve health care. They are intended for reports that describe system-level work to improve the quality, safety, and value of health care.

Team competencies: Competencies needed to enable good team function. The term may also refer to competencies that teams (as opposed to individuals) demonstrate.

CHAPTER TEN

THE NEW FRONTIER OF SYSTEM IMPROVEMENT – MESOSYSTEMS

Marjorie M. Godfrey, Tom Downes, Steve Harrison, Julie K. Johnson, Tina C. Foster

AIM

In this chapter, we will share experiences, lessons learned, and important tips to move beyond improving the microsystem of care to improving the mesosystem of care, which often consists of a collection of microsystems that many patients encounter in their course of care. Each of the previous chapters have included important considerations for improving the mesosystem of care. Recognizing most care and services occur across multiple microsystems to create a system of care that can be well organized or not will help improvers assess and identify system improvement opportunities as illustrated in the two case examples – from Sheffield, UK and the Cystic Fibrosis Foundation (CFF) in the USA.

LEARNING OBJECTIVES

1. Compare and contrast clinical microsystem and mesosystems to identify what is similar and what is different in assessments and improvement processes.
2. Identify key members of the mesosystem team, which represents multidisciplinary members, patient or family partners, leadership, and team coaches to support successful mesosystem improvement.

Quality by Design: A Clinical Microsystems Approach, Second Edition. Edited by Marjorie M. Godfrey, Tina C. Foster, Julie K. Johnson, Eugene C. Nelson and Paul B. Batalden.

3. Describe multi-microsystem leadership significance to mesosystem leadership operations and creating the conditions for mesosystem improvement success.
4. Discuss the two case studies to identify key principles and cultural considerations for mesosystem improvement.
5. Design a mesosystem plan and strategy for a population or pathway based on the case studies to improve processes and outcomes.

Introduction

Nelson, Batalden, and Godfrey remind us that the "places" where patients, families, and care teams meet are called the clinical microsystem (Nelson and others, 2011). As the basic building blocks of health care, they can function in isolation or in concert with other microsystems to make it easy to do the right thing. They remind us that at the end of the day, each patient's care is only as good as the care that is actually delivered by frontline staff.

Our conventional way of organizing health care into separate departments and specialties can make it difficult to see how clinical microsystems truly function as connected, interdependent units. This traditional focus on individual disciplines often creates obstacles that hinder the daily work of both microsystem (smallest building block of health care) and mesosystems (networks of interconnected units).

Health care frequently occurs in multiple microsystems that may be well coordinated or not for the benefit of patients and families. People, who may be known as patients, and families have needs that extend beyond just one microsystem. Their care and service needs may include clinical microsystems, for example, emergency department, intensive care unit, medical-surgical units, *and* supporting microsystems, for example, laboratory, diagnostic, information, dietary, and finance units in the course of care delivery. Collectively, this is called the mesosystem. The mesosystem may be called a **clinical pathway**, a care path, **care pathway**, **integrated care pathway**, **critical pathway**, or **care map**.

No matter what it is called, a mesosystem is a collection of microsystems that come together intentionally or unintentionally and can be recognized *or not* as a system of care to provide care and services to an identified population. Knowledge of the details of the multiple systems and multiple cultures that exist in a mesosystem can help inform process, structure, and outcomes.

Previous examples that illuminate not only microsystem, but mesosystems of care (and macrosystems) include the Bladyka case that highlights how individual microsystems can be tightly or loosely connected with one another and perform better or worse under different operating conditions (Quality by Design, 2007, 57–59). When multiple interdependent microsystems form a "mesosystem," semipermeable boundaries are present that mediate relationships with patients and family and with many support services and other microsystems. These boundaries are not often recognized, studied, or intentionally improved. Instead of collaborating to understand the entire care system and improve it together, people on both sides of the boundaries often resort to blaming each other's processes and staff. Mesosystem efforts can tackle system-wide challenges, identify how care is coordinated or not across different units, and pinpoint missing or ineffective connections communication between those microsystems.

A second mesosystem example is about Amy and the comprehensive breast care program where handoffs and the space between microsystems are emphasized (Value by Design, 2011, 57–60). Both case studies underscore the critical role of communication and relationships in the functioning of mesosystems. These interpersonal connections are crucial not only for fostering collaboration and problem-solving but also for driving system-wide improvements (Value by Design, 2011, 271 and 297).

Leaders at all levels of the healthcare system can support these "places" to create conditions of excellence in the frontlines of care delivery. High-reliability organizations described by Weick and colleagues are "mindful" of their interdependent interactions (Weick, 2002a,b; Weick and Sutcliffe, 2001). To support "**mindfulness**" of mesosystems and interdependent interactions, the M3 matrix (Quality by Design, 2007, 206–209) highlights specific actions leaders can take to ensure the expectations and conditions of excellence are in place to support not only individual microsystem excellence but multiple microsystems (mesosystems) to meet together to increase their mindfulness about their interdependent interactions. Leaders within the mesosystem can create a shared vision and align microsystem goals with mesosystem improvement through seeing the "balcony (30,000-foot system view) and the dance floor (frontline care delivery)" (Heifetz and others, 2009). Identifying barriers and addressing obstacles that hinder collaboration and improvement efforts is also a leader's role in the mesosystem. Leaders can ensure protected time for improvement teams to assess microsystems and mesosystems using standard improvement processes along with facilitating access to needed data and information.

Avedis Donabedian proposed using the triad of **structure, process, and outcome** to evaluate the quality of health care. He further wrote we cannot achieve real excellence without seeing and acting upon health care as a system. To see and act upon health care helps to understand that health system activities are enabled (and constrained) by the system's structure and functional capabilities (Donabedian, 1966).

The Donabedian triad of structure, process, and outcomes provides a structured guide for the initial assessment of a clinical microsystem using the **5Ps** (modified structure, process, and outcomes) to help interprofessional teams "see" the system of health care to collectively make improvements and become **high-performing frontline teams**. We have used this approach for over 20 years for the clinical microsystem.

Over this period of time, we have gained a great deal of experience and knowledge about the benefits of helping frontline teams see and improve their systems of health care often resulting in a sense of **"ownership" of the workplace**. Furthermore, we recognize that health care often involves multiple microsystems, and whether these systems are well-coordinated significantly impacts the quality of care for patients and families.

Recall the story of Ken Bladyka in chapter one of Quality by Design where Ken's care traversed multiple microsystems, mesosystems, and macrosystems. One meso-system of care included primary care, inpatient care unit, laboratory, diagnostic services within the Dartmouth-Hitchcock Medical Center (DHMC) macrosystem (Figure 10.1). Another macrosystem of care was the Fred Hutchinson Cancer Research Center where the Bone Marrow Transplant mesosystem was located (Quality by Design, 2007, 8–10).

These multiple clinical and supporting microsystems together are called a **mesosystem** that meets the particular needs of an identified person or population. Often, a collection of clinical and supporting microsystems who provide care and services to meet people's needs do not function as a mesosystem. The mesosystem members frequently do not see themselves as contributing to a larger system of care in a pathway for a population of patients. Rather, they see themselves as individual independent units or silos and not as an interdependent and connected "pathway" equally interested in helping each unique microsystem to be the best they can to provide the best care and services for those being served.

Bronfenbrenner emphasized that it is the way in which members of the system perceive these relationships that is crucial (Bronfenbrenner, 1981). Effective microsystems can facilitate optimal development of the mesosystem and are charac-terized by a network of enduring and reciprocal caring relationships. Conversely, high-risk microsystems are characterized by a lack of mutually rewarding relation-ships and/or the presence of destructive interactions.

To help improvement teams learn about and assess clinical mesosystems to "see" the mesosystems of care and the larger system of care, we have developed and tested a Clinical Mesosystem Action Guide over the past 10 years which can be found in Appendix A.

Two Case Studies

These two case examples have adapted the Clinical Microsystem Action Guide framework to assess, diagnose, and treat clinical mesosystems of care. In the first case example from Sheffield UK, the FLOW Academy added new strategies to

FIGURE 10.1 FLOWCHART OF KEN BLADYKA'S JOURNEY THROUGH MULTIPLE MESOSYSTEMS OF CARE IN TWO MACROSYSTEMS.

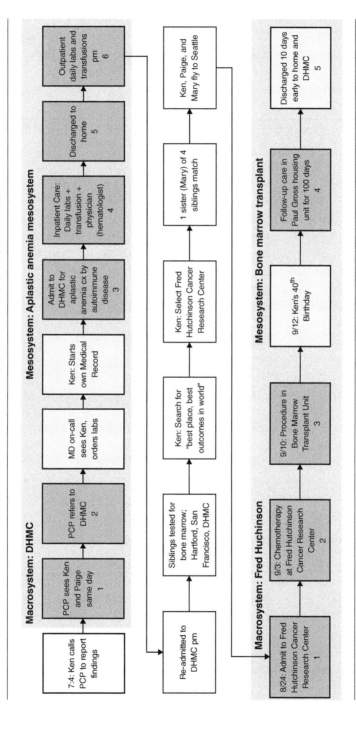

Source: Adapted from Quality by Design, 2007, p. 8–10.

improve care for the population of **frail older patients**. The second case example from the CFF in the USA provides examples of applying the Mesosystem Action guide to improve care for people with **Advanced Cystic Fibrosis Lung Disease (ACFLD)** exploring lung transplant.

Case Example One: Acute Care Flow of Frail Older Patients

A Mesosystem Improvement Journey

This case study describes the work undertaken with Sheffield Teaching Hospitals (STH) and the wider Sheffield health and social care systems. Sheffield is a major city in the UK with a population of around 560,000. Due to its industrial heritage, it has significant urban deprivation with pockets of wealth. A local authority, a health commissioner, and a single coterminous adult hospital provider serve the city. STH is a **vertically integrated provider** operating out of two main acute hospital campuses totaling over 1,800 acute beds and in combination with the community teams employs over 16,000 staff.

First established at STH in 2016 with support from The Health Foundation, the Flow Coaching Academy (FCA) builds on the success of Sheffield Microsystems Coaching Academy, which was developed with support of The Dartmouth Institute Microsystem Academy (www.clinicalmicrosystem.org). Using team co-coaching, pairs of coaches (one improvement coach and one clinical expert) were trained over a one-year action learning program to coach their colleagues to make improvements to care with a focus on people and relationships and practical improvement methods within a specific pathway. The program did this by combining improvement and team coaching skills following the **Flow Coaching Methodology** (https://flowcoaching.academy/).

The Initial Stimulus and Early Work

In 2009, STH started a program of improvement with The Health Foundation (called Flow, Cost, Quality (FCQ)) (The Health Foundation, 2013). The premise of FCQ was to determine whether the **principles of systems engineering** could be applied at a high level across a hospital system. Detailed patient flow analysis was undertaken to understand the profile of patients attending the emergency department and those who were admitted into medical specialties.

The program identified that for frail people, there was potential to reduce the time to being seen by a consultant geriatrician and have a care plan established.

An analysis of long stays in the hospital found opportunities were missed to discharge the patients after rapid assessment and senior clinician review because the services involved in discharge were unable to respond in a timely way.

The use of sharing data and telling patient stories in a structured engaging manner gradually led to a social movement starting across the city. From this period through to the summer of 2011, the team continued to understand the larger system beyond the hospital and made contacts with the community teams, social services, and commissioners. All the work to understand the problem was captured using an **A3 problem-solving methodology**. A significant number of different staff groups were engaged from the acute hospital, primary, and community care to form the "flow" improvement team. Senior leaders formed the "Right First Time" group to mandate citywide enablement of improvement of older people's services.

The Beginning

One early piece of work gained a deeper understanding of the process that a patient experienced when they arrived at the acute medical admissions unit. At that time, patients were sent from the Emergency Department (ED) to a mixed-specialty admissions ward where they were held overnight until a specialty post-take ward round (PTWR) occurred the following morning. A number of these processes were observed in March 2011 and the information was used to design the first **Plan-Do-Study-Act (PDSA) cycle**. This PDSA tested the concept of achieving senior clinician review for patients close to real time rather than batching for the PTWR. This was achieved by the senior clinician moving the day's work forward, reducing the time from arrival at hospital to senior review from 20 hours down to 10 hours. This was followed by two more PDSAs measuring and demonstrating that the time difference was clinically meaningful. The learning from these tests was brought back to each monthly "all flow" team meeting. By the fall of 2011, it became obvious that the monthly meeting did not have the scale and pace required and, in addition, the use of the **A3 method** did not provide the structure for the number of PDSA cycles being planned; an alternative method was explored called the "**Big Room**."

The Evolution of the Big Room

The improvement leaders sought a methodology suitable for improving **a complex adaptive system.** Two of the core principles at the time were to be inclusive of staff from across the whole pathway process and to ensure that the data was visible to everyone. Toyota had been using an **Obeya methodology** for design and launch of high-quality complex cars (https://www.lean.org/lexicon-terms/obeya/). It was recognized that there were similarities in complexity, technology, and scale of a modern car and a modern healthcare system. Having researched Obeya, it was concluded that the approach had merit although a direct translation would be inappropriate, both due to the change from manufacturing to the service sector and the use of Japanese words. "Obeya" was translated to "Big Room" and adapted the room structure to one for health care in the UK (Figure 10.2).

New weekly one hour "Big Room" meetings began in September 2011 in a staff room on the main administrative corridor. The decision was made to use **A0 size display boards** on flipchart stands to display processes and data. An example is shown in Figure 10.3.

The meeting was coached by two coaches using a **co-coaching methodology**. One of the coaches was a senior clinician from the care pathway, the other an improvement manager with no operational responsibility for the care pathway. One or both of the co-coaches were trained as improvement coaches. This coach combination of emotional engagement and independent perspective was shown to be effective in coaching the Big Room. Every meeting started with a patient story (often from a PDSA cycle testing) and most meetings included a patient representative. The goal was to ensure everyone had an equal voice in the Big Room. Patient involvement encouraged a flat hierarchy.

FIGURE 10.2 THE "BIG ROOM" TRANSLATED FROM TOYOTA OBEYA.

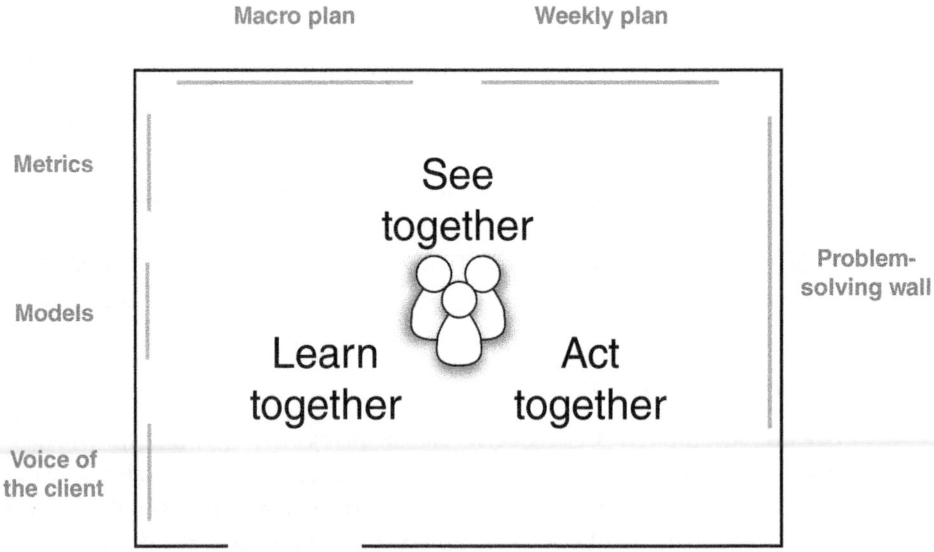

Source: Adapted from The Health Foundation, UK.

FIGURE 10.3 A DISPLAY BOARD IN THE "BIG ROOM."

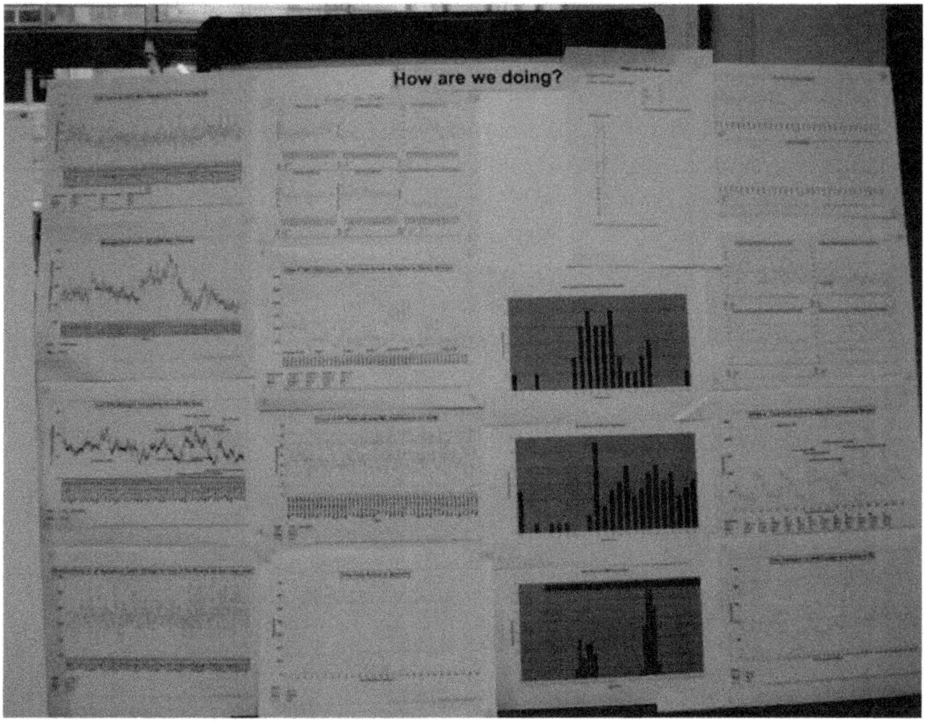

Source: Sheffield Teaching Hospitals NHS Trust, UK.

First Product Launch – Frailty Unit

The initial system assessment of the frailty pathway showed delays on the first day of admission, which led staff to focus the initial aim on improving the first few hours in hospital. **High-level process maps** were developed with learning from the earlier PDSA tests combined with system-level data. Based upon the knowledge gained in the early monthly meetings and associated testing, it was decided to increase the scale of iterative testing. The initial tests had been a series of single-day tests with a single consultant, so it was decided to plan a three-day test involving four consultants. The plans were discussed in the Big Room meetings and all staff were part of the decision-making and planning processes. In November 2011, a three-day test of the new process was undertaken. The results were studied in the Big Room and the scale of testing increased to a whole week involving doctors, nurses, and therapists delivering a novel timely process of specialist geriatric acute assessment. Medical students measured timings and patient experience while staff wore pedometers that showed the team walked several miles each day in the new process. This test was successful with a decrease in average time to complete assessment to six hours with an increased ownership of the pathway by the wider staff group involved.

It had become clear that the system change being tested was beneficial for patients, and staff felt that they were more able to deliver the care that the patients and staff wanted. Data collected over the multiple PDSA cycles confirmed a significant reduction in patient wait time to be seen from 20 hours to four hours. Of significance, three quarters of the consultant staff had been directly involved in the planning, delivery, and discussions surrounding the tests, so the ownership of these potential changes was very high. In a short period of time, all consultants agreed to change their job plans to allow the introduction of the new way of working. Thus, the concept of the **Frailty Assessment Unit** was discovered. When the Frailty Assessment Unit was implemented, the system showed a 60-bed reduction with significantly decreased length of stay by frontloading a timely specialist process (Figure 10.4).

FIGURE 10.4 GSM BED OCCUPANCY FROM JANUARY 1, 2012.

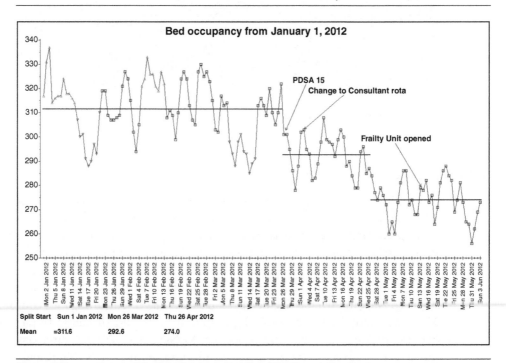

Source: With permission of Sheffield Teaching Hospitals NHS Foundation Trust.

Second Product Launch – Discharge to Assess (D2A)

Through the journey of improving the new Frailty Unit processes, an additional process of the medical decision to discharge a patient required improvement, which included assessment of the patient's needs at home. This involved a separate team of nurses, therapists, and social workers who collectively or individually assessed the patient and then attempted to negotiate with health and social care teams in the community to enable the discharge. The outcomes of this assessment ranged from being able to source the necessary services within an hour, up to delays of many days. During discussions in the Big Room, someone asked why the patient home assessment was done in the hospital, when potentially the best place to assess a patient's future support needs was in the place where they would be delivered – their actual home. The answer was that this system outcome was "perfectly" designed to deliver! The Big Room discussed an alternative hypothesis to test; could a patient be sent home when they were declared ready to leave and undertake the assessment at home with any services required initiated in real time? This felt like a big challenge to everyone in the Big Room. After extensive discussion, over a few weeks, between hospital staff, community health staff, and social services staff (mesosystem members), the decision was made to undertake a PDSA cycle on a single patient. The test would involve a patient being taken home by a staff member with appropriate assessment skills who, following the assessment, could enable the care to be put in place. The community teams agreed to the small-scale test (Figure 10.5).

FIGURE 10.5 CURRENT DESIGN – ASSESS TO DISCHARGE AND FLIPPED TEST.

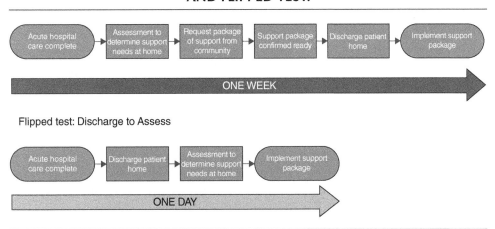

Source: With permission of Sheffield Teaching Hospitals NHS Foundation Trust.

Potential barriers were raised including the issue of transporting the patient and staff member to the home, which required a dedicated ambulance to guarantee time-liness. The service manager facilitated this by agreeing to pay for the additional resource. The test was undertaken, and results were reported back at the Big Room the following Monday as the patient story to start the meeting. The physiotherapist who was part of the PDSA cycle reported that she initially had doubts about the new change as the patient had moderate dementia. During the ambulance journey, she engaged with the patient and when the ambulance arrived outside her house, the patient "visibly brightened." The assessment ended with the patient asking if she could make the physiotherapist a cup of tea. Hearing this story from one of their peers had a profound effect on the staff. After additional successful PDSA cycles with two patients, staff increased the PDSA cycles to include a full day's worth of discharged patients. Finally, after a further full week of discharged patients' PDSA cycles, the team decided to adopt this solution for all discharges from the new Frailty Unit.

In early 2013, the PDSA cycles were discussed, and the question was asked why this new process could not work on a base ward (diagnostic specific ward, for exam-ple, orthopedics, endocrinology, respiratory). A new ward was chosen and the PDSA cycles were attempted but were not successful. On reflection, there were a number of issues that were not addressed. First, *a ward was chosen*, rather than the ward vol-unteering to participate. The lack of ownership meant that any small problem was an excuse not to progress the work.

During a Big Room discussion about the discharge process in August 2013, one of the other wards who had consistently participated in the Big Room shared that they were having problems discharging patients and expressed interest to adapt the tested PDSA cycle to improve their discharge process. This coincided with a management change within the Community team and the new manager of the community team wished to improve the service. Reflecting on the previous PDSA cycles where issues regarding transportation of patients home with staff were perceived to be a barrier, a new barrier was identified concerning what would happen if the patient was unable to remain at home. This new concern raised the possibility that this might require readmission through the ED. The Clinical Director gave permission for the hospital to keep the bed empty until a phone call was received from the community team to either release the bed or arrange for the patient to return directly to the ward, thereby avoiding the ED. There were some levels of mistrust or misinformation between the ward and the community teams, which was resolved by members of the community team visiting the ward, having open team discussions, and building relationships. Following these activities, the Big Room tested a single patient "Discharge to Assess" PDSA cycle. The patient was successfully identified early one morning and was at home fully assessed with a care package in place by tea-time. There were a number of issues that arose during the PDSA cycle about the paperwork complexity and time needed to process the paperwork. After discussing these at the following Big Room weekly meeting, revisions were made, and the teams decided to repeat the PDSA with

FIGURE 10.6 PILOT WARD MEAN SPELL LENGTH OF STAY FOR ALL DISCHARGES FROM JANUARY 2013.

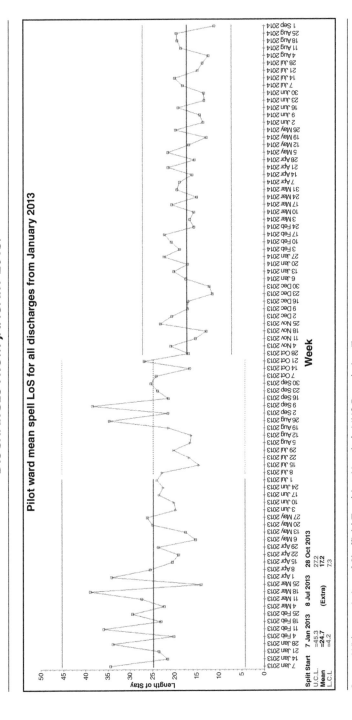

Source: With permission of Sheffield Teaching Hospitals NHS Foundation Trust.

FIGURE 10.7 MEAN DELAY FROM REFERRAL TO ASSESSMENT FOR ALL AR – BY WEEK.

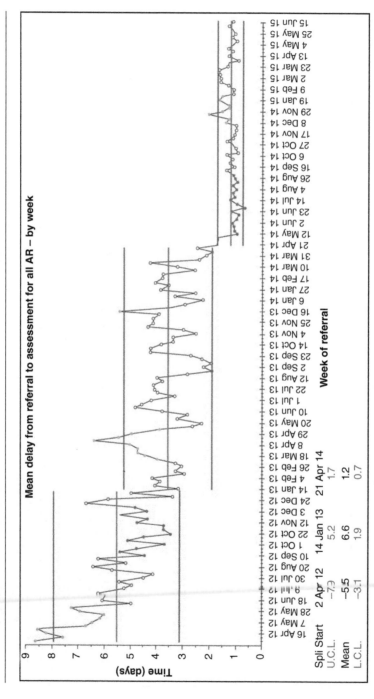

Source: With permission of Sheffield Teaching Hospitals NHS Foundation Trust.

two more patients. The modified PDSA cycles were both successful and the patients were discharged and home by early afternoon. Again, the modified PDSA cycles were discussed at the following Big Room weekly meeting, and the decision was made to repeat the two-patient test. The modified PDSA cycle worked, received positive feedback, and the decision was made to undertake a full-week test of all discharge patients from the ward. The additional PDSA cycles for the full week were successful and at the Big Room meeting the following week, the decision was made not to go back to the previous system and to adopt the new "**Discharge to Assess**" **(D2A)** process (Downes, 2017). Data during this period showed a dramatic reduction in excess stay (Figure 10.6).

This information was then used, with a system simulation model, to raise the discussion of the benefits of this approach across the health and social care system of Sheffield. The result of this was a major injection of funding, which allowed, over the following six months, an increase in community support capacity to enable this new way of mesosystem work. The implementation of D2A across STH significantly decreased the length of stay of frail patients needing support at home after discharge (Figure 10.7).

The Big Room continues to meet every Monday at lunchtime and staff are currently focusing on more complex patients who often require 24-hour care in care homes. Building on the learning of D2A, staff are exploring how to optimize the opportunity for continued independent living. **The FCA** approach captured and formalized the method of improvement described to train others to replicate the key principles to improve mesosystems.

Case Example Two: Improving the Cystic Fibrosis Lung Transplant Mesosystem

The launch of a CFF program aimed to improve the transfer and transition of care for people with ACFLD exploring lung transplant was part of an Advanced Lung Disease initiative at the CFF. This specific program originated from concerns raised by the CF community who had been transferred from Adult CF care programs to lung transplant programs for transplant (Smith and others 2020). Reports of confusion and frustration from people with CF and families resulted in the CF leadership developing a program to improve the mesosystem of care. First, a **CF Lung Transplant Consortium (CFLTC)** of 10 academic centers across North America was convened to research and explore the state of ACFLD lung transplant. The members of the consortium agreed the process of referral, transfer, and transition of people with ACFLD from Adult CF programs to Transplant programs was inconsistent, lacked clarity, and presented opportunities for improvement. Each of the 10 individual consortium lung transplant programs invited a partner Adult CF referring program to join them in a CF Lung

Transplant Transition **Learning and Leadership Collaborative** (CF LTT LLC), which launched in October 2017 (see sidebar on Learning and Leadership Collaborative).

The Cystic Fibrosis Learning and Leadership Collaborative (CF LLC)

The CF LLC was designed to support Cystic Fibrosis centers' response to variation in CF outcomes in the USA. Development of the methodology was based on the need to have a program that was practical, adaptable, and applicable for busy novice improvers in a variety of contextual settings across the USA. The Dartmouth Microsystem Improvement Curriculum was selected as the methodology to develop a 12-month experiential learning improvement collaborative. Using the popular **Improvement Breakthrough Series** developed by the **Institute for Healthcare Improvement** in the late 1990s, and Kolb's experiential learning theory as the initial framework, the LLC was launched in 2002 (Kilo, 1998; Kolb, 1984).

During the LLC, selected interprofessional improvement teams who had applied to be included in the LLC, learned to assess the current state of their CF program and processes, identify strengths and improvement opportunities in their delivery of care, and make improvements. Over the course of 12 months, each improvement team participated in web-based learning sessions and three face-to-face meetings to learn improvement science, practice skills in their daily work, test change ideas, and reflect on the results with the guidance of an assigned CF Quality Team Coach. Using the **Dartmouth microsystem improvement ramp** found in Chapter 11, of Quality by Design, each improvement team completed the 5P assessment (available in Chapter 13 of Quality by Design) to gain new knowledge and perspectives about their CF program. Based on data and lived experiences, the improvement team narrowed their focus to an improvement theme that would address clinical outcomes or processes and systems. A global improvement aim was created from the theme with a high-level flowchart of the identified process created by the team. **Cause and effect diagrams** were created to understand potential causes of the current results. **Change ideas** (interventions) based on evidence-based guidelines and benchmarking were then adapted and tested using PDSA cycles. Successful change ideas and improved processes were "standardized" through **Standardize-Do-Study-Act (SDSA)** processes including a "**playbook**" illustrating new processes.

The CF LLC evolved over 10 years and was informed by participant verbal and internet-based survey feedback, LLC results, the changing teaching and electronic environment, the economy, and faculty and leadership reflection on action. Consistent national CF leadership participation in all aspects of the LLC planning, execution, and evaluation along with a dedicated national LLC coordinator and faculty contributed to a disciplined approach to improvement. Additional information can be reviewed in: Godfrey, M. M. and Oliver, B. J. *BMJ Quality & Safety*, 2014, *23, i23–i32.* doi: 10.1136/bmjqs-2014-002804.

The CF LLC program was adapted to meet the unique needs of the CF Lung Transplant Transition population who received care from the CF Lung Transplant Transition Mesosystem. The improvement discipline of the **Microsystem Improvement Curriculum** remained the same with several notable additions.

1. The CF LTT LLC program lasted 18 months and consisted of action periods of assess, diagnose, treat (improve), standardize, and sustain with specific activities that occurred in each period (see Figure 10.8).
2. Instead of focusing and assessing on one clinical microsystem, the mesosystem consisted of two clinical microsystems: The adult CF referring program and the Lung Transplant program. Each microsystem convened an interprofessional improvement team including a person with CF who had or was waiting for a lung transplant and or family member partner. Each microsystem conducted independent weekly or biweekly improvement meetings, utilizing **effective meeting skills** (Quality by Design, Chapter 12, 20) and the Microsystem Improvement Curriculum (Quality by Design, Chapter 10), to focus on their own specific processes and challenges. A single CF Quality Team Coach was assigned to both the CF referring and Lung Transplant Transition programs. This coach was responsible for reinforcing improvement efforts, providing support and encouragement, and ensuring progress for each individual microsystem as well as the overarching mesosystem.
3. A simplified overview of the entire process of referring someone with CF to the lung transplant program (the "mesosystem") was divided into eight phases. This provided a framework for both the CF and transplant programs to map out their

FIGURE 10.8 CF LUNG TRANSPLANT LEARNING AND LEADERSHIP TIMELINE OF ACTIVITIES.

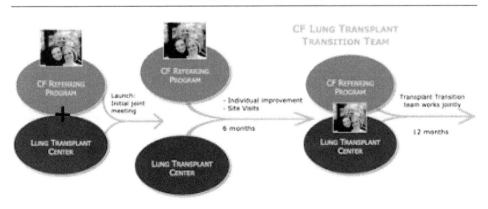

Source: With permission of CF LTT Program.

specific roles and responsibilities, and to identify areas where their processes might overlap or intersect (see Figure 10.9).

4. During the initial six months of the collaborative, each microsystem (CF referring and Lung Transplant) concentrated on their own internal processes. This enabled staff members to gain a deeper understanding of their specific roles and responsibilities within the broader CF lung transplant mesosystem. It also enhanced team dynamics and strengthened their knowledge and skills in quality improvement.

5. On a monthly basis, the CF referring and Lung Transplant programs convened to share updates on their individual progress. These meetings provided a platform for both programs to exchange insights and learnings about their own processes within the framework of the eight-phase model, fostering a collaborative understanding of the entire care journey.

6. Seven months into the collaborative, the CF referring and lung transplant programs began holding monthly meetings as a unified mesosystem. These meetings focused on evaluating the eight phases of the CF lung transplant process, identifying areas of overlapping care, and clarifying roles, functions, and accountabilities. The goal was to streamline the process, eliminate redundancies, and identify opportunities for improvement and redesign. In addition, communication and relationships across the mesosystem were developed and reinforced. While these mesosystem meetings took place, the individual microsystems continued their separate meetings to focus on enhancing their own internal processes.

Prior to the start of the mesosystem improvement, all members of the two programs completed baseline surveys to assess each program's team quality improvement capabilities – **Quality Improvement Assessment Tool (QIA)** (see Table 10.1) and completed a **Relational Coordination (RC)** survey to assess communication and relationships within each program (microsystem) and between the two programs (mesosystem) as it related to the specific lung transplant transition process of care (see Table 10.2).

The aggregate results of each of the QIA and RC surveys provided valuable insights for the CF Quality Team Coach. This information was used to create tailored team coaching plans to support both the individual program improvement teams and the overall mesosystem throughout their improvement journey. The CF Quality Team Coach joined the weekly or biweekly improvement meetings and individual leader meetings virtually to coach the teams and leaders in improvement, leadership of quality improvement, and meeting skills. Over time, with the improvement teams increasing their improvement capabilities, the CF Quality Team Coach frequency of interactions decreased.

FIGURE 10.9 30,000-FOOT VIEW – THE EIGHT PHASES OF CF LUNG TRANSPLANT AND TRANSITION MESOSYSTEM.

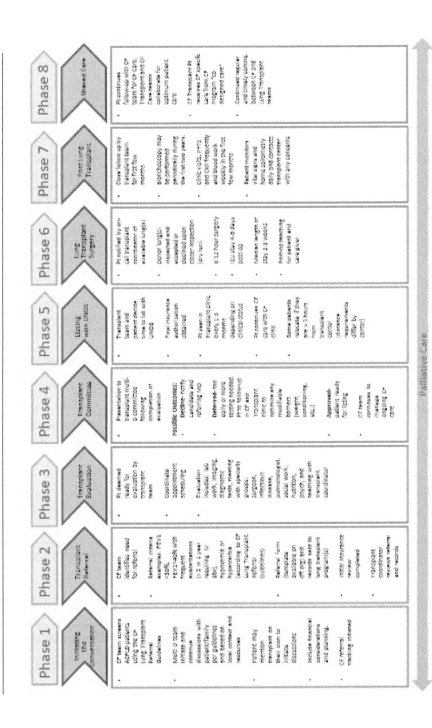

Source: Marjorie M. Godfrey (Author).

TABLE 10.1 QUALITY IMPROVEMENT ASSESSMENT (QIA) CATEGORIES.

1. Quality Improvement Tools and Skills
2. Quality Improvement Measurement
3. Communication and Team Dynamics
4. Organizational Context and Leadership

Source: Adapted from Godfrey, M. M. and others, 2018

TABLE 10.2 RELATIONAL COORDINATION SURVEY DIMENSIONS.

RC is most important when there are multiple stakeholders whose work is highly interdependent, uncertain, and time constrained such as in the CF Lung Transplant Mesosystem.

1. Frequent Communication	**During the CF lung transplant transfer and transition process**, how **frequently** do people in these roles communicate with you?
2. Timely Communication	Do they communicate with you in a **timely** way **during the CF lung transplant transfer and transition process?**
3. Accurate Communication	Do they communicate with you **accurately during the CF lung transplant transfer and transition process?**
4. Problem-Solving Communication	When a problem occurs with the **CF lung transplant transfer and transition process**, do people in these roles blame others or work with you to **solve** the problem?
5. Shared Goals	Do people in these roles **share your goals** for the **CF lung transplant transfer and transition process?**
6. Shared Knowledge	Do people in these roles **know** about the work you do as part of the **CF lung transplant transfer and transition process?**
7. Mutual Respect	Do people in these roles **respect** the work you do as part of the **CF lung transplant transfer and transition process?**
8. CF and Lung Transplant Program Perspective	CF and Lung Transplant perspective.
9. CF and Lung Transplant Program	Site Selection.

Source: Adapted from https://heller.brandeis.edu/relational-coordination/

The Team Coaching Model

The Team Coaching Model research emphasizes the importance of the Team Coach visiting the clinical microsystem they are assigned to coach (Godfrey, 2013). After multiple virtual meetings with the two individual program leaders and the two improvement teams, the team coach and each improvement team developed an agenda for the CF Quality Coach site visit to their clinical microsystems. The purpose of the team coach's site visit was to gain firsthand insight into the improvement team and leaders' activities, both in their clinical work and their improvement efforts. Additionally, the visit aimed to immerse the coach in the unique culture and practices of each microsystem, allowing for a deeper understanding of their specific context. The site visit had two main goals for the CF Quality Coach:

1. **Building Relationships:** The coach aimed to establish stronger connections with each improvement team and their leaders through face-to-face interactions. This would foster trust and open communication, essential for effective coaching and collaboration.
2. **Facilitating an "Exchange Program":** The coach would physically accompany each clinical microsystem (CF and Lung Transplant) to their partner program's location. This "walk in each other's shoes" experience allowed staff from both teams to meet in person, understand each other's roles and challenges, and ultimately enhance their collaboration in caring for patients. The exchange program included the two improvement teams sharing meals together, participating in discipline-specific meetings, engaging in social activities and improved communication, which provided the foundation for their new relationships.

During the site visit or "exchange program," the clinical microsystems (CF and Lung Transplant) would have the opportunity to observe each other's physical spaces and operational workflows. They would then hold a joint mesosystem improvement meeting to discuss their respective roles in each of the eight phases of the CF lung transplant process.

The objectives of these meetings were to:

- **Identify overlaps:** Pinpoint areas where both programs were involved in the same phase of care, highlighting potential redundancies or inefficiencies.
- **Clarify roles:** Clearly define each program's responsibilities within each phase, ensuring smooth transitions and reducing confusion.
- **Improve communication:** Develop strategies for consistent and effective communication between the two programs throughout the patient journey.
- **Enhance efficiency:** Identify opportunities to streamline processes, eliminate unnecessary steps, and improve overall coordination of care.

- **Co-create resources:** Collaboratively develop educational materials and resources for both patients and staff, ensuring consistent messaging and reducing confusion.

Together the partner programs identified strengths, opportunities for improvement, and developed a shared purpose for caring for people with Advanced CF lung disease (ACFLD) exploring lung transplantation. This approach aimed to create a more seamless and patient-centered experience by optimizing the interactions between the two microsystems.

Early in the program, it became apparent that the two clinical microsystems (CF and Lung Transplant) had distinct cultures and primary objectives. Each operated with its own unique purpose, characteristics, and varying levels of experience with quality improvement. Initially, there was a tendency for each team to blame the other for issues, particularly before they had the opportunity to meet, understand their respective roles in the care of ACFLD patients, and establish regular communication channels. It was evident that these "partner" teams had rarely collaborated on planning, improvement efforts, or information sharing. The "exchange program," facilitated by the quality team coach, proved crucial in bridging this gap by allowing both teams to learn more about each other's perspectives and processes.

Following the team coach site visit, the coaches continued coaching the individual programs to ensure improvements in their own programs were made following the Microsystem Improvement Curriculum. Monthly virtual learning sessions involving both the CF referring and Lung Transplant programs ("mesosystem") facilitated the exchange of new ideas and discoveries. These sessions encouraged mutual learning between the improvement teams and provided a dedicated forum for discussing both the technical aspects of their processes and the interpersonal dynamics of their relationships. Shared common themes of improvement included agreed upon co-designed CF Lung Transplant education for staff, patients, and families, and predictable consistent communication with patients, families, and staff within and between each microsystem to demonstrate mesosystem coordination of care. Simple actions such as providing current staff directories with names, emails, and phone numbers to connect with each other provided early gains in communication improvement and energized relationships while improving care coordination. The exchange program contributed to increasing knowledge about each other's program and deeper understanding about the aims and values of the staff while highlighting opportunities to coproduce care to achieve better outcomes. It became clear that to design the best processes and systems for people with ACFLD exploring lung transplant, uncovering behaviors and values of the people involved in the care delivery helped to build a shared purpose for the mesosystem. The need to recognize the communication, relationships, and social aspects of improving systems emerged.

The RC-validated survey results provided an assessment of communication and relationships within and between each clinical microsystem to begin a conversation of improvement. The "within" microsystem results were presented at the LLC in person meeting to learn about communication and relationships "within" and "between" workgroups such as nursing, physicians, social workers, transplant coordinators, psychologist, pharmacist, and so on. Each microsystem discussed the RC findings and identified interventions to strengthen RC within their microsystem. Next, the RC results between the two partner programs were shared. Assessment results consistently showed low RC between the two clinical microsystems (the CF and Lung Transplant programs) in the areas of shared knowledge and timely communication during the lung transplant transition process. This prompted both programs to discuss these findings and collaboratively identify interventions to strengthen their communication and relationships within the mesosystem (Table 10.3).

In the seventh month, dedicated meetings between the CF referring and Lung Transplant programs' professional counterparts from each program were established, fostering deeper understanding and collaboration. A diverse group of professionals from both the CF referring and Lung Transplant programs, including

TABLE 10.3 CF LTT LLC RELATIONAL COORDINATION INTERVENTIONS – EXAMPLES.

Structural Interventions	Relational Interventions	Work Process Interventions
Joint partner program regular meetings	Patient/family partners fully engaged	Invite CF program to attend "patient selection committee meeting."
Shared access to ACFLD patient information	"Walk in each other's shoes" – job shadowing to understand roles, responsibility, and interdependence	Co-develop patient and staff CF Lung Transplant education materials, FAQs
Urgent virtual huddles in real time for patient/family concerns	"Shout outs" to publicly celebrate mesosystem colleagues and reinforce positive behavior	Co-designed/coproduced care pathways, playbooks/standard operating procedures
Shared goals for CF Lung Transplant	Social events such as mesosystem lunch, dinner, celebrations, "date nights" to meet each other in discipline roles	Develop "Roadmap to Transplant" educational pamphlet
Current roles, names, emails, cell phone number directory	Partner together to improve processes of care	Refer to all members of the mesosystem as "our team"

social workers, nurses, coordinators, physicians, pharmacists, patients, families, psychologists, respiratory therapists, and physical therapists, convened to share insights and discuss their respective practices. Significantly, many of these individuals were meeting their counterparts from the other program for the first time. These meetings between professional counterparts from different programs ignited a sense of excitement and energy, highlighting the potential for enhanced collaboration and communication within each professional discipline group involved in the care process.

Importantly, the QIA and RC surveys were conducted again one year after the initial baseline assessments. The results demonstrated a positive impact of the quality improvement efforts. After a year of micro and mesosystem teams testing and implementing changes, as outlined in Table 10.3, both the QIA scores (measuring quality improvement capabilities) and RC scores (measuring RC) showed improvement. This suggests that the interventions and collaborative efforts successfully enhanced the teams' ability to change and strengthen communication and relationships between the two programs.

Discussion

Both case studies offer real-world examples of successful collaboration within a mesosystem to improve care for a specific patient population. However, it is important to acknowledge that mesosystems or pathways often lack dedicated time for meetings focused on assessing and improving the microsystem or the entire system of care (mesosystem). When improvement teams do have opportunities to meet, their attention tends to be directed towards their individual microsystem rather than the broader system-wide perspective. Most members of microsystems were accustomed to focusing on their specific role within the care pathway, rather than understanding the whole system. Engaging patient and family partners can be a valuable strategy to overcome this limitation, as they can offer a unique perspective on the overall patient journey and help identify areas for improvement across the entire system.

The two case studies provide different approaches to achieve this important mesosystem activity through a "Big Room" approach or a "Mesosystem Learning and Leading Collaborative" (see Table 10.4).

Similarities and differences in the two approaches can be highlighted to provide some guidance when there is interest to improve multiple microsystems of a pathway or mesosystem. The key similarities of both cases is they both utilized an adapted clinical microsystem process including rigorous assessments, PDSA cycles, and QI

TABLE 10.4 COMPARISON OF TWO CASE STUDIES

	Case Study 1 – Sheffield	**Case Study 2 – Cystic Fibrosis Lung Transplant**
Population	Frail older patients in acute care	Patients with advanced cystic fibrosis lung disease exploring lung transplant
Setting	Sheffield Teaching Hospitals (STH), and wider Sheffield health and social care systems in United Kingdom (UK)	Cystic Fibrosis Lung Transplant Consortium (CFLTC) across North America
Methodology	Flow Coaching Academy (FCA), based on microsystem improvement, team co-coaching of mesosystem improvement, teams including patients and family members as partners	Cystic Fibrosis Learning and Leadership Collaborative (CF LTT LLC), based on Microsystem Improvement Curriculum, team coaching of micro and mesosystem improvement teams that included patients and family members as partners
Key Intervention	Big Room meetings for collaboration and problem-solving	CF LTT LLC program with structured phases, assessments, and interventions
Assessment Tools	**5Vs**, A3 problem-solving, patient flow analysis, PDSA cycles	5Ps, Quality Improvement Assessment Tool (QIA), Relational Coordination (RC) survey
Outcomes	Reduced time to consultant review, decreased length of stay, successful Discharge to Assess (D2A) implementation	Improved communication, co-designed care pathways, standardized processes, improved care coordination
Key Principles	Inclusivity, patient-centeredness, data-driven decision-making, collaboration, continuous improvement	Collaboration, structured improvement, assessment-driven interventions, improved communication, relationship building
Challenges	Overcoming system inertia, resistance to change, coordinating across multiple teams	Different cultures and purposes of microsystems, initial finger-pointing and blaming
Success Factors	Strong leadership support, engaged staff, patient involvement, data transparency	Dedicated team coaches, structured program, focus on relationships and shared goals

team coaches. An important difference between Sheffield and the CF Lung Transplant mesosystem improvement design was Sheffield focused immediately on convening the mesosystem members to learn improvement together while the CF program executed a staged approach, developing improvement capabilities and mesosystem awareness within each microsystem before convening the mesosystem. This approach helped the microsystems practice improvement knowledge and skills in their own setting and to develop improvement knowledge and experience before joining together with their Lung Transplant program to form the mesosystem of improvement.

Key Differences

- Timing of Convening the Mesosystem:
  - Sheffield: Focused immediately on bringing together all members of the mesosystem (acute care and community teams) to learn and improve collectively.
  - CF Lung Transplant: Adopted a staged approach, first building improvement capabilities and mesosystem awareness within each individual microsystem (CF and Lung Transplant) before bringing them together.
- The patient populations and healthcare settings were different.
- Sheffield focused more on the physical flow of patients and system-level changes, while CF Lung Transplant emphasized communication, relationships, and coordination between microsystems.
- Sheffield utilized a more organic, emergent approach to improvement, while CF Lung Transplant followed a more structured, phased program with specific assessments and interventions.

Similarities

- Adapted Clinical Microsystem Process: Both Sheffield and the CF Lung Transplant program adapted clinical microsystem improvement principles, emphasizing rigorous assessments (for example, process mapping, data analysis) and PDSA cycles for testing changes.
- Quality Improvement (QI) Team Coaches: Both initiatives utilized QI coaches to provide guidance, support, and expertise in improvement methodologies.
- Quality Improvement process and methods: Both cases focused on improving the quality and efficiency of care for a specific patient population and included patients in the improvement journey.
- Both cases emphasized collaboration, data-driven decision-making, and continuous improvement.

- Both cases illustrated the "misunderstandings" that can exist between microsystems within a mesosystem when regular efforts to meet to understand each other's role and contribution to the population mesosystem have not occurred.
- Both demonstrated successful outcomes in terms of improved processes, decreased length of stay, enhanced patient experiences and improved communication and relationships.

Guidance for Improving Multiple Microsystems

The choice between these approaches depends on the specific context, needs, and strategy of the organization:

- **Immediate Mesosystem Focus (Sheffield Model):** This approach may be suitable when there is a strong sense of urgency, a shared vision for improvement, and existing relationships between microsystem members. It fosters rapid collaboration and system-wide thinking from the outset.
  - **Strategic Planning:** This top-down approach begins with a high-level overview of the entire mesosystem, creating a strategic plan that outlines the desired outcomes and key goals. The plan then guides the improvement work within each microsystem, ensuring alignment with the broader mesosystem objectives. (Sheffield)
- **Staged Approach (CF Model):** This approach may be preferable when microsystems have varying levels of improvement readiness or when there is a need to build trust and relationships between teams before tackling system-wide issues. It allows each microsystem to develop its internal capabilities and gain a deeper understanding of its role within the larger system.
  - **Inside out improvement:** This approach focuses on continuous improvement within individual microsystems first. Teams learn and apply improvement methodologies within their own unit before expanding their efforts to collaborate across microsystems in mesosystems. This bottom-up approach empowers frontline staff and builds a culture of continuous improvement from the ground up. (CF Lung Transplant)

Additional Considerations

- *Organizational culture:* Assess the organization's readiness for change and the existing level of collaboration between teams.
- *Resources:* Ensure adequate resources (time, funding, expertise) are available to support both individual microsystem and mesosystem improvement efforts.

- *Leadership support:* Strong leadership commitment and engagement are essential for both approaches to succeed.
- *Flexibility:* Be prepared to adapt the chosen approach as needed based on the evolving needs of the organization and the progress of the improvement efforts.

By carefully considering these factors, healthcare leaders can select the most appropriate approach to effectively improve multiple microsystems within a pathway or mesosystem, leading to better patient care and outcomes.

Guiding Principles from the Two Case Examples

"Healthcare improvement often risks being too "technocratic" and losing sight of the *people who provide* care and services and *people who receive* the care and services." Edgar H. Schein (Schein, 2013)

Improvement programs often prioritize technical aspects like process mapping and data analysis but overlook the human element of response to change among frontline staff. To achieve sustainable change, organizations must actively address staff reluctance by building relationships, fostering open communication, and developing everyone's improvement capabilities. This means meeting staff where they are, listening to concerns, and celebrating successes to create a more positive environment for change. This approach not only reduces resistance but also boosts energy, engagement, and the likelihood of lasting improvement.

Key Strategies for Mesosystem Improvement

1. *Patient and family partnership:* Patients and families are vital partners in improvement teams, offering unique insights and co-creating solutions for better care.
2. *Leadership engagement:* Leaders at all levels must create the conditions for successful mesosystem improvement by consistently communicating expectations and maintaining a patient-centered focus.
3. *Multidisciplinary improvement teams:* Each microsystem should have a diverse team representing the entire care pathway. Using a standard improvement method and language helps foster ownership of the mesosystem.
4. *"Balcony, dance floor, and catwalk" perspectives:* Leaders and improvers need to "dance" on the frontlines, gain a broader view from the "balcony," and see the big picture from the "catwalk" to understand the system and identify improvement opportunities (Heifetz and others, 2009). Paul B. Batalden, M.D. quipped, "If people do not see the process, they cannot improve it. Anyone needs to see the process as a catwalk, a flow diagram" (Deming, 2018).

5. *Building knowledge and relationships:* Understanding the contributions of all team members and fostering relationships through meetings, "exchange" visits, and social activities are foundational to mesosystem improvement.

6. *The role of the QI team coach:* Quality improvement team coaches, whether individually or as part of a co-coaching dyad, can catalyze change and empower staff to drive improvement initiatives.

Additional Considerations

- *Time for reflection:* Dedicated time for reflection and sharing experiences is crucial for staff to develop and contribute ideas for improvement.
- *Communication and trust:* Open communication and trust-building are essential for effective collaboration within and between microsystems.
- *Shared goals and mutual respect:* Fostering shared goals and mutual respect among team members is essential for successful mesosystem improvement.

By incorporating these strategies and embracing a patient-centered approach that empowers staff, healthcare organizations can effectively improve care while addressing the human element of change. This approach fosters improvements at both the microsystem and mesosystem levels, resulting in better patient care, outcomes, and experiences. It also enhances the capabilities of multidisciplinary staff, feeds a sense of "ownership" of the micro and mesosystem and leads to more sustainable improvements overall.

Key Principle

Regardless of the approach, keeping the patient and population central to the improvement process is crucial. Co-production of care, where patients and families actively participate in designing and improving care processes, ensures that the changes truly meet their needs and enhance their experience. Mindfulness of the "boundaries" between microsystems in the mesosystem can lead to increased interdependence, communication, and relationships.

Conclusion

Patients navigate through various interconnected healthcare teams (mesosystems) throughout their care journey. While mesosystems have the potential for better organization, achieving high performance requires a dual focus: attention to both the frontline care delivery and the overarching system design. Ultimately, the quality of patient care hinges on the effectiveness of frontline staff. To optimize this care, it is crucial to assess all microsystems within the mesosystem, with a focus on strengthening interdependencies and fostering robust communication and relationships between them. As Nelson and colleagues highlight, the success of individual microsystems, and consequently the entire mesosystem, is influenced by their ability to facilitate or hinder doing what is best for the patient. By enhancing awareness and relationships within and across microsystems, healthcare organizations can cultivate shared goals, mutual respect, and effective problem-solving, ultimately leading to better patient care.

Review Questions

1. Define microsystem and mesosystems.
2. Compare and contrast the Sheffield and CF Lung Transplant mesosystem improvement models in relation to your own context to determine which process would be best in your context.
3. How can microsystem leaders enhance mesosystem improvement?
4. What is the role of a QI Team Coach in microsystem/mesosystem improvement?

Discussion Questions

1. What forces are driving and blocking improvement of mesosystems in your health system?
2. Discuss technical and human aspects of improvement and implications in your setting.
3. Provide a story of a patient pathway experience and create a flowchart of the experience across multiple microsystem to identify mesosystems. Discuss gaps and inefficiencies in processes and consider the seven dimensions of RC.

Additional Activities

1. Pick a particular type of patient – for example, person with diabetes, or heart failure, pregnant woman, person who had a heart attack, joint replacements.
2. What microsystems will this person encounter on his/her journey? Create a flowchart of the patient pathway identifying the microsystems.
3. What support microsystems contribute services to the person as his/her journey progresses?
4. Does this collection of microsystems – direct and support – recognize themselves as a mesosystem that share the work of helping this type of patient get the best outcomes at the lowest cost?

References

Batalden, P.B. (2018). Conversation with Edward Deming. In: *The New Economics for Industry, Government, Education*, 3e (ed. W.E. Deming), 22. Cambridge MA: The MIT Press.

Bronfenbrenner, U. (1981). *The Ecology of Human Development*. Cambridge MA: Harvard University Press.

Donabedian, A. (1966). *Evaluating the Quality of Medical Care. Milbank Memorial Fund Quarterly* 44: 166–206.

Downes, T. (2017). *What If We Flipped the Patient Discharge Process?* Institute for Healthcare Improvement, April https://www.youtube.com/watch?v=KJEyZ1Y5O0w

Godfrey, M. M. "Improvement capability at the front lines of healthcare: Helping through leading and coaching." Unpublished doctoral dissertation, School of Health Sciences, Jonkoping University, Dissertation Series No. 46, 2013.

Godfrey, M. M., Foster, V. L., and Mats, N. "Validation of the quality improvement assessment (QIA) tool." *BMJ Open Quality*, 2018, 7 (1), A1-A36. doi: https://doi.org/10.1136/ihisciabs.22.

The Health Foundation. "Improving the flow of older people Sheffield Teaching Hospital NHS Trust's experience of the flow cost of quality improvement programme." *The Health Foundation Inspiring Improvement*, 2013. http://www.health.org.uk/sites/default/files/ImprovingTheFlowOfOlderPeople_casestudy_1.pdf.

Heifetz, R.A., Linsky, M., and Grashow, A. (2009). *The Practice of Adaptive Leadership: Tools and Tactics for Changing your Organization and the World*. Brighton, MA: Harvard Business Press.

Kilo, C. M. "A framework for collaborative improvement: Lessons from the Institute for Healthcare Improvement's breakthrough series." *Quality Management in Health Care*, 1998. doi: https://doi.org/10.1097/00019514-199806040-00001.

Kolb, D.A. (1984). *Experiential Learning: Experience as the Source of Learning and Development*. Englewood Cliffs, NJ: Prentice-Hall.

Nelson, E.C., Batalden, P.B., and Huber, T.P., and others(2007). *Quality by Design: A Clinical Microsystems Approach*. San Francisco: Jossey-Bass.

Nelson, E.C., Lazar, J.S., Godfrey, M.M., and Batalden, P.B. (2011). *Value by Design: Developing Clinical Microsystems to Achieve Organizational Excellence*. San Francisco, CA: Jossey-Bass.

Schein, Edgar H. Personal conversation with M. Godfrey, Cambridge MA, June 2013.

Smith, P. J., Dunitz, J. M., Lucy, A., and others. "Incorporating Patient and Caregiver Feedback into Lung Transplant Referral Guidelines for Individual with Cystic Fibrosis – Preliminary Findings from a Novel Paradigm." *Clinical Transplant*, 2020, 00, e14038. doi: https://doi.org/10.1111/ctr.14038.

Weick, K.E. and Sutcliffe, K.M. (2001). *Managing the Unexpected: Assuring High Performance in an Age of Complexity*. San Francisco, CA: Jossey-Bass.

Weick, K.E. "Essai: Real-Time Reflexivity: Prods to Reflection." *European Group for Organizational Studies*, 2002a. doi: https://doi.org/10.1177/0170840602236011.

Weick, K.E. "Puzzles in Organizational Learning: An Exercise in Disciplined Imagination." *British Journal of Management*, 2002b, 13, s2.2. doi: https://doi.org/10.1111/1467-8551.

Key Words/Terms

5Ps: An assessment process that evaluates the anatomy and current performance of the clinical microsystem, **for example**, primary care practice. Donabedian's structure, process, and outcome framework provides the foundation to the microsystem purpose, patients, professionals, process, and patterns evaluation (Donabedian, 1966).

5Vs: (Value, Vision, inVolve, eVidence, Visualization): A modified conceptual model of the 5Ps utilized by the Sheffield Flow Academy to assess a mesosystem.

A3 method: A structured approach to problem-solving developed by Toyota in which one large (A3) sheet of paper, which includes analysis, corrective actions, and action plan.

A3 problem-solving: See A3 method.

Advanced Cystic Fibrosis Lung Disease (ACFLD): Multisystem disorder caused by pathogenic mutations of the *CFTR* gene (CF transmembrane conductance regulator). Pulmonary disease remains the leading cause of morbidity and mortality in patients with CF. When CF lung disease becomes severe, additional evaluation and treatment are overlaid onto the standard therapies that are applicable to all patients with CF lung disease. A person with Cystic Fibrosis who has a lung function of forced expiratory volume (FEV1) <40% and other severity markers may consider lung transplant.

"Big Room": Adapted from the Japanese Obeya. Multidisciplinary team members including those being served, meet together in one large room for collaboration, problem-solving using visual representations of data and processes of a mesosystem and everyone's unique perspectives.

Care map: A tool to assist families and the professionals they partner with in a person-centered process, which highlights a patient and family strengths and communicates both the big picture and the small details of all of the resources needed to support a patient and their family.

Care pathway: A care pathway is a complex intervention for the mutual decision-making and organization of care processes for a well-defined group of patients during a well-defined period.

Cause and effect diagram: A term used interchangeably with fishbone diagram, often called an Ishikawa diagram. Used to identify the causes of an effect that the microsystem is interested in.

Change ideas: Generated from literature review, best practices, benchmarking, and change concepts to select a change idea to test.

Clinical pathway: Clinical pathways (CPWs) are tools used to guide evidence-based health care. CPWs widely used since the 1980s, aim to translate clinical practice guideline recommendations into clinical processes of care within the unique culture and environment of the health-care institution, thereby maximizing patient safety and clinical efficiency.

Co-coaching methodology: A structured model of coaching an improvement team where two individual coaches form a co-coaching relationship with the team being coached. Identification of each coach's strengths and interests support the partners to coach technique, subject matter, and behavioral processes to support improvement success.

Complex adaptive system: A system in which many independent elements or agents interact, leading to emergent outcomes that are often difficult (or impossible) to predict simply by looking at the individual interactions.

Critical pathway: A clinical management tool that helps medical care providers coordinate the delivery of patient care for a particular case type or condition. As a guide to usual treatment patterns, a CP gives a view of the "big picture."

Cystic Fibrosis Transplant Consortium (CFLTC): A network of 10 academic lung transplant programs whose mission is to advance outcomes in cystic fibrosis patients who may need or have received a lung transplant.

Dartmouth Microsystem Improvement Ramp: A systematic approach which helps guide improvement teams gain an understanding of their core and supporting processes, identify global and specific aims, understand "causation" with fishbones, generate change ideas, and conduct rapid tests of change (PDSA cycles), and sustain improvement using SDSA cycles, and measures.

Discharge to assess (D2A): A care process to assess patient's needs after discharge in the patient's own home rather than in the hospital.

Effective meeting skills: Organized and structed meeting process consisting of timed agenda, meeting roles, **for example**, meeting leader, recorder, facilitator, and a timekeeper to ensure all members equally participate by creating and using ground rules, practice communication skills, and increase productive and value of meetings.

Exchange program: Clinical microsystems who belong to a "mesosystem" of care visit each other's microsystem, to observe work and delivery of care processes while developing relationships and new perspectives.

Flow coaching academy (FCA): Developed within the National Health Service (NHS) in the UK based on the Dartmouth Institute Microsystem Academy model and processes. The academy exists to provide a learning and development academy for healthcare professionals to increase improvement capabilities and successful improvement of processes and systems of care.

Flow coaching methodology: A model of replicable training in team coaching and technical improvement skills that equips staff at all levels to make sustained improvements to health and care outcomes, experience, and cost-effectiveness.

Frail people: A person who meets three or more criteria: unintentional loss of 10 or more pounds in the past year, weakness, exhaustion, trouble standing without assistance, or reduced grip strength.

Frailty assessment unit: Frail patients and elderly that present to an emergency department are comprehensively assessed by a multidisciplinary team to perform a comprehensive geriatric assessment in order to reduce unnecessary hospital admissions and reduce length of stay.

High-level process maps: Graphic representation using standard symbols to depict high-level steps in a selected process.

High-performing frontline teams: A multidisciplinary group of individuals who care for patients who have shared vision, defined roles and responsibilities, clear and respectful communication with mutual trust and respect in an environment of continuous learning and improvement (see Quality by Design, Chapter 1).

Improvement breakthrough series: A collaborative learning model of the IHI, which blends improvement and subject matter expertise in a shared learning system.

Institute for Healthcare Improvement (IHI): Founded in 1991, with a commitment to redesigning health care into a system without errors, waste, delays, and unsustainable costs, which has evolved to meet current and future health care challenges.

Integrated care pathway: Structured multidisciplinary care plans, which detail essential steps in the care of patients with a specific clinical problem.

Mesosystem: Two or more microsystems – **for example,** a patient pathway.

Microsystem improvement curriculum: See Dartmouth Microsystem Improvement Curriculum.

Mindfulness: The act of being attentive, aware, or careful.

Obeya methodology: In Japanese, a workspace where multidisciplinary teams gather to collaborate and coordinate. The walls of Obeyas are traditionally covered with paper boards, notes, sticky notes, and other materialization of the collective intelligence that emerges in this place. This method includes communication, cross-functional cooperation, and decision-making over time.

"Ownership" of the workplace: The sense of personal responsibility and accountability that employees have for their work, which involves taking the initiative to make a difference.

Plan-Do-Study-Act (PDSA): A model of continuous quality improvement that uses scientific approach, plan-do-study-act. Originally developed by Walter Shewhart and made popular by W. Edwards Deming, who ascribed inherent variation in processes to chance and intermittent variation to assignable causes. The PDSA cycle is a four-part method for discovering and correcting assignable causes to improve the quality of processes.

Playbook: The "how we do things" book. Written directions or "plays" for how different activities (usually standardized best practices) are completed on the unit. Consists of primarily a collection of best practice process maps to standardize care and processes that all staff are aware of and accountable for. Similar to "Standard Operating Procedure" SOP book.

Principles of systems engineering: Design, integration, and management of complex systems over their life cycle utilizing systems thinking principles.

Quality improvement assessment tool (QIA): The QIA is a validated survey to assess individual and aggregate team changes in quality improvement skill growth QI Importance and Confidence, QI Tools and Skills, Improvement Measurement, Communication and Team Dynamics, and Organizational Context and Leadership.

Relational coordination (RC): The theory of relational coordination proposes that highly interdependent work is most effectively coordinated through relationships of shared goals, shared knowledge, and mutual respect, and supported by frequent, timely, accurate, and problem-solving communication.

Standardize-Do-Study-Act (SDSA): A model for standardizing improvement, standardize-do-study-act. The steps taken when PDSA Cycle has been successfully done to achieve the original aim consistently- "best it can be" now. The purpose is to hold the gains that were made using PDSA cycles and standardize the process in daily work.

Structure, process, and outcome: A conceptual model by Donabedian (1980) for evaluating the quality of health care.

Vertically integrated provider: Providers fulfilling different functions along the care continuum.

AFTERWORD

Göran Henriks

Chief Executive of Learning and Innovation at Qulturum,
Region Jönköping County, Sweden

L et me first say that it is a great privilege to have the opportunity to contribute in such a profound context and writing. I admire all the authors in this book; they are my stars and role models. Thank you so much for summarizing 30 years of experience where Quality as Business Strategy has been in the forefront. The theory of Microsystems and Quality as a fundamental design process has given us so many improvement efforts, strong methods, and good tools in daily care to help us strengthen the relationship between the caregiver and the care recipient. Now to the focus of this afterword.

To Take Perspective Is to Take Charge of Tomorrow

A Search for Better Ways of Engaging for Complex Healthy Collaboration in Community and Care Organizations

Perspective-taking is the act of viewing a situation or understanding of a concept from an alternate point-of-view (Wikipedia, 2020).

Quality by Design: A Clinical Microsystems Approach, Second Edition. Edited by Marjorie M. Godfrey, Tina C. Foster, Julie K. Johnson, Eugene C. Nelson and Paul B. Batalden.
© 2025 John Wiley & Sons, Inc. Published 2025 by John Wiley & Sons, Inc.

Please consider my afterword as a positive provocation.

We can all recognize that digitalization and specialization/knowledge acceleration bring new challenges as well as great opportunities for modernizing our microsystems perspective. It will take new leadership actions, new ways of integrating learning into daily work, new metaphors, and the courage to *take perspective*. So, is it possible to see the wholeness of microsystems and teams with fresh eyes?

> *En este muno traidor*
>
> *No hay verdad ni mentira,*
>
> *Que todo esta en el color*
>
> *Del cristal con que se mira.*
>
> *(In this world of many mazes*
>
> *There is nothing false or true,*
>
> *All depends upon the hue*
>
> *Of the glass through which one gazes.)*
>
> ~ Sixteenth-century Spanish quatrain (Bell, 1924, p. 12)

We, as improvement advisers, managers, leaders, or quality designers are seeking to create better value in our processes and relationships. To make this happen, we must understand how complex systems adapt and evolve in response to the direct and indirect interactions of all stakeholders, the different goals they have, the diversity of resources they can access and use, the outcomes they prioritize and often, the widely different (and sometimes conflicting) values that drive their actions. So . . .

- What will be required to "take perspective" on microsystems in a fast-changing world?
- Can we combine the benefits of modern learning ideas in both micro-, meso-, and macrosystems to create the value we seek for our patients and communities?
- What does the new perspective look like?

What Will Be Required to "Take Perspective" on Microsystems in a Fast-Changing World?

The era of the Internet and the personal health record greatly expand the types of information and evidence available to patients. Importantly, in a true learning healthcare system, learning is bidirectional: working not only to support better-informed patients but also to ensure that patient preference is incorporated for "best care." These perspectives introduce the complexities and possibilities of a truly patient-centered healthcare system, one which seeks to learn from patients and provide the means for collaboration in the delivery of care.

To "take perspective" means for us to develop a deeper understanding of the concepts inherent in coproduction. This open doors to new research areas and drives the development of new scientific platforms. It will not be enough to use traditional biological and medical sciences; the social sciences and their research methods will become ever more important. Social science and research will influence our thinking and require us to collaborate with informed and educated individuals who live with chronic diseases. The microsystem and mesosystem tools and methods described in this book come in very handy as we seek to make these important changes in the clinical setting. Well used, these models and methods can also improve our ability to develop and coproduce services with the whole population as equal partners in health decision-making.

To "take perspective" also means the efforts we put into thinking about our services. It is service design models that provide the types of information needed. These models can give the patients and families ownership of the care processes, as "service-givers" become guests in the data warehouses owned by the patients about themselves. A new level of reliability develops, one which will require us to develop new rules of engagement about accountability for the integrity of data, communication and response, and safeguarding privacy. Reliability and safety are, as described in the book, key quality components for the modern complex healthcare system.

Can We Combine the Benefits of Modern Learning Ideas at Both Micro-, Meso-, and Macrosystems to Create the Value We Seek for Our Patients and Communities?

Learning has transformational power. Learning is a qualitative change in the way we perceive and understand something, rather than a simple quantitative change (that you know more than before). Learning allows us to understand different phenomena in new ways. According to John Dewey (1997), an education reformer, experiential learning occurs through reflective activities. One can have experiences, but without reflection, there is no learning.

This is why microsystems and small teams have many advantages. They can respond quickly, communicate freely, and make decisions without layers of bureaucracy. But this is not enough for the fast-developing, steep learning curves of our new systems. Without a systemic culture of learning, our services will become insufficient and outdated. A first sign of this may be when systems focus more on productivity than the main purpose of the work. The response must be learning how to promote patients' and relatives' opportunities to interact, integrate needed information, and improve their knowledge.

Today, the context moves so quickly that we need everybody to act as if they have "two jobs." The first job is to deliver the daily work processes and services to a level that is expected. The second job is for everyone to improve the work processes and improve their own competence in the daily work (Batalden and Davidoff, 2007). This means we must recognize two challenges at the same time for micro-, meso-, and macrosystems – knowledge use and knowledge development.

What Does It Look Like to "Take Perspective" of Coproduction and Digitalization?

The microsystem is where people (patients) with a need and the professionals have both become experts in working "upstream" in a spirit of collaboration. They both see how the modern digital world helps them better understand the "now" much better and to anticipate the future.

Both patients and professionals work and learn together in new learning improvement practices where the two learners' partnership feels natural and anticipating and planning the future has a natural place. The awareness of data and facts is beneficial for everyone and with that come expectations of competence and relevance. Healthcare services are becoming more and more "digi-physical" (a combination of virtual connections with physical meetings) where feedback loops are quick and require timely reactions and responses. This develops a "stronger customer" who can both know more and own more data (the "digi world"). The expectation of trustworthy relations, continuity, and an equally current service provider becomes crucial for the results of a therapy or a treatment.

We have good examples where systems and management test tomorrow's solutions and make them today's opportunities. These organizations have transformed their business strategies to recognize:

- Health is the strategy
- Care from hospital to "homespital," with more and more service provided in the local setting
- Responsibility and knowledge-based services

These systems have management that talk about a paradigm shift: daily work needs a mind-space for proactivity and upstream actions. Three systems that exemplify this are Southcentral Foundation, Alaska (https://www.southcentralfoundation.com/), Cincinnati Children's (https://www.cincinnatichildrens.org/), and Public Health

Scotland (formerly NHS Health Scotland; http://www.healthscotland.scot/). They promise person-centeredness, trustworthy relationships, improved knowledge about the health of the local community, and they try hard to see the wholeness of the individuals and families they serve. They have improved the digital processes of the work and invest in how work can be improved with daily feedback systems added to traditional patient records.

A world of increased socioeconomic polarization provides a new context of job disruption for health and care and a demand for new skills. Primary and specialty care systems in close partnership with public health have a critical role to play in preparing themselves as partner service organizations for coproduction and competent organizations for the global citizens where health, homespitals, and measures of success in changing outcomes becomes central. To inspire and make this happen, it is good to remember what Scotland's retiring chief medical officer Harry Burns stated, "We need compassion, not judgements about poor people" (Hetherington, 2014). He continued on to describe the risk of poor living circumstances and why compassion and being together are so essential.

A Third Revolution

Health care has become global. When a pandemic hits the globe, we immediately connect with friends working in the same area of interest all over the world at the same time. We learn from people in Taiwan, Australia, Singapore, England, Brazil, USA, and Scandinavia using digital platforms. Experiences are compared, data exchanged, and the conclusions are reached together. We harmonize not only our perspectives on opportunities but also our platforms of possible solutions. Today, most countries in the world share the same language of needs, ideas, and what is important for success. The world becomes a learning improvement community.

We understand the need of a service system to move toward a vision of "health happens at home and hospitals repair." The tempo is increased and the preparation of the transformation happens digitally across borders. All systems share the value that in order for trust in a service to develop, open access to a primary care must be promised. They strive to achieve the best possible outcome by strengthening the pathways (mesosystems) for the patients. Patients and professionals codesigning models of care, both in primary and specialty care, build trust during the process of learning and improving. The system and all those in it can see the person, not just the diagnosis and can co-create a common, holistic view of the patient journey.

Another ambition is to minimize the time in hospital for patients who do not need intensive care. Management and leaders are "pushed" into system thinking on all levels at the same time when strong polarities are parts of the daily leadership performance. Examples of these polarities that we can see today are:

- Invest in upstream preventive care and intensive care at the same time.
- Develop more and more self-screening processes and increase the speed and accuracy of medical diagnosis (think artificial intelligence).
- Promote more and more self-learning and ensure that ever greater competence develops.
- We know the importance of Public Health and we still need Specialist Care for knowledge.

These polarities will be managed when systems have a learning organization culture on all levels – where daily work is viewed as the school where each employee has the power and the capacity to minimize gaps in performance and improve competence in the work processes and effectively coproduce care with patients and families.

To achieve all this, coaching becomes key for all managers and process leaders. A team coaching approach allows the language and communication to be both diagnostic and dialogic. It creates places and moments in daily work where the good questions can come to the fore as a coach helps individuals reflect on their work. In such a community of practice, collaborative, or new model of organization, it is fun to increase the opportunities to make breakthrough results. Daily feedback systems with huddles and dashboards keep the focus on how we are doing from the patient's point of view. Togetherness can be achieved through "taking perspective," "thinking upstream," and "acting proactively" across all organizations, at all levels and by all individuals with a shared purpose. The microsystem approach provides a superior and strong model to help achieve these ideas and enables us to focus on the individual, micro-, meso-, and macrosystems to learn what is best for the populations we care for.

References

Batalden, P.B. and Davidoff, F. (2007). What is "quality improvement" and how can it transform healthcare? *Quality & Safety in Health Care* 16 (1); 2–3, doi: 10.1136/qshc.2006.022046.

Dell, A.F.G. (1924). *A Pilgrim in Spain*, 12. Boston, MA: Little, Brown, and Company.

Dewey, J. (1997). *Democracy and Education: An Introduction to the Philosophy of Education.* New York, NY: The Free Press.

Hetherington, P. "Harry Burns: 'We need compassion, not judgments about poor people.'" [https://www.theguardian.com/society/2014/mar/12/harry-burns-scotland-chief-medical-officer-health]. *The Guardian*, Mar. 12, 2014.

Wikipedia. "Perspective-taking." [https://en.wikipedia.org/wiki/Perspective-taking]. Apr. 2020.

Additional Resources

Cincinnati Children's Hospital Medical Center, https://www.cincinnatichildrens.org/

Public Health Scotland (previously NHS Health Scotland), http://www.healths cotland.scot/

Southcentral Foundation, Alaska, https://www.southcentralfoundation.com/

APPENDIX: ACCELERATING IMPROVEMENT IN CLINICAL MESOSYSTEMS

Action Guide

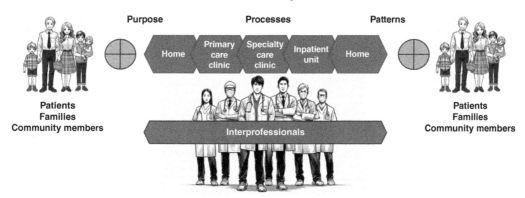

Marjorie M. Godfrey, PhD, MS, BSN, FAAN and Coua Early, MS

© 2024, Marjorie M. Godfrey, all rights reserved.

Quality by Design: A Clinical Microsystems Approach, Second Edition. Edited by Marjorie M. Godfrey, Tina C. Foster, Julie K. Johnson, Eugene C. Nelson and Paul B. Batalden.
© 2025 John Wiley & Sons, Inc. Published 2025 by John Wiley & Sons, Inc.

An instructional video and additional materials to guide you in
Accelerating Improvement in Clinical Mesosystems Action Guide
can be found at
clinicalmicrosystem.org.

The video provides a high-level roadmap of the improvement process along with step-by-step instructions and details for this Action Guide.

Additional worksheets, examples, and the fundamental improvement electronic learning modules are also available.

NOTE: We have developed this Action Guide to give ideas to those interested in improving health care in micro- and mesosystems. The Microsystem Academy and the developers of this Action Guide are pleased to grant use of these materials without charge, provided recognition is given for their development, and that use is limited to an individual's own use and not for resale.

Table of Contents

Aim: The aim of *Accelerating Improvement in Clinical Mesosystems Action Guide* is to increase microsystem/mesosystem awareness and attention to the larger system of care – the mesosystem processes, communication, and relationships between individual microsystems that form a "pathway" of care for a population of patients. This Action Guide can support improvers to see the "forest" or 30,000-ft view of the pathway of care (mesosystem) and identify the "trees" (microsystems) that contribute to the mesosystem.

Important References and Resources

This "Quality by Design: A Clinical Microsystems Approach, 2nd Edition" dedicates significant attention to the mesosystem level of a health system, recognizing its crucial role in healthcare quality improvement. (Godfrey, M. M., Foster, T., Johnson, J. K., et al. San Francisco, CA: Jossey-Bass, 2025)

Key Resources in "Quality by Design" (2nd Edition)

- **Co-Production of care with those providing care and those receiving care:** Regularly practicing partnership with those being served to inform improvement and innovation.
- **Mesosystem Leadership and Team Coaching:** The book emphasizes the importance of leadership at all levels of the organization – microsystem, mesosystem, and macrosystem levels. The book provides guidance on how leaders can foster collaboration, communication, and alignment across microsystems to achieve shared mesosystem goals. Additionally, the behavior and skills of a Team Coach are introduced to help busy multidisciplinary improvement teams.
- **Data and Information Technology:** It highlights the vital role of data and information technology in mesosystem improvement, discussing how data and measurement can provide feed forward-feedback systems, data tracking with dashboards to track performance of micro- and mesosystems and identify improvement opportunities to sustain improvement.
- **Value-Based Care Models:** The book explores how value-based care models can be implemented at the mesosystem level to improve outcomes and reduce costs, providing examples and case studies of successful implementations.
- **Expanded Case Studies:** The 2nd edition includes international case studies that illustrate the principles and practices of mesosystem improvement in a variety of healthcare settings.
- **Worksheets:** The suggested worksheets in this Action Guide can be digital worksheets as well as hard copy depending on local capabilities.

By utilizing the resources and strategies outlined in "Quality by Design, 2nd Edition" healthcare organizations can gain valuable insights into how to optimize their mesosystem systems and ultimately deliver higher quality care to their patients.

The original textbook, *"Quality by Design: A Clinical Microsystems Approach"* by Nelson, Batalden, and Godfrey (2007), provides a strong theoretical foundation and practical guidance for improving healthcare quality at the microsystem level that can be adapted at the mesosystem level.

* _"Assess, Diagnose and Treat"_ form the structure for improvement.

Accelerating the Rate of Improvement in Clinical Mesosystems

Mesosystem improvement is like improving microsystems but more complex. Connecting healthcare professionals from multiple microsystems to assess and "see" the whole system of mesosystem care can be challenging.

Learning about the details of the multiple systems and multiple cultures that exist in a mesosystem can help inform process, structure, outcomes, and improvement strategies. Mesosystem members can increase their sense of "ownership" and result in an "awakening" about the mesosystem and the opportunities to learn more about the overall system of care to support continuous improvement for those being served.

When multiple interdependent microsystems form a "mesosystem," semipermeable boundaries are present that mediate relationships with patients and family and with many support services and other microsystems. These boundaries are not often recognized, studied, or intentionally improved. Instead of collaborating to understand the entire care system and improve it together, people on both sides of the boundaries often resort to blaming each other's processes and staff.

When systems are well-coordinated, care transitions smoothly, information is readily shared, and patients feel supported and empowered throughout their healthcare journey. This leads to improved patient satisfaction, better health outcomes, reduced healthcare costs, and improved staff sense of engagement. In addition, mesosystem improvement efforts can tackle system wide challenges, identify how care is coordinated or not across different units, pinpoint missing or ineffective connections communication between those microsystems, and enhance relationships between microsystem members presenting a mesosystem "team" approach to care and services to those being served.

Edgar Schein cautioned improvers that "health care improvement often risks being too 'technocratic' and losing sight of the people who provide care and services and the people who receive the care and services." Mesosystem improvement efforts show improved communication and relationships within and between multiple microsystems in a mesosystem, illustrating that mesosystems can achieve impressive improvement outcomes with a strong emphasis on the people receiving and providing care and services. Mesosystem members report the importance of regular communication, meeting in person, sharing specific patient knowledge and engaging in shared care of the population being served. Further, mesosystem members acknowledge the importance of a standard improvement methodology, protected time to assess, improve and reflect on how care and services are provided, and the role of patient and family partners to coproduce care.

The "Forest" (30,000 Foot View)

This Action Guide helps healthcare professionals visualize the entire patient care journey, from initial contact to post-treatment follow-up. This "big picture" view allows for the identification of key milestones, transitions, and potential bottlenecks in the care process. By understanding the overall flow of care, improvers can identify opportunities to streamline processes, improve coordination, communication and relationships between microsystems to enhance the patient experience.

The "Trees" (Microsystems within the Mesosystem)

Within the larger "forest" of the care pathway, this Action Guide also helps identify the individual "trees," which represent the various microsystems that contribute to the mesosystem. These microsystems could include specific clinical departments, teams, or units that interact with the patient at different stages of their care journey. Every microsystem has its own distinct culture which can be explored to find shared purpose for populations of patients and facilitate improved communication and relationships. By examining each microsystem, improvers can pinpoint areas for improvement in communication, collaboration, processes, and care delivery.

Key Benefits of This Approach

- **Holistic Understanding:** By seeing both the forest and the trees, healthcare professionals gain a more holistic understanding of the complex interactions within the care pathway.
- **Targeted Interventions:** This understanding enables the identification of specific areas where interventions can have the most significant impact on patient outcomes and system performance.
- **Enhanced Collaboration:** This Action Guide fosters collaboration between different microsystems by highlighting their interconnectedness, handoffs, transitions, and shared goals.
- **Continuous Improvement:** This approach supports a culture of continuous improvement by encouraging multidisciplinary multi-microsystem members to meet regularly and learn about their contributions to the overall pathway of care.

Overall, this Action Guide empowers healthcare improvers to **see the big picture while also focusing on the details**, enhances the effectiveness and patient-centeredness of care, and plays a crucial role in eliminating waste, rework, poor communication and relationships, and misunderstandings within the workforce.

Bronfenbrenner emphasized that it is the way in which members of the system perceive relationships that is crucial (Bronfenbrenner, 1979). Effective microsystems can facilitate optimal development of the mesosystem and are characterized by a network of enduring and reciprocal caring relationships. Conversely, high-risk microsystems are characterized by a lack of mutually rewarding relationships and/ or the presence of destructive interactions.

Reference

Bronfenbrenner, U. (1979). *The ecology of human development: Experiments by nature and design.* Cambridge, MA: Harvard University Press.

Mesosystem Assessment

We have gained a great deal of experience and knowledge about the benefits of helping frontline teams see and improve their clinical microsystem, often resulting in a sense of **"ownership" of the workplace**. The reality is healthcare frequently occurs in multiple microsystems (not just one microsystem) that may be well coordinated or not for the benefit of patients and families. People, who may be known as patients, families, and community members may have needs that extend beyond just one microsystem. Their care and service needs may include clinical microsystems, e.g., emergency department, intensive care unit; medical-surgical units *and* supporting multiple microsystems, e.g., laboratory, diagnostic, information, dietary; and finance units during care delivery. Collectively, this is called the mesosystem. The mesosystem may be called a **clinical pathway**, a **care path**, **care pathway**, **integrated care pathway**, **critical pathway**, a service line, or **care map** that meets the particular needs of an identified person or population.

No matter what it is called, a mesosystem is a collection of microsystems that come together intentionally or unintentionally and can be recognized *or not* as a system of care to provide care and services to an identified population. Often a collection of clinical and supporting microsystems who provide care and services to meet people's needs do not function as a mesosystem. The mesosystem members frequently do not see themselves as contributing to a larger system of care in a pathway for a population of patients. Rather, they see themselves as individual independent units or silos and not as an interdependent and connected "pathway" equally interested in helping each unique microsystem to be the best they can to provide the best care and services for those being served.

Identifying representatives from each microsystem within a mesosystem to form a mesosystem improvement team can begin the improvement efforts to improve the larger system while simultaneously improving the individual microsystems. The mesosystem improvement team can begin to place the spotlight on the "whole system" and help individual microsystem members begin to see their role in the overall patient/family community member experience of care. This holistic perspective is essential for identifying bottlenecks, inefficiencies, and opportunities for collaboration across the entire care pathway.

As the team delves deeper into this process, people begin to connect with people beyond their usual professional circles and microsystems. Individuals in different roles start to see commonalities and opportunities to collaborate, becoming more efficient and consistent. In many cases, these connections even blossom into friendships, fostering a positive and supportive work environment.

Mesosystem Leadership

Leaders at all levels of the healthcare system can support these "places" to create conditions of excellence in the frontlines of care delivery. High-reliability organizations described by Weick and colleagues are "mindful" of their interdependent interactions (Weick, 2002; Weick and Sutcliffe, 2001). To support "**mindfulness**" of mesosystems and interdependent interactions, the **M3 matrix** (Quality by Design, 2007, 206–209) (see pg. 64) highlights specific actions leaders can take to ensure the expectations and conditions of excellence are in place. This not only supports individual microsystem excellence but also fosters collaboration among multiple microsystems (mesosystems) to increase their awareness of their interdependent interactions. When improvement teams do have opportunities to meet, their attention tends to be directed toward their individual microsystem rather than the broader system-wide perspective. Most members of microsystems are accustomed to focusing on their specific role within the care pathway, rather than understanding the whole system. Engaging patient and family partners can be a valuable strategy to overcome this limitation, as they can offer a unique perspective on the overall patient journey and help identify areas for improvement across the entire system.

Leaders within the mesosystem can:

- ensure protected time for multidisciplinary improvement teams which include those being served (patients, families, members of the community) to assess and improve microsystems and mesosystems using standard improvement processes.
- create a shared vision.
- facilitate access to needed data and information.
- align microsystem goals with mesosystem improvement by seeing the view of the "forest and the trees" from the "balcony (30,000-foot system view) and the dance floor (frontline care delivery)" (Heifetz et al., 2009).
- identify barriers and address obstacles that hinder collaboration and improvement efforts.
- role model and set expectations of relationship building communication and partnership.
- meet regularly to review mesosystem improvement progress and problem solve.

References

Weick, K. E. (2001). *Making sense of the organization.* Malden, MA: Blackwell.

Weick, K. E., & Sutcliffe, K. M. (2001). *Managing the unexpected: Assuring high performance in an age of complexity.* San Francisco, CA: Jossey-Bass.

Nelson, E. C., Batalden, P. B., & Godfrey, M. M. (2007). *Quality by design: A clinical microsystems approach.* San Francisco, CA: Jossey-Bass.

Heifetz, R. A., Grashow, A., & Linsky, M. (2009). *The practice of adaptive leadership: Tools and tactics for changing your organization and the world.* Cambridge, MA: Harvard Business Press.

To help improvement teams learn about and assess clinical mesosystems and the larger system of care, the **Accelerating Improvement in Clinical Mesosystems Action Guide** empowers multidisciplinary improvement teams across multiple microsystems in the mesosystem to take a holistic approach to healthcare improvement, resulting in better outcomes for patients, families, and the healthcare workforce. Improvement teams can gain a deeper understanding of their healthcare system's microsystem and mesosystem strengths and opportunities for improvement. This knowledge can empower data-driven improvement decisions and implement targeted interventions that result in meaningful improvements in care delivery and improved communication and relationships.

This action guide serves as a valuable resource for multidisciplinary improvement teams to:

1. **Visualize:** Clearly depict the entire care pathway, highlighting the interactions between microsystems and the larger mesosystem. (Forest-trees or Balcony-dance floor metaphors).
2. **Assess:** Evaluate the performance of both microsystems and the overall care pathway (mesosystem), identifying strengths and improvement opportunities.
3. **Optimize:** Develop and implement targeted interventions to enhance system coordination, communication, relationships, streamline processes, and improve patient care.

The Action Guide's **dual focus** allows improvement teams to:

1. **Understand the Big Picture:** Visualize the entire care pathway (mesosystem) to identify bottlenecks, redundancies, and opportunities for improvement.
2. **Zoom in on Details:** Assess individual microsystems to understand their unique contributions to the overall care process and identify areas for targeted interventions.
3. **Improve System Coordination:** By understanding the interactions between microsystems and the larger care pathway, teams can identify and address communication breakdowns, information gaps, and other barriers to effective coordination between parts of the mesosystem.
4. **Enhance Patient Care:** Ultimately, by optimizing both microsystems and mesosystems, healthcare organizations can deliver more efficient, effective, and patient-centered care.

5. **Improve Staff Efficiency:** Streamline workflows, eliminate redundancies, and optimize resource utilization to maximize staff productivity and reduce burnout.

Designing an Approach for Mesosystem Improvement

Leaders can consider multiple approaches for mesosystem improvement. Quality by Design, 2nd Edition, highlights case examples of two different approaches to improve mesosystem performance and outcomes (Sheffield Big Room and Lung Transplant Mesosystem Improvement).

There are many other approaches to consider within the local context, organization strategic plans, and available resources. A few examples include:

- C Suite-driven (Executive leaders) initiatives to improve subpopulation/diagnosis pathways using taskforces to conduct most of the preliminary performance data analysis, identify specific "best practices," identify key performance indicators of the selected pathway and strategically implement change with the microsystems involved in the pathway mesosystem.
- Local frontline mesosystem improvement led by microsystem leaders implemented by convening representatives of each microsystem as a lead improvement team to review pathway mesosystem performance data, identify strengths and improvement opportunities, and prioritize improvement cycles with frontline staff.

Any mesosystem improvement approach is dependent on the specific context, needs and available resources, and strategy of the organization. Leadership must be deeply involved in selecting an improvement approach, ensuring it aligns with the organization's strategic goals. This includes fostering a culture of continuous learning and improvement, building staff capacity to participate in improvement initiatives, developing leadership skills for change management, partnering with patients and families, promoting diversity and inclusion, and addressing staff burnout. By considering these factors, leaders can increase ownership and engagement, ensure sustainability, maximize resources, and ultimately achieve meaningful improvements in quality, safety, and patient experience. This requires clear communication of strategic goals, careful evaluation of potential approaches, provision of necessary resources and support, ongoing monitoring and evaluation, and a willingness to adapt as needed.

The desired timeline for results will also influence the choice of the improvement approach. Some approaches may yield quicker results, while others may require a longer-term commitment. It is important to balance the need for immediate improvements with the desire for sustainable, long-term change.

- **Immediate Mesosystem Focus (Sheffield Model):** This approach may be suitable when there's a strong sense of urgency, a shared vision for improvement, and existing relationships between microsystem members. It fosters rapid collaboration and system-wide thinking from the outset.

o **Strategic Planning:** This top-down approach begins with a high-level overview of the entire mesosystem, creating a strategic plan that outlines the desired outcomes and key goals. The plan then guides the improvement work within each microsystem, ensuring alignment with the broader mesosystem objectives.

o **Key Intervention:** "Big Room" meetings for multidisciplinary collaboration, problem-solving, and tests of change. Focused immediately on bringing together all members of the mesosystem (acute care and community teams) to learn and improve collectively.

- **Staged Approach (Lung Transplant Mesosystem):** This "inside-out improvement" approach may be preferable when microsystems have varying levels of improvement readiness or when there's a need to build trust and relationships between teams before tackling system-wide issues. It allows each microsystem to develop its internal capabilities and gain a deeper understanding of its role within the larger system. This approach focuses on continuous improvement within individual microsystems first. Teams learn and apply improvement methodologies within their own unit before expanding their efforts to collaborate across microsystems in mesosystems. This bottom-up approach empowers frontline staff and builds a culture of continuous improvement from the ground up.

o **Key Intervention:** Structured phases of assessment and interventions in a dual approach including local "microsystem" assessment to practice improvement language and processes to lead to "mesosystem" assessment and improvement.

- An important difference between Sheffield and the Lung Transplant mesosystem improvement design is Sheffield focused immediately on convening the mesosystem members to learn improvement together while the Lung Transplant program executed a staged approach, developing improvement capabilities and mesosystem awareness within each microsystem before convening the mesosystem.

o Sheffield focused more on the physical flow of patients and system-level changes, while Lung Transplant emphasized communication, relationships, and coordination between microsystems with process flows.

Key Similarities of both cases:

- Focused on improving the quality and efficiency of care for a specific patient population and included patients in the improvement journey.
- Utilized an adapted clinical microsystem process including rigorous assessments of systems and performance (e.g., process mapping, data analysis).
- Emphasized collaboration, data-driven decision-making, and continuous improvement.
- Effective meeting skills and roles resulted in efficient and productive meetings.

Developing Staged Improvement from Microsystems to the Mesosystem

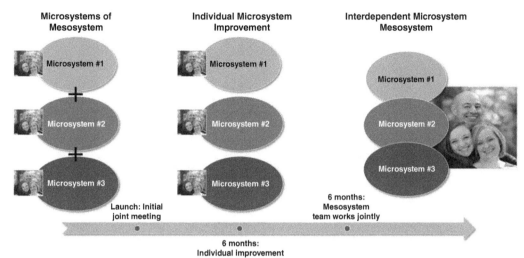

- Plan-Do-Study-Act (PDSA) cycles for testing changes.
- Multidisciplinary improvement teams including patients and families.
- QI team coaches provided guidance, support, and expertise in improvement methodologies.
- Both cases illustrated the "misunderstandings" that can exist between microsystems within a mesosystem when regular efforts to meet to understand each other's role and contribution to the population mesosystem have not occurred.
- Both demonstrated successful outcomes in terms of improved processes, decreased length of stay, enhanced patient experiences, and improved communication and relationships.

Guidance for Improving Mesosystems

This Action Guide, with its focus on visualizing and optimizing the entire care pathway," the whole system" offers a powerful tool for improving system coordination. By identifying bottlenecks, clarifying roles and responsibilities, and promoting relationship building communication, this guide can help healthcare organizations create a more seamless and patient-centered experience. This can lead to better health outcomes, increased patient satisfaction, and a more efficient and effective healthcare system with a happier multidisciplinary mesosystem team.

Recommendations for Using Both Quality by Design 1st and 2nd Editions

- **Start with Quality by Design, 1st Edition:**
  - o   If you are new to the concept of clinical microsystems, we recommend starting with the original textbook to gain a solid understanding of the theory and principles behind this approach.
  - o   As you work through the action guide, refer to Quality by Design, 1st Edition, for additional guidance and support. The textbook can serve as a valuable reference resource as you navigate the challenges of disciplined quality improvement.

    NOTE: Part Two of the first edition of Quality by Design can be found at www.clinicalmicrosystem.org

- **Use the Action Guide:** Once you have a grasp of the theoretical foundation, use the action guide to put the principles into practice. The guide provides practical steps and tools to help you implement quality improvement initiatives in your own microsystem and across a mesosystem.

By using both resources in tandem, you can equip yourself with the knowledge and skills needed to drive meaningful change in your healthcare organization.

Your Mesosystem and Interdependent Microsystems

Assess, Diagnose, and Treat Your Mesosystem Which Consists of Interdependent Microsystems. Strategies for improving "The place where patients, families, and care teams meet."

AN OVERVIEW

People have many interdisciplinary health professionals coming together with them and their families to create care and services across the pathway of care. We call this place where patients, families, and care teams come together from many microsystems of care, the *Clinical Mesosystem*.

Clinical mesosystem

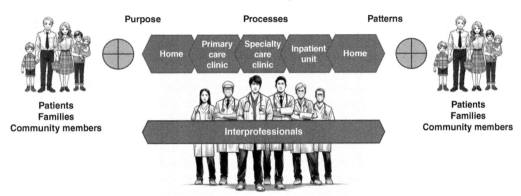

Your ***clinical mesosystem*** consists of individual ***microsystems*** as shown in the diagram. Collectively, these microsystems come together to form a mesosystem that provides comprehensive care for a specific pathway or subpopulation. Your mesosystem has essential functions that can be assessed and improved to achieve the best possible outcomes, not only for each individual microsystem but also for the overall quality of care within the entire mesosystem.

The quality of care each person receives depends on both the effectiveness of each microsystem and the seamlessness of the "handoffs" between microsystems within the mesosystem. Mesosystems encompass not only patients and families but also staff, processes, technology, and recurring patterns of information, behavior, and results.

The microsystem and mesosystem are where:

- Care is delivered.
- Quality, safety, reliability, efficiency, and innovation are realized.
- Staff morale and patient satisfaction are cultivated.
- Handoff and transitions are smooth (or not).
- Communication and relationships are productive and add value (or not).

Clinical mesosystems are the frontline units that provide day-to-day health care. The mesosystem can most easily be thought of as the "multiple places where patients, families, and healthcare professionals meet."

Technically, clinical microsystems are seen as the smallest replicable units and basic building blocks of the mesosystem and ultimately the macrosystem:

> "A small group of people who work together on a regular basis to provide care to discrete **subpopulations of patients**. It has clinical and business aims, linked processes, and a shared information environment and it produces performance **outcomes**."

Clinical microsystems (the places where care is delivered within home care, a specialty program, or an inpatient unit) are the building blocks that form the system of care (mesosystems) and macrosystems.

For quality of care to be improved and sustained, continuous work is required both within individual microsystems and across the entire mesosystem. Therefore, all healthcare professionals – including everyone working within the mesosystem as a whole – have two essential jobs.

Job One: Provide high-quality, safe, patient, and family centered care.

Job Two: Continually improve coproduced care with patients, families, and interprofessionals.

To effectively accomplish both the delivery of care and continuous improvement, these efforts must be seamlessly integrated into the everyday activities of everyone involved. Without this dedicated focus on continually enhancing both work processes and care provision, optimal quality cannot be achieved, and neither the mesosystem nor its individual microsystems will perform at their highest potential.

How Might We "See" the Mesosystem of Care?

Convene a few microsystem leaders/clinicians from the microsystems within the mesosystem to map out a "high-level" 30,000 "forest view" or Catwalk view of the pathway of care. This small group will then draft the high-level pathway of the process of care for the individual microsystems to review and "customize" to their own context. Each microsystem will identify transitions between each step or phase in the overall mesosystem including communication, education, handoffs, and processes.

An example is the Cystic Fibrosis Lung Transplant Transition Mesosystem 30,000 Foot view: 8 Phase Model

Cystic fibrosis lung transplant eight phases

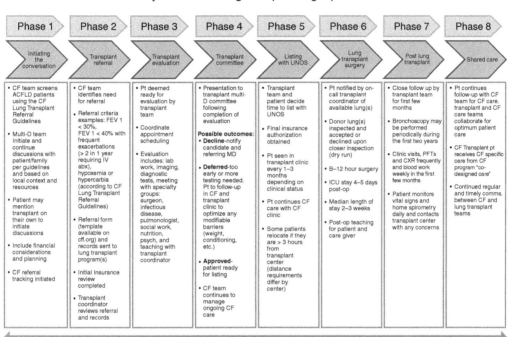

Phase 1	Phase 2	Phase 3	Phase 4	Phase 5	Phase 6	Phase 7	Phase 8
Initiating the conversation	Transplant referral	Transplant evaluation	Transplant committee	Listing with UNOS	Lung transplant surgery	Post lung transplant	Shared care
• CF team screens ACFLD patients using the CF Lung Transplant Referral Guidelines • Multi-D team Initiate and continue discussions with patient/family per guidelines and based on local context and resources • Patient may mention transplant on their own to initiate discussions • Include financial considerations and planning • CF referral tracking initiated	• CF team identifies need for referral • Referral criteria examples: FEV 1 < 30%, FEV 1 < 40% with frequent exacerbations (> 2 in 1 year requiring IV abx), hypoxemia or hypercarbia (according to CF Lung Transplant Referral Guidelines) • Referral form (template available on cff.org) and records sent to lung transplant program(s) • Initial Insurance review completed • Transplant coordinator reviews referral and records	• Pt deemed ready for evaluation by transplant team • Coordinate appointment scheduling • Evaluation includes: lab work, imaging, diagnostic tests, meeting with specialty groups: surgeon, infectious disease, pulmonologist, social work, nutrition, psych, and teaching with transplant coordinator	• Presentation to transplant multi-D committee following completion of evaluation **Possible outcomes:** • **Decline**-notify candidate and referring MD • **Deferred**-too early or more testing needed. Pt to follow-up in CF and transplant clinic to optimize any modifiable barriers (weight, conditioning, etc.) • **Approved**-patient ready for listing • CF team continues to manage ongoing CF care	• Transplant team and patient decide time to list with UNOS • Final insurance authorization obtained • Pt seen in transplant clinic every 1–3 months depending on clinical status • Pt continues CF care with CF clinic • Some patients relocate if they are > 3 hours from transplant center (distance requirements differ by center)	• Pt notified by on-call transplant coordinator of available lung(s) • Donor lung(s) inspected and accepted or declined upon closer inspection (dry run) • 8–12 hour surgery • ICU stay 4–5 days post-op • Median length of stay 2–3 weeks • Post-op teaching for patient and care giver	• Close follow up by transplant team for first few months • Bronchoscopy may be performed periodically during the first two years • Clinic visits, PFTs and CXR frequently and blood work weekly in the first few months • Patient monitors vital signs and home spirometry daily and contacts transplant center with any concerns	• Pt continues follow-up with CF team for CF care. transplant and CF care teams collaborate for optimum patient care • CF Transplant pt receives CF specific care from CF program "co-designed care" • Continued regular and timely comms. between CF and lung transplant teams

Palliative care

Shared, co-designed and coproduced care, relational coordination

Overview of Accelerating Mesosystem Improvement

A Path Forward

This Action Guide provides a path forward for you and those who work with you to a higher level of performance. Just as you can assess, diagnose, and treat patients, you can assess, diagnose, and treat your mesosystem (pathway) and clinical microsystems (e.g., Primary Care, Specialty Care clinics, ED, OR, Inpatient units).

The steps in this Action Guide help you evaluate how your mesosystem functions and how it can be improved. The tools and forms are based upon the experiences and research of individuals and clinical teams including programs around the United States and the world. Although this is not the only way in which improvement can be achieved, it is a way that has been demonstrated to be effective in achieving higher quality and value care, enhanced workforce morale, satisfaction, and partnerships with patients and their families.

All Action Guide forms, and additional information, tools, and examples are available at clinicalmicrosystem.org.

For a clinical microsystem and a mesosystem to achieve optimal performance, the steps for enabling improvement are ones that are never ending. Once one cycle of improvement is completed, another cycle can begin and then many more cycles will follow. Opportunities for improvement are never ending as patient care and the work – life experience can always be improved.

Selecting the Mesosystem Method to Guide Improvements

Before embarking on the path forward, leadership should determine the mesosystem method that will best guide their improvement efforts. There are several options to consider:

1. **The "Big Room" Approach:** Leaders regularly convene representatives from each microsystem in the mesosystem/pathway "big room" to learn improvement methodology together, assess the mesosystem as a whole, and collaboratively test changes (https://flowcoaching.academy).
2. **Individual Microsystem Focus:** Leaders provide an overarching vision for the mesosystem/pathway, but initially support improvement efforts within each individual microsystem. Microsystem members learn and practice improvement methods in their own context, developing a shared language and process before coming together to address the larger mesosystem (clinicalmicrosystem.org).
3. **Alternative Methods:** Leaders may choose to explore other approaches tailored to their specific needs and resources. These could include hybrid models, external consultation, or innovative strategies developed within their own organization.

Utilize the Clinical Microsystem/Mesosystem Approach

Part Two in Quality by Design, 1st Edition, provides a step-by-step process to assess, diagnose, and treat the clinical microsystem using the Dartmouth Microsystem Improvement Curriculum (DMIC) as a "ramp of improvement." (Pages 197–386). The same method can be used for mesosystem improvement once a theme is selected for the microsystems to work on together. Part Two is also available at clinicalmicrosystem.org.

Dartmouth Microsystem Improvement Curriculum Improvement Ramp

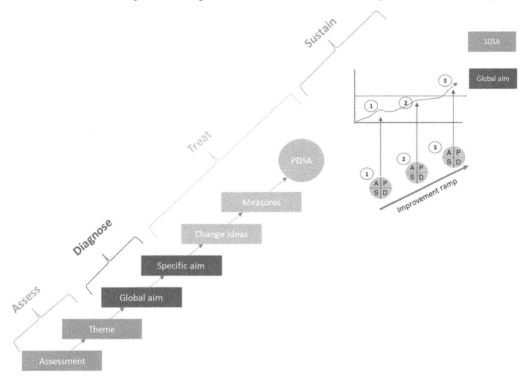

Based on improvement colleagues in the field over the past decade, the DMIC ramp of improvement has been updated as a "Microsystem Improvement Process (MIP) Spiral." As the "MIP" figure illustrates, the central focus of improvement in the micro- or mesosystem is patients and families, forming the "spine" of the spiral.

The grey shades of ribbon define the "assess, diagnose, improve, disseminate/ sustain, and then repeat" phases of the MIP. The MIP is adaptable for microsystem and mesosystem improvement.

Each phase includes key improvement tools to utilize during each specific phase. For example, the assess phase includes practicing effective meeting skills and assessing the 5Ps of the microsystem/mesosystem while creating a 30,000-foot view of the process. The high-level view of the process combined with performance assessments and related current data help inform improvement themes to then select one to focus on for the first improvement initiative.

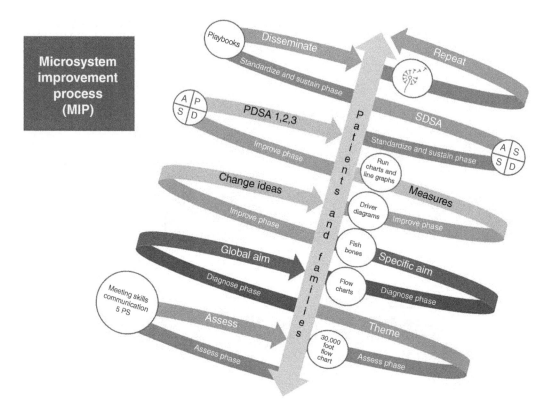

Steps in the Path

Before embarking on the path forward, leadership should carefully consider the mesosystem perspectives of the "forest and trees/balcony and dance floor" and determine the mesosystem method best suited for their organization's unique needs and capabilities.

The following steps walk you through the process of evaluating and improving your mesosystem. Once a decision is made, **we encourage you to read the case study at the end of this Action Guide.** This real-world example will provide valuable insights into how a mesosystem successfully implemented improvement strategies, offering inspiration and practical guidance for your own journey.

GETTING STARTED

1. Identify a subpopulation to improve care for, e.g.:
   a. Heart failure, joint replacement, head and neck cancer surgery patients – based on diagnosis.

   b. Service lines such as perioperative services, comprehensive breast care program, emergency services, and processes.
2. Map a high-level general flow of patients from the selected subpopulation care or service line, e.g., emergency services:
   a. Emergency Department through diagnostic studies to inpatient care to the operating room to the recovery room to the inpatient unit to home with home health services [service line].
3. Explore the community of the mesosystem [*Who are the microsystems and members?*]. Create a BIG ROOM where data and information can be shared. With the members of the mesosystem, create a process map of the patient journey [*include patients, families, community members*].
4. Enhance the process map by adding value stream mapping measurement of cycle times, information, and data flow (digital, in person, telephone, text, portals, faxes etc.).
5. Identify key measures across the mesosystem and at the end of the process.
6. Consider "walking the mesosystem" if possible, through the "eyes of the patients" to make observations and validate the processes within and between microsystems. Identify and assess transitions and handoffs of plans of care, information, and data between microsystems. This may take multiple days to complete the full process.
7. Assess the communication and relationships within and between the clinical microsystems in the mesosystem using Relational Mapping (see pg. 426).
8. Assess and identify WASTE including waits, delays, redundancies, rework, extra motion/movement, and information gaps.

Use data, information, and organization strategic goals to inform improvement themes and follow the pathway of the MIP Spiral to engage in disciplined, organized, and sustainable improvement.

STEP 1: Creating a Mesosystem Community

The principal task of the mesosystem is to
enable the work of microsystems for the population(s) of patients served.
—Paul Batalden

1. Identify the microsystems that form the mesosystem to gain insight of the larger care system – the between activities and processes where hand-offs occur – and identify processes and systems to improve the mesosystem to provide a smooth, safe patient care journey (one microsystem at a time).

2. Review what the mesosystem itself is doing to foster/develop the leadership and performance of the microsystem(s) to achieve a seamless, high quality/value, safe patient care experience.
3. Identify, recognize, and enhance mesosystem community, communication, and relationships. What infrastructure can encourage and support communication and relationships between microsystems?

Becoming Aware of the Mesosystem

Mesosystem Awareness Worksheet	
Mesosystem Name/Diagnosis:	
Aim of Mesosystem:	
Identify and name the person(s) who is (are) ultimately responsible for the functioning of the mesosystem	
Does the mesosystem utilize care paths or clinical paths? If yes, how is the path monitored and feedback provided?	
What does the literature reveal about evidence-based care and best practice? What does benchmarking reveal? Who does the care best?	
Do the microsystems in the mesosystem meet regularly to discuss care delivery, results and challenges?	

Microsystems Involved				
Microsystem	**Leaders**	**Core Process in Mesosystem**	**Handoffs**	**Processes to Improve**
(add rows as needed)				
Notes:				

Engage the Microsystem and Mesosystem Leaders

Microsystem and Mesosystem Leadership Engagement	
1. How often does the mesosystem meet to review and discuss patient/family care, processes, safety, errors, near misses, and transition handoffs? Who attends this meeting?	
2. Describe how 2 or more microsystems join together to improve the care and services and processes for patients, families, staff, and outcomes.	
3. Who is ultimately responsible and accountable to ensure safe, effective, and smooth patient care?	
4. Are the roles in the mesosystem optimized? Does each role make full use of education, license, and scope of practice? If there are multiple people in professional roles across the mesosystem (e.g., social workers, RNs, MDs, etc.), do they meet regularly to share their professional experiences and insights?	
5. Can you name a person or people in each of the involved microsystems in the mesosystem you can easily contact related to patient care and flow?	
6. When there is conflict within the mesosystem, how does it get resolved? a. Are there usual patterns of conflicts?	
7. How do the mesosystem and the microsystems learn about and track outcomes?	

Create Your Obeya Room (Big Room)

One of the mesosystem improvement methods is the "Big Room" and is described in Quality by Design, 2nd Edition, chapter 10. As a guiding mesosystem method, the "Big Room" can bring the microsystem members together regularly for learning and improving together (https://flowcoaching.academy).

Or a "Big Room" can provide a space to collect and provide visual data and information displays for the microsystem and mesosystem teams to review assessments and improvement while engaged in individual improvement efforts to help stimulate mesosystem curiosity and improvement.

Inspired by Toyota's success, the Obeya (Oobeya), or "Big Room," approach was introduced in the 1990s, as a collaborative workspace to bring teams together to coordinate and improve. The walls of "Big Rooms" are traditionally covered with visual representations of collective intelligence, including paper boards, notes, sticky notes, and increasingly, digital displays.

While traditionally a physical workspace where teams gather to collaborate, many mesosystems now utilize digital "share spaces" as a modern alternative. These online platforms offer convenience and efficiency by centralizing data and information, accessible to all members. However, the importance of physical visual displays in the workplace should not be overlooked. These tangible reminders reinforce the necessity of improvement efforts and foster a culture of continuous progress.

Whether through a physical "Big Room," a digital share space, or a combination of both, the centralization of information remains crucial. It promotes collaboration, streamlines project execution, and ultimately drives the improvement process forward.

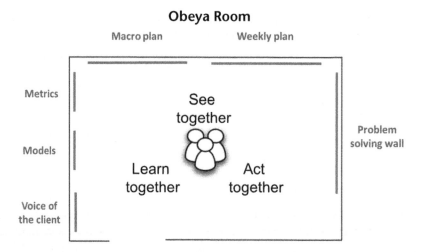

Ideal Future State

Once a decision is made, interprofessional members of the mesosystem should come together to assess the high-level path flow and envision an ideal future state. This involves identifying clear goals and objectives, informed by the insights of patients, families, and community members. Key performance indicators should be established to measure progress toward these goals.

The use of patient/family/community member stories can be a powerful tool in shaping this future state vision. These narratives often reveal pain points, unmet needs, and opportunities for improvement, providing invaluable guidance for the mesosystem team.

What does a review of the literature or benchmarking efforts to high performing paths provide for ideas and innovation?

Some tips to consider in designing the future state.

- Focus on the patient.
- Standardize the work to be customized.
- Consider the 5S method (Sort, Set, Shine, Standardize, Sustain), a core element of the Toyota Production System (TPS), to organize the workplace in an organized way (The 5S's of Lean (n.d.). ASQ. https://asq.org/quality-resources/five-s-tutorial).
- Reduce non-value-added clinician work.

STEP 2: Assess Your Mesosystem

Assessing the 5Ps of Your Mesosystem

To begin to increase awareness of the systems and processes of care in mesosystems and to assess the unique features of any microsystem, use the 5P framework. The 5P framework can be thought of as a structured and organized method of discovering the anatomy of a mesosystem. Every complex system has a structure, process, patterns, and outcomes the members may or may not be aware of.

Identification of data sources, including the Registries, Electronic Health Records, Data Repositories, and Manual Sampling, helps to discover the inner workings of the mesosystem. If data cannot be identified from data sources, members of the microsystem can help collect data and information using the worksheets and processes within this Action Guide.

This figure provides an example of the 30,000-ft view of the CF Lung Transplant Mesosystem.

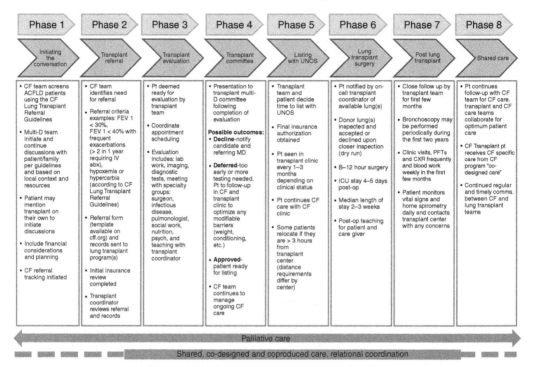

Cystic fibrosis lung transplant eight phases

Phase 1	Phase 2	Phase 3	Phase 4	Phase 5	Phase 6	Phase 7	Phase 8
Initiating the conversation	Transplant referral	Transplant evaluation	Transplant committee	Listing with UNOS	Lung transplant surgery	Post lung transplant	Shared care
• CF team screens ACFLD patients using the CF Lung Transplant Referral Guidelines • Multi-D team initiate and continue discussions with patient/family per guidelines and based on local context and resources • Patient may mention transplant on their own to initiate discussions • Include financial considerations and planning • CF referral tracking initiated	• CF team identifies need for referral • Referral criteria examples: FEV 1 < 30%, FEV 1 < 40% with frequent exacerbations (> 2 in 1 year requiring IV abx), hypoxemia or hypercarbia (according to CF Lung Transplant Referral Guidelines) • Referral form (template available on cff.org) and records sent to lung transplant program(s) • Initial insurance review completed • Transplant coordinator reviews referral and records	• Pt deemed ready for evaluation by transplant team • Coordinate appointment scheduling • Evaluation includes: lab work, imaging, diagnostic tests, meeting with specialty groups: surgeon, infectious disease, pulmonologist, social work, nutrition, psych, and teaching with transplant coordinator	• Presentation to transplant multi-D committee following completion of evaluation **Possible outcomes:** • **Decline**-notify candidate and referring MD • **Deferred**-too early or more testing needed. Pt to follow-up in CF and transplant clinic to optimize any modifiable barriers (weight, conditioning, etc.) • **Approved**-patient ready for listing • CF team continues to manage ongoing CF care	• Transplant team and patient decide time to list with UNOS • Final insurance authorization obtained • Pt seen in transplant clinic every 1–3 months depending on clinical status • Pt continues CF care with CF clinic • Some patients relocate if they are > 3 hours from transplant center (distance requirements differ by center)	• Pt notified by on-call transplant coordinator of available lung(s) • Donor lung(s) inspected and accepted or declined upon closer inspection (dry run) • 8–12 hour surgery • ICU stay 4–5 days post-op • Median length of stay 2–3 weeks • Post-op teaching for patient and care giver	• Close follow up by transplant team for first few months • Bronchoscopy may be performed periodically during the first two years • Clinic visits, PFTs and CXR frequently and blood work weekly in the first few months • Patient monitors vital signs and home spirometry daily and contacts transplant center with any concerns	• Pt continues follow-up with CF team for CF care. transplant and CF care teams collaborate for optimum patient care • CF Transplant pt receives CF specific care from CF program "co-designed care" • Continued regular and timely comms. between CF and lung transplant teams

Palliative care

Shared, co-designed and coproduced care, relational coordination

Join your interprofessional mesosystem colleagues with your patients and families on the catwalk – what do you see in the processes transitions, handoffs, relationships, and measured results?

How might you regularly review and discuss the processes of care to create a community with a shared purpose to achieve desired goals and targets? What processes are currently in place? Huddles? Shift reports? Monthly review of processes and outcomes?

The 5Ps have provided a tested organized and disciplined framework to assess microsystems. A modified 5Ps for mesosystems can provide a similar assessment of the "whole system" specific to a population, pathway, or service line to help identify strengths and improvement opportunities. Many of the assessment tools are similar and some new ones help focus on the handoffs between microsystems in the mesosystem.

A reminder of the 5Ps diagram.

Clinical mesosystem

PURPOSE: Why Does Your Mesosystem/Pathway Exist?

Raise this question with EVERYONE: include patients and families to create the best statement of purpose everyone can relate to. This engages everyone in meaningful conversation that isn't achieved by just taking out a mission statement. What does this mesosystem/pathway mean to you? Use your purpose statement to guide decision-making and improvement planning.

Who oversees the pathway?

Who are the leaders?

PATIENTS/POPULATION AND COMMUNITY MEMBERS: Know Your Patients/Population, Families, and Community Members

Take a close look at your mesosystem/pathway, create a "high-level" picture of the PATIENT POPULATION that you serve. Who are they? What resources do they use? How do patients view the care they receive?

Use the profile to know your patients/population, families, and community members (if part of the high-level flowchart). Determine if there is information you need to collect or if you can obtain this data from existing sources. Remember, the goal is to collect and review data and information about patients, families, or population that might lead to new designs in care models, processes, and services. Example: diabetes, lung transplant, frail elderly care, perioperative care returning to the community would benefit from partnership with the community.

Add other essential information about those being served that will provide critical information to standardize care and services to the unique population, patients, family, and community member needs.

MESOSYSTEM PROFILE Population/service line, patients, families

Aim: *Review and list population/service line information to help understand those being served with more facts*

Population/Service Line (insert)	

Age	Percent (%)
Birth–5 years	
6–20 years	
21–40 years	
41–60 years	
61–70 years	
71+	

List primary diagnoses and additional co-morbidities
1.
2.
3.
4.
5.
6.
7.
8.
9.
10.

Satisfaction or Experience of Care Scores
Does the macrosystem have an overall patient satisfaction/experience of care survey evaluating the entire mesosystem/pathway/ service line?
❑ Yes
❑ No
If yes, document scores here:
Do patients/families, populations report experiencing a cohesive approach to care or fragmented care process?
❑ Yes
❑ No
If no, do each microsystem in the mesosystem evaluate their own contribution to the mesosystem with their own individual surveys?
❑ Yes
❑ No
List which microsystems have their own evaluations

Health Outcomes

List related health outcomes currently being measured.

List top 5 resources used e.g. PT, Hospice, etc.
1.
2.
3.
4.
5.

Mental Health Survey Scores (if used)		
Mental Health Survey	Total Patients Screened	Score Range
PHQ-9		
GAD-7		
The PHQ-9 and GAD-7 detail can be found at phqscreeners.com		

Patient Population Census	#	Y/N
# Pts seen per day		
# Pts seen in the past week		
# New Pts in the past month		
# Encounters per		
Do these # vary throughout the year?		
Can you identify peak and low volume Periods?		

population

Patient Family Population Experience

Patient Family Population Experience Worksheet	
1. Assess safety, errors, near miss incidences that have occurred across the mesosystem that you are aware of. What are the themes?	
2. Assess patient/family feedback related to mesosystem performance e.g., handoffs. Consider compliments and complaints.	
3. How do members (microsystems) of the mesosystem learn about the compliments and complaints?	

4. Assess staff feedback related to mesosystem performance, e.g., handoffs and transitions in care. What processes go well? What processes need improvement?	
5. Identify one or more family members to interview about the whole process of care in the mesosystem using the 30,000-ft high level flowchart. Focus discussion on: a. Entering the mesosystem b. Transition between microsystems c. Discharge/Transition from the mesosystem d. Communications and explanations of pending transitions and expectations	

Through the Eyes of Patients and Families

Follow the path of a patient from the time they enter your mesosystem through the various microsystems until they exit the mesosystem. This may take multiple days/weeks. Create a tracking form to ensure complete tracking of the patient experience is documented.

*Some tips: **Enter the mesosystem as a patient** and experience the journey **or follow a patient/family** experience from the first encounter until discharge. Consider digital pictures and/or video to capture the experience.*

Patient Journey Planning	
Dates to Complete	
Who?	
How?	
Where?	

Imagine standing on an elevated "catwalk" overlooking the microsystem or mesosystem of care with your interprofessional mesosystem colleagues and patients and families. Gathering input from interprofessional colleagues, patients, and families enriches this "catwalk" view with each group bringing unique insights and perspectives. From this vantage point process flow, handoffs, transitions, relationships, and measured results can be observed.

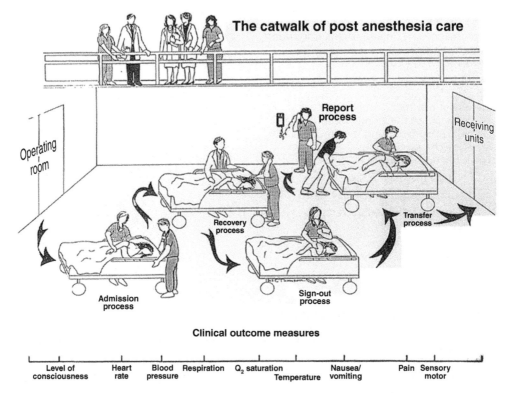

Once the data and observations are collected, take time with the Mesosystem Improvement Team to review the data to see patterns, variation in practice, and connections between the Patients, Professionals, Processes, and Patterns to find improvement opportunities. Discuss how the mesosystem members might regularly review and discuss processes of care to create a community with a shared purpose to achieve desired goals and targets that are valued by those being served.

PROFESSIONALS: **Know Your Professionals**

Assessing Your Pathway/Mesosystem Use the following template to create a comprehensive summary picture of your mesosystem. Who does what and when? Is the right person doing the right activity? List all roles, total FTEs, and overtime by role. Are the roles being optimized? Are all roles that contribute to the patient experience listed? What days and hours are the professionals at the mesosystem? Create a worksheet for each microsystem in the mesosystem.

Mesosystem "Know Your Professionals" Worksheet			
Microsystem Name:			
Current Staff	**FTE**	**Hours worked**	**Notes**
MDs – Total			
NP/PAs – Total			
RNs – Total			
LPN/NA/MAs – Total			
PT/RT/RD - Total			
Case Workers - Total			
Social/Case Workers – Total			
Secretaries – Total			
Pathway Facilitators - Total			
Others – Total			
Do you use on-call staff?	☐ Yes		☐ No
Do you use a float pool?	☐ Yes		☐ No
Do you use Travelers/Agency staff? If yes, which roles and how frequently?	☐ Yes		☐ No
How often do discipline-specific roles within the mesosystem meet to discuss care and process improvement? E.g. MDs, Nurses, Social Workers, meet as professional groups?			
How often do the microsystems within the mesosystem meet to discuss the processes, outcomes, patient experiences to engage in continuous improvement?			

Staff Satisfaction Scores

How stressful is the mesosystem?   (% Very Stressful) _____

Would you recommend the mesosystem as
a great place to work   (% Strongly Agree) _____

Supporting Microsystems, such as finance, pharmacy, others.

_____

_____

_____

Professionals: Staff Satisfaction

- Creating a joyful work environment starts with a basic understanding of staff perceptions of the mesosystem. You may have an organization-wide survey in place that you can use to replace this survey, but be sure it is CURRENT data, not months or years old, and that you are able to capture the data from all professionals specific to your mesosystem.
- If you do not have a current organizational staff satisfaction survey, ask mesosystem staff members to complete this survey thinking specifically about the MESOSYSTEM.
- Often you can distribute this survey to any professional who spends time in the mesosystem. Set a deadline of 1–2 weeks and designate a place for the survey to be dropped off. An alternative is to use an electronic survey such as Survey Monkey to invite staff to respond to the staff satisfaction questions.
- It is important to emphasize that this survey is anonymous and is a voluntary activity.
- Consider assessing Team burnout, resilience, and well-being.
- If you have Employee Engagement Scores for each Microsystem, please enter here:
  o Employee Engagement Scores:

Staff Satisfaction Survey- Mesosystem
1. I am treated with respect every day by everyone that works in the mesosystem. ☐ Strongly agree　　☐ Agree　　　　　　☐ Disagree　　　　☐ Strongly Disagree
2. I am given everything I need – tools, equipment, and encouragement to make work meaningful to my life ☐ Strongly agree　　☐ Agree　　　　　　☐ Disagree　　　　☐ Strongly Disagree
3. When I do good work, someone in this mesosystem notices that I did it. ☐ Strongly agree　　☐ Agree　　　　　　☐ Disagree　　　　☐ Strongly Disagree
4. How stressful would you say it is to work in this mesosystem? ☐ Very Stressful　　☐ Somewhat Stressful　☐ A Little Stressful　☐ Strongly Disagree
5. How easy is it to ask anyone a question about the care we provide? ☐ Very Easy　　　　☐ Easy　　　　　　　☐ Difficult　　　　☐ Very Difficult
6. How would you rate other people's morale and their attitudes about working here? ☐ Excellent　　☐ Very Good　　☐ Good　　☐ Fair　　☐ Poor

7. This mesosystem is a better place to work than it was 12 months ago.

☐ Strongly agree ☐ Agree ☐ Disagree ☐ Strongly Disagree

8. I would strongly recommend this mesosystem as a great place to work.

☐ Strongly agree ☐ Agree ☐ Disagree ☐ Strongly Disagree

9. What would make this mesosystem better for patients and their families?

_____

_____

_____

10. What would make this mesosystem better for those who work here?

_____

_____

_____

Professionals: Activities

- What do you spend YOUR time doing in the mesosystem? What is your best estimation of how much time you spend doing it? The goal is to have the right person doing the right thing at the right time in the mesosystem. The group can discuss which activities are or are not appropriate for the individual's level of education, training, and licensure and explore role-optimization efforts.

- You can start with one group of professionals such as MDs, NPs, RNs, or clerical staff, assessing their activities using the Activity Survey. This estimate of who does within the mesosystem or specific to a population of patients is what is intended to reveal, at a high level, to identify mismatches between education, training, licensure, and actual activities. It is good to eventually have all roles and functions within the mesosystem complete this survey for review and consideration. Be sure to create the same categories for each functional role. Some groups may hesitate to make time estimates; if this happens, just ask them to list their activities for the first review.

- Electronic versions, blank sheets, and examples can be found at clinicalmicrosystem.org

Example: Activity Tracking (Ambulatory Clinical Microsystem)

Position: MD	% of Time
Activity: See patients in the program Specific Items involved: • Review chart history • Assess/diagnose patient • Determine treatment plan	30%
Activity: Minor procedures	9%
Activity: OR procedures	10%
Activity: See patients in hospital	2%
Activity: Write prescriptions	5%
Activity: Dictate/document patient encounter Specific items involved: • Dictate encounter/use scribe • Review transcriptions and sign off	20%
Activity: Complete forms Specific items involved • Referrals • Prior authorizations	5%
Activity: Follow-up phone calls/emails	5%
Activity: Manage charts	5%
Activity: Evaluate test results Specific items involved • Review results/determine next actions	5%
Activity: See patients in outreach clinics	2%
Activity: Miscellaneous Specific items involved • CME; attend seminars; attend meetings	2%
Total	**100%**

Position: RN	% of Time
Activity: Triage patient issues/concerns Specific items involved: • Phone • Face to face	15%
Activity: Patient/family education	3%
Activity: Direct patient care Specific items involved: • See patients in the program • Assist provider with patients • Infusions	30%
Activity: Follow-up phone calls/emails	22%
Activity: Review and notify patients of lab results Specific items involved • Normal with follow-up • Drug adjustments	5%
Activity: Complete forms Specific items involved: • Referrals • Prior authorizations	18%
Activity: Call in prescriptions	5%
Activity: Miscellaneous Specific items involved • CME; attend seminars; attend meetings	2%
Total	**100%**

Activity Occurrence Sheet and Example

What's the next step? Insert the mesosystem activities from the activity survey here.

Activities are combined by role from the data collected above. This creates a master list of activities by role. Fill in THE NUMBER OF TIMES AM and PM THAT YOU PERFORM THE ACTIVITY. Make a mark by the activity each time it happens, per session. Use one sheet for each day of the week. Once the frequency of activities is collected, the mesosystem team should review the volumes and variations by session, day of week, and month of year.

This evaluation increases knowledge of predictable variation and supports improved matching of resources on the basis of demand. The blank activity occurrence sheet can be found on pg. 28.

Role:		Date:		Day of week:	
Visit activities		AM		PM	Total
Triage patient concerns					
Family/patient education					
Direct patient care					
Non-visit activities		AM		PM	
Follow-up phone calls/emails					
Complete forms					
Call in prescriptions					
Miscellaneous					
Total					

Role: RN	Date July 1	Date of Week: Monday	
Visit Activities	**AM**	**PM**	**Total**
Triage Patient Concerns	7	7	14
Family/Patient Concerns	4	3	7
Direct Patient Care	21	21	42
Non-Visit Activities	**AM**	**PM**	
Follow Up Phone Calls/Emails	10	16	26
Complete Forms	11	6	17
Call in Prescriptions	6	10	16
Miscellaneous	5	10	15
Total	**64**	**73**	**137**

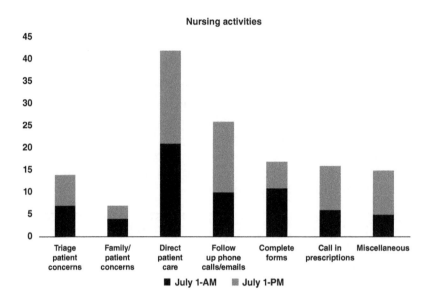

Activity Survey Sheet (Customize for Each Meso/Microsystem)

The blank template for an ambulatory clinical microsystem below allows roles to customize the Activity Survey Sheet for the positions (e.g., MD, NP, RN, RD, RT, SW, and others) of members of your Mesosystem and create activities that are relevant to that position. Using the template to customize the survey sheet provides the team with insight into each member's role and what they spend their time doing. This information will help when the team begins to plan for PDSA. The example above shows how data can be manually collected and displayed as a bar chart. To create a hospital-based mesosystem Activity Survey sheet, identify the key activities such as admissions, transfers, discharges, medication distribution, huddles, answering call bells, interprofessional bedside rounds as a few examples to then create the survey sheet for staff to complete.

Activity Survey Sheet	
Position	**% of Time**
Activity: Specific Items Involved: •	
Activity: Specific Items Involved: •	

Activity: Specific Items Involved: •	
Activity: Specific Items Involved: •	
Activity: Specific Items Involved: •	
Activity: Specific Items Involved: •	
Activity: Specific Items Involved: •	
Total	**100%**

Activity Occurrence Sheet			
Role:	**Date:**	**Day of Week:**	
Visit Activities	**AM**	**PM**	**Total**
Triage Patient Concerns			
Patient/Family Education			
Direct Patient Care			
Other:			
Non-Visit Activities	**AM**	**PM**	
Follow-Up Phone Calls/Emails			
Complete Forms			
Call in Prescriptions			
Miscellaneous			
Total			

Processes: Access, Transitions, and Discharge

Transitions and Handoffs

A high-risk time during a patient journey in a mesosystem is the transition and handoff periods between microsystems. Miscommunications and errors are more likely to occur during these periods. Plans of care may not be clearly described including where in the care plan patients are, their preferences that have been identified and the next steps for the care plan to move forward.

This worksheet helps to raise awareness of patient volumes, transfer frequencies, and the various microsystems involved in sending and receiving patients. What are the processes for handoffs? How is safe and reliable care ensured? How does technology and/or electronic medical records help or hinder the process? How do mesosystem members ensure "smooth and warm handoffs?"

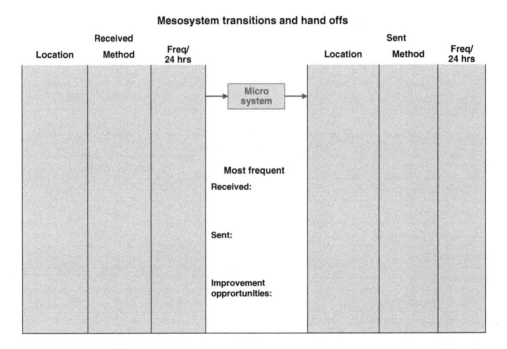

Make notes about the transitions in your mesosystem.

Process: Access, Transfer, Transitions, and Discharge: Where do the "Handoffs" Occur?

Cystic fibrosis lung transplant eight phases

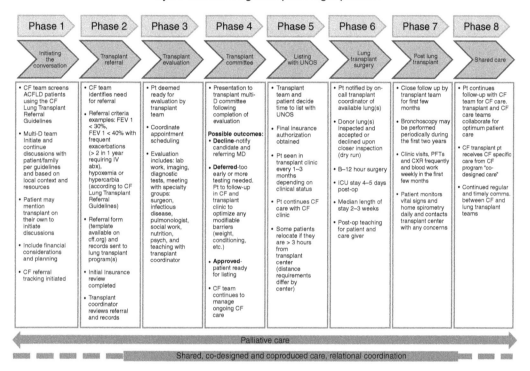

Example: Cystic Fibrosis Lung Transplant Phases

Process: Cycle Time Tools

One key measure of clinical microsystem efficiency is the patient *cycle time*. It is important to understand that cycle time is a result of systems, processes, and individual style. This is defined as the time from when a patient enters the mesosystem until they leave. The Patient Cycle Time Tool can be administered in several ways in a mesosystem and if often challenging when applying to pathways of care that occur over multiple days/weeks or months:

Mesosystem Cycle Time Worksheet		
Who completed form?	☐ **Patient**	☐ **Family Member**
Instructions: Please follow a patient pathway through the mesosystem.		
Patient entered mesosystem:	**Date:**	**Time:**
Date/Time Entered Mesosystem	**Microsystem and Activity**	**Date/Time Handsoff to Next Microsystem**
Comments:		
_____		
_____		
_____		

Beginning to increase staff understanding of the processes of care and services in the mesosystem is key to developing a common "system" understanding and focus for improvement.

Start with the high-level process of a patient entering the pathway/mesosystem by using the Patient Cycle Time Tool.

1. If the mesosystem pathway journey is over multiple days, weeks, months or even years, developing a Mesosystem Tracker is a helpful tool to track the patient over the mesosystem and over time. An example is the Advanced Lung Disease Tracker for Lung Transplant that can be adapted in many settings.

Advanced Lung Disease Tracking Sheet

CFF ID	Last Name	First Name	Transplant Center	Journey Outcome	Oxygen	Modulator	Obstacles	BMI <17	G-tube	DOB	Gender	Notes	

Cycle Time Example

Below is a cycle time example provided by **Loyola University Medical Center** and used with their permission. The Loyola Lead Improvement team collected cycle time data from both a tool completed by people with CF and a tool completed by their staff, and then compared the cycle time data. The tools and data are provided below.

By utilizing a cycle time tracking tool, the Mesosystem Improvement Team uncovered valuable insights into the patient care experience. Data revealed that time spent in radiology and phlebotomy added nearly an hour to the total visit duration. Additionally, significant variations were observed in clinic time between Microsystem #1 and Microsystem #2, prompting further investigation into the underlying causes of these discrepancies.

All data collection forms used in this analysis can be found at clinicalmicrosystem.org.

Clinic flow data collection

CF multidisciplinary clinic

	Time in	Time out
Vitals		
Respiratory therapist		
RN clinic coordinator		
Dietitian		
Social worker		
Physician		
Other		
RN checkout		

Schedule for LTX clinic appointment day

Date: _____ Time of appointment: _____ Physician: _____

Location (circle one):   Maywood   Oakbrook

Time arrived at clinic: _____   Time left clinic: _____

Comments: _____

_____

_____

Timeline: Please document the time spent in each department and/or with each provider (include lab, radiology, nurse, doctor, respiratory, dietitian, social worker, everything!).

Time	Action/provider	Comment
Example: 10:00–10:20	Nurse	
10:25–10:35	Dietitian	

Clinic timeline data – initial averages

Legend:
- Phlebotomy
- Radiology
- Downtime
- MD
- SW
- Dietitian
- RN
- RT
- RN vitals

Minutes spent in clinic

Patient collected data | Staff collected data

n = 5 patients *n* = 18 patients

Clinic timeline data – four months of data

— Downtime — Total

Time spent in clinic (min)	Clinic #1	Clinic #2
Arrival to room	11.1 min	15.8 min
Vitals	9.7 min	7.3 min
RT	11.8 min	10.0 min
RN	12.0 min	15.9 min
Dietitian	12.0 min	11.5 min
SW	9.3 min	9.6 min
M.D.	10.2 min	21.9 min
Downtime	13.6 min	22.3 min

Processes: MESOSYSTEM Core and Supporting Processes

Review, adapt, and distribute the *Core and Supporting Processes* Assessment form to ALL mesosystem staff. Be sure the list is accurate for the mesosystem and then ask staff to evaluate the CURRENT state of these processes. Rate each process by putting a tally mark under the heading that most closely matches your understanding of the process. Also mark if the process is a source of patient complaints. Tally the results to give the Mesosystem Improvement Team an idea as to where to begin to focus on improvement from the staff perspective.

- Some mesosystems create and display a wall-sized version of the Core and Supporting Process Assessment chart and ask all staff to select choices by using different colored dots for each role. This creates a *scatter plot display* of the ratings and priorities for all staff to see.
- **Steps for Improvement:** Explore improvements for each process based on the outcomes of this assessment tool. Each of the processes below should be flowcharted in its current state. Based on the flowcharts of the current state of your processes and determinations of your *Change Ideas* (pg. 43–45), you will use the PDSA (Plan-Do-Study-Act) cycle worksheet (pg. 51–54) to run tests of change and to measure your change ideas.

Mesosystem Core and Supporting Processes Assessment

Processes	Works Well	Small Problem	Real Problem	Totally Broken	Cannot Rate	We're Working on it	Source of Patient/ Family Complaint
Orient patients/families to Mesosystem of care							
Admit to microsystems							
Orientation of patients/families to microsystem including rhythm of rounds and daily activities							
Coproducing care plans							
Writing orders for care plans							
Diagnostic studies processes and reporting							
Medication orders and distribution							
Making referrals							
Nutrition processes							
Transfer to other microsystems in the mesosystem processes							
Handoff process between microsystems							
Patient/Family Education							
Patient/Family Feedback							
Experiencing individual microsystems as a mesosystem care team							
Others:							

Patient Flow in the Mesosystem

Questions to consider regarding patient flow:

1. Which areas in your pathway experience prolonged wait times with or between microsystems?
2. When and where are healthcare professionals waiting for patient arrival?
3. Where are the opportunities to optimize flow?
4. Can the service be provided closer to the patient (e.g., can lab work be performed near the patient rather than sending the patient to central lab?)
5. Are there delays in handoffs and transitions between microsystems in the mesosystem? What types of delays exist?
6. Are there errors or missing information in handoff and transitions?

PATTERNS: **Know your Patterns**

Patterns are present in our daily work and we may or may not be aware of them. Patterns can offer hints and clues to our work that inform us of possible improvement ideas.

What patterns are present but not acknowledged in your mesosystem? What are the leadership and social patterns? How often does the mesosystem meet to discuss patient care? Are patients and families involved? What are your results and outcomes?

- How often does your mesosystem meet to discuss patient care?
- How do leaders across the mesosystem relate to one another?
- Do the members of the mesosystem regularly review and discuss quality, safety, and reliability issues?
- Are patients and their families involved? (Use clinicalmicrosystem.org)
- What is the most significant pattern of variation in the mesosystem? Does patient volume and flow in the mesosystem vary by day of week or season? Do professionals vary their schedules? What other variations can be found?
- What has the mesosystem successfully changed?
- What is the mesosystem most proud of?
- What is the financial trend for the mesosystem?
- What are the mesosystem results and outcomes?
- How do leaders relate to mesosystem staff?

Relationships Within the Mesosystem

Mesosystem Relationship Worksheet	
1. Describe the relationships between	
a. Microsystem leaders	
b. Microsystem staff to staff	
c. Support units to the mesosystem	
d. External agencies to the mesosystem	
e. Senior leaders and the mesosystem	
2. Describe how the microsystems within the mesosystem communicate and co-design systems of care	

Create a Relational Map of Your Mesosystem

Relational Coordination provides a validated theory to assess communication and relationships within a microsystem or across a mesosystem using seven dimensions (https://heller.brandeis.edu/relational-coordination/index.html).

Relational Coordination:

- Measures the quality of relationships and communication involved in the coordination of work.
- Matters most for work that is complex, uncertain, and time constrained.
- Drives quality, efficiency, satisfaction, and engagement outcomes.
- Is supported and reinforced by relational, structural, and process improvements.

The Seven Dimensions of Relational Coordination

Frequent Communication
During the **identified mesosystem process**, how **frequently** do people in these roles **communicate** with you?
Timely Communication
Do people in these roles **communicate** with you in a **timely** manner during the **identified mesosystem process**?
Accurate Communication
Do they **communicate accurately** with you during the **identified mesosystem process**?
Problem-Solving Communication
When a **problem** occurs with the **identified mesosystem process**, do people in these roles blame others or work with you to **solve** the problem?

Shared Goals
Do people in these roles **share** your **goals** for the **identified mesosystem process**?
Shared Knowledge
Do people in these roles **know** about the **work** you do as part of the **identified mesosystem process**?
Mutual Respect
Do people in these roles **respect** the **work you do** as part of the **identified mesosystem process**?

Relational Coordination Mapping is an opportunity for people to understand their own and each other's work in the context of the whole (mesosystems perspective).

The process of mapping multiple microsystems, fostering open and constructive dialogue about their collaboration (utilizing the seven dimensions framework), can unearth strengths and pinpoint improvement opportunities within the mesosystem. This deeper understanding cultivates stronger communication and relationships, ultimately leading to enhanced systems of care.

1. From a mesosystem perspective, microsystems can reflect on:

   - Where does communication and relationships work well in this mesosystem?
   - Where does it work poorly?

2. Create the relational map, by individual microsystems initially thinking about the other microsystems they work with in the mesosystem and using the Seven dimensions, assessing an overall relational coordination score about the process and the workgroups. Mapping is not about rating individuals in the mesosystem. It is about rating the identified process of care and the workgroups relational coordination between microsystems.

3. Once each microsystem completes its relational mapping for other microsystems, a mesosystem meeting can be organized to share and discuss perspectives in the spirit of improving the processes of care. Celebrating strengths is essential in this meeting.

4. To complete the relational mapping:

   - Use a **GREEN** pen to note the high relational coordination (RC),
   - Use a **RED** pen to note the low RC, and
   - Use a **BLUE** pen to note neutral RC.
   - The relationships move in both directions. Notice when there are differences in the rated RC between microsystems to explore the communication and relationships more closely.

Relationship Map Example: Perioperative Mesosystem

Note: In the example above, the darkest shade represents a high score, the medium shade represents a neutral score, and the lightest shade represents a low relational score.

Interventions to Increase Relational Coordination – "Intervention Toolbox"

Once assessments are completed, discussed, and in the spirit of improvement, the mesosystem can design PDSA cycles to test to improve the identified relational coordination low scores. Using relationship mutual respect, shared goals and shared knowledge consider the following:

RC Dimension-Specific Interventions

Mutual respect: What will help people speak up and harness their differences?

- Ground rules (created and maintained by group).
- Skills for listening and multiple perspective-taking.
- Storytelling-especially from patient/family/community member perspectives.

Shared goals and identity: What fosters alignment?

- Stories – founding, key moments.
- Mission statement, strategy (organizational and team).
- Huddles.
- Visual indicators.

Shared knowledge: How do people learn about each other's work?

- Huddles.
- Shadowing and process mapping.
- Conversations of interdependence.

Consider the three categories of structural, relational and work process interventions below to jump start their thinking.

Structural Interventions

- Individual microsystem meetings to continuously improve processes and care.
- Joint microsystem improvement meetings to review and improve mesosystem processes.
- Urgent virtual huddles in real-time care and processes.
- Timely communication/time management across the mesosystem.
- Team members rotate through each quality improvement role in meetings.
- Sharing responsibility and relationship building to improve seamless care delivery.
- Shared access to reporting about the mesosystem performance and outcomes.
- Training and professional development for building relational and team competencies (retreat, workshops, simulations, etc.).
- Use of templates to track and monitoring metrics, progress, and action items for cascaded goals.
- Visual displays posted in common areas or digital shared drives to track and monitor goals.
- Shared accountability and rewards for all microsystems in the mesosystem.

Relational Interventions

- "Walk in our shoes" Plan "exchange" activities where each microsystem observes and spends time in each other's microsystem to gain more insight into their daily activities and experiences.
- Shared job description to better understand relationships.
- Improved communication through program participation.
- Job shadowing to understand roles, responsibilities, and interdependence.
- Social events – staff BBQ, volunteer opportunities, quarterly summits, virtual game night, professional "date nights."
- Create a safe space – e.g., safe words to freeze/unfreeze discussion, physical object to signify violation of agreed upon norms for respectful interaction, etc.
- "Shout-outs" – publicly celebrating colleagues and reinforcing positive behavior, core values, and common decency.

Work Process Interventions

- Develop PDSAs to track mesosystem patients.
- Develop institutional policies that reflect guidelines for population care.
- Development of client-facing brochures to demystify the care process, educate, or address frequently asked or commonly misunderstood topics.
- Interdisciplinary application of Lean and Six Sigma – value stream mapping, process mapping, Plan-Do-Study-Act (PDSA) cycles with emphasis on cross-functional visibility.
- Co-designed care pathways and/or standard operating procedures (SOPS) and playbooks.
- Commit to creating and sharing process maps/flowcharts to make care delivery visible to everyone.

Patterns: Unplanned Activity

- Patterns can be found through tracking the volumes and types of activities across the mesosystem.
- Communication and meetings between microsystems, patient flow and handoffs, and transfer of patients between microsystems which include delays in processes are a few of the patterns to look for in the mesosystem.
- Identify core and supporting activities across the mesosystem to create a worksheet to sample frequency and associated challenges and barriers. Ask staff to track selected activities over the course of a week to find the patterns of successes, delays, barriers, and problems along with the volume peaks and valleys.
- Be alert for new design possibilities to consider tracking volumes and root causes.
- Note the changes in volume by the day of the week and AM/PM. Remember, this example can be modified for other activities such as "missing orders" or delays from time to ready to be transferred to the next microsystem to actual transfer to learn about patterns to consider if new designs might eliminate the volumes, failed processes, and frequencies.
- An example from the mesosystem is when patients are transferred to the next microsystem and the type of "handoff" report varied depending on who the staff were involved in the process. This resulted in missing personalized information about the patient and family, gaps in care, missed orders and delays in care delivery. The frequency of this unplanned activity decreased when the mesosystem improvement team identified how frequently this happened and the consequences of individual variation in "handoff" reports. The multiple microsystems in the mesosystem tested the "SBAR" (Situation, Background, Assessment, and Recommendation) handoff communication process resulting in less missing information and smoother transitions in care (https://www.ahrq.gov/teamstepps-program/curriculum/communication/tools/

sbar.html). Identification and improvement discussions and planning were held during the every other week "mesosystem" improvement team meetings.

Mesosystem Unplanned Activity Tracking Sheet					
Week of:	**Day of Week:**		**Day of Week:**		**Week Total**
	AM	**PM**	**AM**	**PM**	
Transfer delays					
Total					
Communication delays between microsystems					
Total					
Communication delays with care team members					
Total					
Order delays					
Total					
Individual patient information missing					
Total					
Care Plan delays					
Total					
Total					
Total					
Total					
Total					
Day Total					

Metrics that Matter – The Mesosystem

- Metrics are essential for microsystems and mesosystems to make and sustain improvements to attain high performance. Review the mesosystem's performance data based on the population being cared for, flowcharts, cycle times, and other collected data to identify what is done well and where there are "gaps" in care and opportunities for improvement. All mesosystems are awash with data but relatively few have rich information environments that feature daily, weekly, and monthly use of Metrics That Matter (MTM). The key to doing this is to get started in a practical, doable way, and to build out your MTM and their vital use over time.
- Some guidelines for consideration are listed below. Remember these are just guidelines and the mesosystem should do what makes sense in the way of collecting, displaying, and using measures and MTM.

1. **What?** Every mesosystem has vital performance characteristics, things that must happen for successful operations specific to the population being served. Metrics That Matter should reflect the mesosystem's vital performance characteristics, including Key Metrics for the mesosystem's population of patients.
2. **Why?** The reason to identify, measure, and track MTM is to ensure that you are not "flying blind." Safe, high-quality, and efficient performance will provide specific, balanced, and timely metrics that show:
   a. When improvements are needed.
   b. If improvements are successful.
   c. If improvements are sustained over time.
   d. The amount of variation in results over time.
3. **How?** Here are steps to take advantage of MTMs

Mesosystem Improvement Team Work with your Mesosystem Improvement Team to establish the need for metrics and their routine use specific to the population being served in the mesosystem. Consider benchmarking the mesosystem outcomes with other similar settings to identify improvement possibilities. Quality begins with the intention to achieve measured excellence.

BALANCED METRICS
- Build a balanced set of metrics to provide insight into what's working and what's not working. Some categories to consider are process flow, delays, clinical/safety outcomes, patient and family perceptions, staff perceptions, operations, and finance/costs. Pick a few measures to start with.

- Every metric should have an *operational definition, data owner,* current value, and *target value.*
- *Conceptual Definition:* tells what will be measured (e.g., patient waiting for clinic visit).
- *Operational Definition:* tells how it will be measured (e.g., time elapsed from patient appointment time until time patient enters exam room in minutes).

DATA WALL DISPLAYS – Consider the "Big Room"

A *data wall* is a designated space to display your Metrics That Matter over time the Mesosystem Improvement Team can review to help prioritize improvement efforts. Use the data wall at daily huddles, weekly meetings, monthly mesosystem team meetings, and annually to assess progress and acknowledge improvement gains that have been achieved and sustained. Your organization may have "electronic" data walls and tracking systems which can help monitor the important data of the mesosystem. Some organizations have electronic display boards on each unit to easily review the data. Gather data for each metric and display it on the "data wall" reporting:

- Current value.
- Target value.
- Action plan to improve or sustain level.
- Display metrics as soon as possible – daily, weekly, and monthly metrics are most useful – using physical visual displays such as *time trend charts* and bar charts OR digital share drives depending on the local context.

DATA OWNER Start small and identify a data wall owner(s) who are guided by the mesosystem team to create a visual display of the MTM and other key metrics.

Consider a data owner(s) for each measure. The owner will be responsible for obtaining and reporting the measure to the mesosystem team. Seek sources of data from organization-wide systems before manually counting.

If the identified mesosystem data are not available, use manual methods to sample and provide a *"snapshot"* of the data. Strive to build data collection into the flow of daily work.

Mesosystem data is often not available because organizations have created data systems by traditional formats such as division, department, unit, and not as a collective mesosystem, so "sampling" will be necessary until organization data processes recognize the mesosystem.

REVIEW AND USE Review your data walls/"Big room" on a regular basis with the microsystem and mesosystems – daily, weekly, monthly, quarterly, and annually – to track the improvement process and determine if process and clinical outcomes are at the desired level of performance.

Make metrics fun, useful, and a lively part of your mesosystem/microsystem development process. Consider including the measures in all staff meeting agendas. Discuss MTM frequently and act on them as needed.

Microsystem Improvement Process with Measurement

Improvement activities and measurement are inextricably connected. To help you "see" this relationship, *The Microsystem Improvement Process Spiral* and the *Measurement Chain* illustrate how improvement measurement can be woven into each step of the MIP Spiral.

Careful consideration of the conceptual and operational definitions will ensure reliable measurement throughout the improvement process.

The development of data collection plans supports the PLAN of PDSA cycles. Together, these models create an improvement process that is grounded in *improvement sciences.*

Microsystem Improvement Process with Measurement

Measurement components

Data overtime and dashboards

Collect, display, assess adapt/adopt/abandon

Detailed measurement plan

Conceptual /operational definition 'what and how will you measure?'

Change ideas 'how do know change is an improvement?'

Global/specific aims and measures

5 Ps Assessing data needs

Repeat

SDSA

Standardize and sustain phase

Measures

Improve phase

Specific aim

Diagnose phase

Theme

Assess phase

Disseminate

Standardize and sustain phase

PDSA 1,2,3

Improve phase

Change ideas

Improve phase

Global aim

Diagnose phase

Assess

Assess phase

Run charts and line graphs

Driver diagrams

Fish bones

Flow charts

30,000 foot flow chart

Playbooks

Meeting skills communication 5 PS

Patients and families

S A
S D

A P
S D

Mesosystem Metrics That Matter

- Review the currently determined "best metrics" for the population being served that the mesosystem should be monitoring.
- List current performance on these metrics and what the targets are.
- List Process Outcome title:
- Clinical Outcome title:

Metrics That Matter Worksheet				
Metrics	**Goal**	**Current and Target Values**	**Definition and Data Owner**	**Action Plan and Process Owner**
Outcome Measures				
Process Measures				
Patient and Family Perceptions				
Collaborative Goal Setting With Patients and Families				
Patient/Family Action Plan				
Access				
Staff resilience/well-being/burnout				
Safety				
Finance				

Measurement Cycle Times

Pay particular attention to waits, delays, rework, missing information, gaps) when completing the flowchart/value stream map of the mesosystem. (Use the Value Stream Mapping Process.)

1. Whole path of care – note waste, bottlenecks, rework.
2. Milestone cycle times e.g., Admission (from time identified to be admitted to actual admission), Transfers (from time ready to transfer to actual transfer). Completion of orders to first treatment.

Professional to Professional Patient Reports/Updates
- MD to MD
- Interdisciplinary Team to Interdisciplinary Team
  - RN to RN
  - Nursing Assistant- Nursing Assistant
  - Secretary to Secretary
  - Transfer reports
- Shift to Shift Reports
  - MD to MD
  - RN to RN
- Transfer from microsystem to microsystem
  - Time identified to be transferred to orders being written
  - Time orders written to report to receiving staff
  - Time patient physically moved to new microsystem
- Discharge of patient
  - Time from identified ready for discharge to time of written order
  - Time from written order to activation of resources needed
  - Time from written order to physical departure
  - Time from discharge preparation to notification of resources
  - Time from initial communication to transfer of information
  - Time from discharge to initial contact and follow-up

Clinical Value Compass

The Clinical Value Compass traditionally has tracked the outcomes for each individual microsystem. Thinking about the mesosystem, the same principles apply to identify and track measures specific to the mesosystem and the population being served over multiple microsystems.

Refer to the Clinical Value Compass Worksheet available at clinicalmicrosystem.org

- Way to link fundamental clinical goals to measured outcomes.
- Links patient case mix variables with real clinical care processes with key outcomes.
- A place (compass point) for everyone – patients, families, doctors, nurses, employers, payors, etc.

Value compass
value + Q/$

- Physical
- Mental
- Social/role
- Risk status
- Perceived well-being

Function and risk status

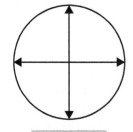

Biological status

- Mortality
- Morbidity
- Complications

Satisfaction versus need

- Health care delivery
- Perceived health benefit

Costs

- Direct medical
- Indirect social

STEP 3: Diagnose Your Mesosystem

With the Mesosystem Improvement Team, review the mesosystem 5Ps assessments including the Metrics That Matter, consider your organizational strategic plan to select a first "theme" (e.g., improved clinical outcomes, improved patient flow through the mesosystem, decreased HAI (hospital acquired infection) rates, reduced return to ED visits) for improvement.

The purpose of completing a mesosystem assessment is to make an informed overall diagnosis of your mesosystem.

- First, identify and celebrate the strengths of your mesosystem.
- Second, identify and consider opportunities to improve your mesosystem.
  o The opportunities to improve may come from your own microsystem based on assessment, staff suggestions, and/or patient and family needs, perceptions, priorities, and concerns to contribute to the overall mesosystem improvements.
  o The opportunities to improve may come from outside your microsystem to other microsystems within the mesosystem or overall system infrastructure and design that improves the whole system performance – based on a strategic project or external performance/quality measures (e.g., The Joint Commission: jointcommission.org).
- Look at the detail of each of the assessment tools, but also synthesize all the assessments and Metrics That Matter to "get the big picture" of the mesosystem. Identify linkages within the data and information. Consider:
  o Waste and delays in the process steps. Look for processes that might be redesigned to result in better functions for roles and better outcomes for patients.
  o Patterns of variation in the mesosystem. Be mindful of smoothing the variations or matching resources with the variation in demand.
  o Patterns of outcomes you wish to improve.
  o Handoffs and transitions between microsystems in the mesosystem.
- It is usually smart to pick or focus on one important theme to improve at a time and to work with all the "players" in the mesosystem to make a big improvement in the area selected.

DIAGNOSE YOUR MESOSYSTEM

Write your theme for improvement _____

_____

_____

"GLOBAL" AIM STATEMENT FOR THEME

Create an aim statement that will help keep your focus clear and your work productive.

We aim to improve _____
                              (Name the process)

In _____
                  (Clinical location in which process is embedded)

The process begins <u>with</u> _____
                              (Name where the process begins)

The process ends <u>with</u> _____
                              (Name where the process ends)

By working on the process, we expect _____
                                          (List benefits)

It is important to work on this now because _____
                                              (List imperatives)

_____

_____

_____

_____

STEP 4: Treat Your Mesosystem

Draft a clear, specific aim statement and way to measure the aim using improvement models – PDSA (Plan-Do-Study-Act; pg. 51–52) and SDSA (Standardize-Do-Study-Act; pg. 55).

- Now that you've made your diagnosis and selected a theme worthy of improving, you are ready to begin using powerful change ideas, improvement tools, and the scientific method to change your mesosystem.
- This begins with making a specific aim and using PDSA, which is known as the "model for improvement." The ***improvement model*** raises three important questions to answer before starting to make changes.

  1. What are we trying to accomplish?
  2. How will we know that a change is an improvement?
  3. What changes can we make that will result in an improvement?

- After you have run your tests of change and have reached your measured aim, the challenge is to maintain the gains that you have made. This can be done using SDSA, which is the other half of making improvement that has "staying power."
- You will be smart to avoid totally reinventing the wheel by taking into consideration best-known practices, "Change Ideas" that other clinical teams and patients and families have found to really work. A list of some of the best Change Ideas that might be adapted and tested in your clinic follows the aim statement worksheet

Specific Aim Statement

SPECIFIC AIM STATEMENT
Instructions: 1. Create a specific aim statement that will help keep your focus clear and your work productive. 2. Use numeric goals, specific dates, and specific measures.
SPECIFIC AIM _____ _____ _____

```
┌─────────────────────────────────────────────────────────────────┐
│ MEASURES                                                          │
│ _____  │
│ _____  │
│ _____  │
└─────────────────────────────────────────────────────────────────┘
```

Specific Aim Example

SPECIFIC AIM STATEMENT
Instructions: 1. Create a specific aim statement that will help keep your focus clear and your work productive. 2. Use numeric goals, specific dates, and specific measures.
SPECIFIC AIM Decrease the variation in the patient/family education materials for patients receiving a hip replacement in our mesosystem to 100% consistent materials and information. _____
MEASURES Measure the number and types of education materials on the 15th of each month across the mesosystem _____ _____ _____

Mesosystem Change Ideas to Consider

- Create a mesosystem improvement team that meets every other week/monthly to lead improvement.
- Hold mesosystem pre-shift huddles to prepare for the day's patients and mesosystem activities.
- Develop and consistently apply evidence base practice for care including guidelines and algorithms.
- Hold patient and family care focus groups to develop short-term and long-range plans of care.
- Coproduce an action plan with mesosystem members and the patient and family to plan care that is mutually agreed upon and meets the patient's and family's goal(s).

Consider the *CHANGE CONCEPTS* (Langley et al., 1996)

A. Eliminate Waste

B. Improve Workflow

C. Optimize Inventory

D. Change the Work Environment

E. Enhance the Producer/Patient, Family, and Health Care Professionals Relationship

F. Manage Time

G. Manage Variation

H. Design Systems to Avoid Mistakes

I. Focus on the Product or Service

Reference

Langley, G. J., Nolan, K. M., Nolan, T. W., Norman, C. L., & Provost, L. P. (1996). *The improvement guide: A practical approach to enhancing organizational performance.* San Francisco, CA: Jossey-Bass Publishers.

Improve Patient Flow

1. Minimize patient walking: bring the services to the patient.
2. Create flexible spaces that can be reconfigured based on the patients and procedure.
3. Stop the process when problems occur to assess the process and understand the problems. May slow down flow initially but flow will speed up in the long run.
4. Implement sequential order of processing. Study your patient processes and flows. Put the patient's process steps in sequential order to eliminate the need for rework or backtracking of patient steps.
5. Use one-piece flow to keep patients on a first-in, first-out system. Handle each patient one at a time, addressing all his needs.
6. Assess between microsystem delays and bottlenecks.

Flow of Information

The efficient and effective flow of information enables timely patient care, high quality of care, enhanced safety, and improved mesosystem relationships. You don't want a break in information flow – for example, a personalize plan of care – to interrupt patient flow. Neither do you want incorrect or missing information (e.g., allergies to medications) to endanger the patient. Share patient preferences and insights as part of the handoffs between microsystems.

Ways to stimulate the flow of information:

1. Electronic medical record documentation can be helpful when current and complete.
2. Consider other "real-time" templates that can be "handed off" during transitions in care.
3. Determine how information will flow when designing a process.
   - Where should information be visual?
   - Where should it travel electronically?
   - When might a hard copy information template be useful? Where should the information be stored and easily retrieved?
4. Implement arrangements that facilitate the flow of information between clinicians and make transferring information at nursing shift change easy.

Questions to consider for information flow:

- Where and how can you make information flow with the patient?
- Are you providing information clinicians don't use and should be removed?
- Where do you find redundancy and rework in information flow?
- What is your process for flow of information? How can you improve this flow to better serve your patients?

Coproduction Change Concepts/Change Ideas

Efforts to ensure effective participation of patients in health care are called by many names-patient centeredness, patient engagement, and patient experience. Improvement initiatives in this domain often resemble the efforts of manufacturers to engage consumers in designing and marketing products. Services, however, are fundamentally different from products; unlike goods, services are always "coproduced." Failure to recognize this unique characteristic of a service and its implications may limit our success in partnering with patients to improve health care.

Some ideas to consider co-production in care improvement.

1. Use pull systems.
2. Reduce choice of features.
3. Increase choice of features.
4. Give people more access to information.
5. Help people understand information.
6. Conduct training.
7. Implement cross-training.
8. Share risks and benefits.

9. Emphasize natural and logical consequences.
10. Develop alliances and cooperative relationships.
11. Listen to patients, families, and healthcare professionals.
12. Coach patients, families, and healthcare professionals to use products or services.
13. Focus on the outcome that matters to the patient, family, and healthcare professionals.
14. Understand contribution made by product or service to outcome that matters to the patient, family, and healthcare professionals.
15. Use a coordinator.
16. Reach agreement on expectations.
17. Standardize.
18. Customize.
19. Attend to emotion, esthetic, and experience.
20. Don't waste the patient, family, and healthcare professionals' time.
21. Provide exactly what is wanted.
22. Provide exactly where it is wanted.
23. Provide exactly when it is wanted.
24. Ensure that goods and services work and that they work together.
25. Aggregate solutions to reduce patient, family, and healthcare professionals' time and hassle.
26. Recognize and invite individual patient and family agency and capacity.
27. Invite patients, families, and healthcare professionals to network and share solutions.
28. Remove barriers to use of product or service.
29. Understand and limit burdens created by product or service.
30. Optimize information technology to enable partnership.
31. Distinguish unique needs of different patients, families, and healthcare professionals.
32. Enable trust.
33. Share power.
34. Optimize time together.
35. Eliminate aspects of the product or service that do not add value.

Reference

Batalden, M., Batalden, P., Margolis, P., Seid, M., Armstrong, G., Opipari-Arrigan, L., and Hartung, H. "Coproduction of Healthcare Services." *BMJ Quality & Safety*, 2016, 25(7), 509–517 doi: 10.1136/bmjqs-2015-004315.

Sustaining Daily Care: Change Concepts/Change Ideas

Change Concept: Person before the patient

<u>Change Ideas</u>

1. During pre-care huddles when the patient list is being reviewed, include discussing something personal and nonmedical about the patient and/or family to help understand the context of managing their condition.
2. Identify member(s) of the care team with the best attributes to discuss an important health goal(s) with a patient/family.
3. Enter the patient's room with a smile and ask what is going on in their life. Share something about yourself to encourage personable connection.

Change Concept: Optimize interactions

<u>Change Ideas</u>

1. To set an agenda, ask your patients what their priorities are for your discussion.
2. Use active listening to explore their thoughts, feelings, and experiences about their condition and their life.
3. Choose nonjudgmental words and use open-ended inquiries to emphasize that you are there for your patients as a partner.
4. Choose words that acknowledge that everyone struggles to do everything at 100%. Setting realistic goals can help someone achieve what is best for them right now (shared humanity).
5. Use the "teach-back" method: Have them "teach" and reflect back what they understood you to say to make sure you are on the same page.
6. When discussing topics with your patients and colleagues, collect and share solutions and stories you've heard from others to help inspire patients to think differently.

Change Concept: Debrief before the handoff

<u>Change Ideas</u>

1. After seeing the patient, quickly debrief with the next team member before they see the patient to share important information in an effort to reduce redundancy and encourage new interactions.
2. Debrief after clinic on the list of patients and update your notes to inform the next visit.

Reference

Cindy George, the Senior Director of Partnerships for Sustaining Daily Care at the Cystic Fibrosis Foundation, offers the following change concepts and ideas to help sustain daily care (Cindy.George@CFF.org).

Mesosystem Huddle Sheet

1. What can we proactively anticipate and plan for in our workday/shift/week? At the beginning of the day or shift, hold a review of today's mesosystem patient volumes, flow, transfers, review of plans for today, and any mesosystem staffing or patient bed concerns.
2. This worksheet can be modified to add more detail to the content and purpose of the mesosystem or microsystem huddles.

MESOSYSTEM HUDDLE SHEET
Date:
Aim: Enable the mesosystem to proactively anticipate and plan actions based on patient need and available resources, and contingency planning.
UPDATES and FOLLOW-UPS/Include Improvement activities. Mesosystem: Microsystem:
"HEADS UP" FOR TODAY: (include special patient needs, sick calls, staff flexibility, contingency plans, supply issues)

Patient Needs:	Meetings:
Staff Needs:	

REVIEW OF NEXT/SHIFT DAY AND PROACTIVE PLANNING	
	Meetings: **Improvement** **Microsystems** **Mesosystem**

Driver Diagrams

The *driver diagram* is a tool to organize and track multiple improvements to achieve the "Global Aim" of the "Theme" of improvement and helps everyone involved in the improvement to:

- **Understand the overall strategy:** See the big picture and how each piece fits together.
- **Identify areas for improvement:** Pinpoint specific areas where changes can be made.
- **Track progress:** Monitor how changes are impacting the desired outcomes.
- **Communicate effectively:** Share the plan in a clear and concise way.

Essentially, a driver diagram acts as a roadmap for your improvement journey, ensuring everyone is on the same page and working toward the same goal.

The driver diagram also shows the relationships between the theme, global aim, specific aims, measures, and PDSA cycles in a quick, visual way. Creating a *"Gantt chart"* to add pace and timing to the improvement is often helpful.

The driver diagram can be used in two ways for improvement teams.

1. It can be used at the beginning of improvement to list and organize the evidence-based, best-known practices and other improvement PDSA cycles to conduct to reach the goals of improvement.

    The PDSA cycles can be conducted one-by-one (especially when you are learning improvement skills).
2. It can be used as a road map when multiple staff have improvement capabilities and multiple PDSA cycles can be conducted simultaneously to achieve improvement goals in a timelier way.

Driver diagram

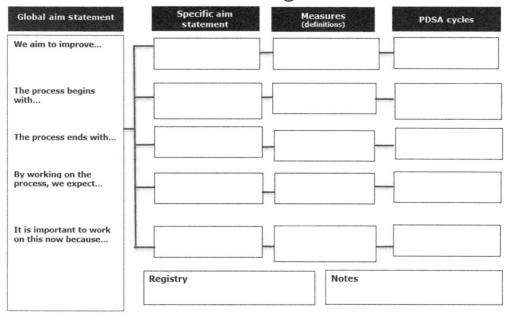

1. Identify the population of interest and associated registry.
2. Define the global aim statement and document the registry-level measure(s), if available.
3. Review evidence-based practice, best practice benchmarking, and other improvement literature information to determine the best change ideas to adapt and test. Define specific aim statements including, improvement targets and deadlines.
4. Define the operational definitions for each of the specific aim statements.
5. List the PDSA cycles.

Driver diagram - example

Pulmonary outcomes driver diagram

Global aim statement (include registry data)	Specific aim statements	Measures (operational definitions)	PDSA cycles
We aim to improve pulmonary outcomes for our patients in the University of Virginia Pediatric Cystic Fibrosis Center. **The process begins with** identifying modifiable factors that impact patients' lung health both in and outside of the clinic setting. **The process ends with** addressing and modifying the factors we have identified as barriers to improving lung health. **By working on the process, we** expect improved pulmonary outcomes for our patients. **It is important to work on this now because** the center report indicates a gap between our patient pulmonary outcomes and the top 10 centers. We have an opportunity and support for improvement through our LLC involvement.	Increase the percentage of patients following out-patient personal infection prevention and control (IP&C) practices (mask and handwashing for clinic entrance and exit) from baseline observation study of 75% wearing masks and 0% washing hands; to 100% adherence by all patients over the age of 2 by August 9, 2016.	• Observation data pre and post; tick and tally	• Sticker on appointment reminder • Mail protocol with newsletter • Verbal reminder • In-clinic education with check-off sheet • Eventually add to EMR • New hygiene stations first and third to supplement sixth floor station
	We will improve the quality of clinic hygiene by monitoring our cleaning practices according to IP&C protocols 100% of the time.	• Measure EVERY Tuesday Clinic • ATP values < 100 = pass for patient contact • ATP values < 150 = pass for bathroom.	• Select swab location narrow to five locations • Change cleaning solution to Virex • Put weekly report on agenda and team troubleshooting • Change bathroom value threshold • Use dice app to randomize room selection • Bathroom magnet protocol
	Aim to improve and sustain FEV$_1$ in patients 6–12 years old (under construction).	• Education module scores (pre/post) • 6 min. walk test (pre/post) • CFQ-R scores (pre/post) • FEV$_1$ • Quittner tool	• Under construction (planning phase) • Projected start date November

Registry data: Median FEV$_1$, percentage of patients 6–17 years below national average since 2008

Source: University of Virginia, Pediatric Program/with permission of Rector and Visitors of the University of Virginia.

Gantt Charts and Action Plans (Rhythm and Pace)

These improvement tools are helpful to support busy Mesosystem Improvement Teams stay on track in their improvement efforts. Field experience has showed us improvement teams who use **action plans** and Gantt charts are more organized and keep a *"rhythm and pace"* of improvement.

A Gantt chart is a useful organizing and management tool to plan and track overall improvement work. The Gantt chart provides a graphical illustration of the improvement activity schedule to be able to plan, coordinate, and track specific activities.

Inserting the driver diagram-specific aim statements and PDSA cycles into the Gantt chart supports the team to plan immediate and long-term improvement actions. The Gantt chart can show estimated times of completion and resources needed and can lay out the order of improvement to balance rhythm and pace of improvement. The Gantt chart often allays team member concerns with having too much to do when improvement is displayed using this tool.

Gantt charts also help to monitor progress and to quickly identify when improvement activities are behind schedule or not progressing to allow quick remedial action.

Gantt charts can be manually made or created through programs such as Microsoft Project or Excel.

Action Plans An action plan is a list of tasks specific to the next steps that need to be completed to achieve current improvement aims. The action plan is a simple and helpful organizing tool often created at the end of an improvement meeting to ensure all action items are captured to be completed before the next meeting. Please note the detail of the action plan includes what the task is, by whom and how it will be completed, and by when.

Reference
Nelson, E.C., Batalden, P.B., and Godfrey, M.M. (2007). *Quality by Design.* Chapter 23. San Francisco, CA: Jossey-Bass.

Gantt Chart

Month #1 _____

Name of activity, theme, aim, test of change	1	2	3	4	5	6	7	8	9	10	11	12	13	14	15	16	17	18	19	20	21	22	23	24	25	26	27	28	29	30	31

Month #1   July 2020 _____

Name of activity, theme, aim, test of change	1	2	3	4	5	6	7	8	9	10	11	12	13	14	15	16	17	18	19	20	21	22	23	24	25	26	27	28	29	30	31
Implement preclinic huddle																															
Requisitions given to patients in clinic																															
Clerical staff input comments																															
Clinic flow coordinator trailed																															
Test a preclinic prep day by multi-disciplinary team																															
Arrival policy letters posted to patients																															
Letter posted in clinic, given to patients in clinic; reinforced verbally																															

Gantt Chart Example

Month #2   August 2020

Name of activity, theme, aim, test of change	1	2	3	4	5	6	7	8	9	10	11	12	13	14	15	16	17	18	19	20	21	22	23	24	25	26	27	28	29	30	31
Implement preclinic huddle																															
Requisitions given to patients in clinic																															
Clerical staff input comments																															
Clinic flow coordinator trailed																															
Test a preclinic prep day by multi-disciplinary team																															
Arrival policy letters posted to patients																															
Letter posted in clinic, given to patients in clinic; reinforced verbally																															

Action Plan

What tasks will be done?	By Whom	By When?	How?	Comments

Plan-Do-Study-Act (PDSA) (Langley et al., 1996)

The Mesosystem Improvement Team should continue to meet regularly to review progress in the design of the PDSA and then during the execution of the test of change in a pilot format to observe and learn about the Change Idea implementation. Remember to always test Change Ideas in *small pilots* to learn what adaptations and adjustments need to be made before implementing on a larger scale. Data collection and review during the testing are important to answer the question: How will we know if the Change Idea is an improvement?

Once the PDSA cycle is completed and the mesosystem team reviews the data and qualitative findings, the plan should be revised or expanded to run another cycle of testing until the aim is achieved.

When the Change Idea has been tested and adapted to the context of the mesosystem and the data demonstrate that the Change Idea makes an improvement, the Mesosystem Improvement Team should design the Standardize- Do-Study-Act (SDSA, pg. 57) process to ensure the process is performed as designed. During this process it is important to continually learn and improve by monitoring the steps and data to identify new opportunities for further improvement. You will move from PDSA to SDSA and back to PDSA in your continuous improvement environment. New methods, tools, technology, or best practice will often signal the need to return to PDSA to achieve the next level of high performance. You want to be able to go from PDSA to SDSA and back to PDSA as needed. The scientific method is a two-way street that uses both experimentation (i.e., PDSA) and standardization (i.e., SDSA).

Reed and Card (2016) reflected on the use of the PDSA cycle and cautioned users not to use PDSA as a "stand-alone" method – it must be included in a suite of QI methods to ensure deeper understanding of the context and the problem. This action guide provides the suite of QI methods and encourages the rigorous use of reflective practice throughout the improvement process.

Reference

Reed, J. E. and Card, A. J. "The Problem with Plan-Do-Study-Act Cycles." *BMJ Quality & Safety*, 2016, 25(3), 147–152. doi: https://doi.org/10.1136/bmjqs-2015-005076

Langley, G. J., Nolan, K. M., Nolan, T. W., Norman, C. L., & Provost, L. P. (1996). *The improvement guide: A practical approach to enhancing organizational performance.* San Francisco, CA: Jossey-Bass Publishers.

Complete the Plan-Do-Study-Act worksheet to execute the Change Idea in a disciplined, measured manner, to reach the specific aim. See clinicalmicrosystem.org for examples. An example of this worksheet can be found on page 53.

Model for improvement

What are we trying to accomplish? (Aim)

How will we know that a change is an improvement? (Measures)

What changes can we make that will result in an improvement? (Changes)

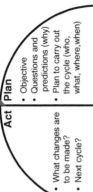

The PDSA cycle

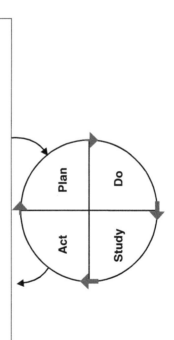

Act	Plan
• What changes are to be made? • Next cycle?	• Objective • Questions and predictions (why) • Plan to carry out the cycle (who, what, where, when)
Study	Do
• Complete the analysis of the data • Compare data to predictions • Summarize what was learned	• Carry out the plan • Document problems and unexpected observations • Begin analysis of the data

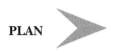 **PLAN** How shall we **PLAN** the pilot test? Who? What is the task? When? With what tools? What baseline data will be collected, over what period of time, to determine if the AIM is being achieved?

Tasks to be completed to run test of change	Who	When	Tools Needed	Measures

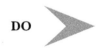 **DO** What are we learning as we **DO** the pilot? What happened when we ran the test? Any Surprises?

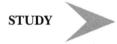 **STUDY** As we **STUDY** what happened, what have we learned? What do the measures show?

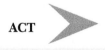 **ACT** As we **Act** to hold the gains or abandon our pilot efforts, what needs to be done? Will we modify the change? Make a **PLAN** for the next cycle of change.

Example of Designing the PDSA Cycle Starting with the Plan

Tasks to be completed to run test of change	Who	When	Tools Needed	Measures
Educate the staff on new algorithms for nutrition screening.	Lead RN Lead MD	Tuesday morning meeting	Measurement plan	Number of staff present at meeting / Total number of staff
Follow up with staff not able to attend meeting via email.	Lead RN	Tuesday afternoon	Measurement plan	Number of staff who received email / Number of staff not present at meeting
Create checklist of topics for dietitian to discuss with patient.	Lead Dietitian	Wednesday afternoon	Checklist (draft)	Completed checklist, reviewed by team
Checklist to be shared and reviewed by Lead Improvement Team.	Team	Thursday morning	Checklist (draft)	Agreement on checklist
Implement and audit new algorithm for nutrition screening.	Lead MD Dietitian	Tuesday afternoon	Tick and tally sheet for prior two weeks	Number of patients being assessed using the new algorithm for nutrition screening from dietitian/ Total number of patients aged 2-20 years seen in clinic each day

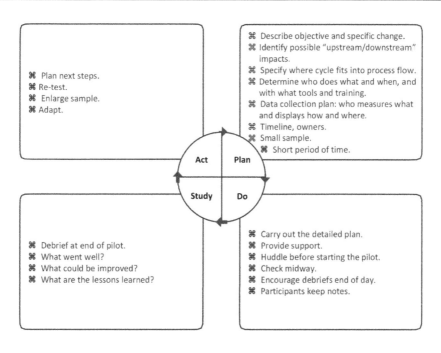

⌘ Plan next steps.
⌘ Re-test.
⌘ Enlarge sample.
⌘ Adapt.

⌘ Describe objective and specific change.
⌘ Identify possible "upstream/downstream" impacts.
⌘ Specify where cycle fits into process flow.
⌘ Determine who does what and when, and with what tools and training.
⌘ Data collection plan: who measures what and displays how and where.
⌘ Timeline, owners.
⌘ Small sample.
⌘ Short period of time.

Act | **Plan**

Study | **Do**

⌘ Debrief at end of pilot.
⌘ What went well?
⌘ What could be improved?
⌘ What are the lessons learned?

⌘ Carry out the detailed plan.
⌘ Provide support.
⌘ Huddle before starting the pilot.
⌘ Check midway.
⌘ Encourage debriefs end of day.
⌘ Participants keep notes.

Measurement Fundamentals: Operational and Conceptual Definitions – Worksheet

Instructions: Complete the following worksheet to derive measurement definitions from your global and specific aims following these five steps.

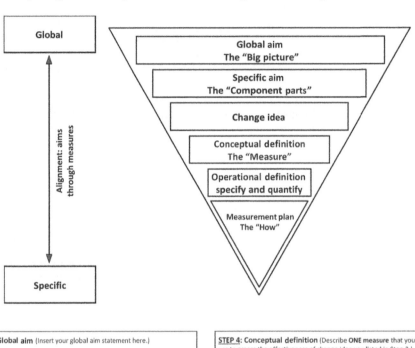

STEP 1: Global aim (Insert your global aim statement here.)

We aim to improve:
In:
The process begins with:
The process ends with:
By working on this process, we expect:
It is important to work on this now because:

STEP 2: Specific aim (List ONE specific aim derived from your global aim in Step 1.)

We aim to (by how much):

By (when):

STEP 3: Change Ideas (List ONE change idea that will appropriately address the specific aim listed in Step 2.)

STEP 4: Conceptual definition (Describe ONE measure that you could use to assess the effectiveness of change idea you listed in Step 3.)

STEP 5: Operational definition (Define very precisely what you conceptually described above in Step 4.)

STEP 6: Measurement Plan (Define HOW you will collect the data described above in Step 5.)

Measurement Fundamentals: Data Collection Plan Worksheet

Instructions: Draft a data collection plan for the measure that you conceptually and operationally defined.

1. List the Operational Definition of your selected measure here (refer to your Definitions worksheet, pg. 53).
2. Complete the table below to create a basic data collection plan for your measure.

Data Collection Worksheet	
Operational Definition:	
WHO? Who will collect and manage the data and how will they be trained? What is the data source (i.e., patients, providers, data registry owners, electronic medical record)?	
WHAT? What data will be collected (i.e., survey, observation, discussions or other techniques).	
WHERE? Where will the data be collected (i.e., inpatient clinic, specialty clinic, or other setting).	
WHEN? When will the data be collected (i.e., pilot test dates, pre-intervention, and post-intervention data collection, frequency of data collection).	
HOW? How will the data be collected, how will you ensure consistency and accuracy of measurement, how will you deal with missing data, and is your plan feasible to implement in the current system at this time?	

Standardize-Do-Study-Act (SDSA)

Standardize Current Best Process and Hold the Gains **STANDARDIZE** the process (specify which roles do what activities in what sequence with what information flow). A good way to track and standardize process is through the creation of a Playbook. The Playbook* is the collection of *process maps* to provide care and services that all mesosystem staff are aware of and accountable for. The Playbook can be used to orient new staff and patient/family advisors, document current processes, contribute to performance appraisals, and formalize the mesosystem improvements that have been achieved.

DO the work to integrate the standard process into daily mesosystem work routines to ensure reliability and repeatability.

STUDY at regular intervals. Consider whether the process is being adhered to and what adjustments are being made. Review the process when innovation, technology, or roles are being considered. Review what the measures of the process are showing. Be particularly mindful when significant staff changes such as when new residents arrive in academic centers to ensure they are oriented to the best practices.

ACT based on the above, maintain or tweak the standard process and continue doing this until the next wave of improvements/innovations takes place with a new series of PDSA cycles.

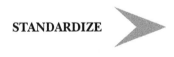

STANDARDIZE

How shall we **STANDARDIZE** the process and embed it into daily practice? Who? What's the task? When? With what tools? What needs to be "unlearned" to allow this new habit? What data will inform us if this is being standardized daily?

Tasks to Be Completed to "Embed" Standardization and Monitor Process	Who	When	Tools Needed	Measures

*Playbook – Create standard process maps to be inserted in your playbook.

DO — What are we learning as we **DO** the standardization? Any problems encountered? Any surprises? Any new insights to lead to another PDSA cycle?

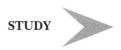

STUDY — As we **STUDY** the standardization, what have we learned? What do the measures show? Are there identified needs for change or new information or "tested" best practice to adapt?

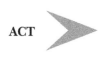

ACT — As we **ACT** to hold the gains or modify the standardization efforts, what needs to be done? Will we modify the standardization? What is the Change Idea? Who will oversee the new PDSA? Design a new PDSA cycle. Make a PLAN for the next cycle of change. Go to PDSA worksheet (pg. 51).

Data Wall (Dashboard) (Nelson et al., 2011)

Performance Dashboards Healthcare delivery systems frequently operate without measured performance systems that monitor performance and population health outcomes in real time. *Performance dashboards* can provide programs key information in real time to do the work of providing care and continuously improve the delivery of care and services. Using performance dashboards, microsystem- and mesosystem-level performance measurements can be employed effectively and efficiently to create rich and actionable information environments that can facilitate continuous improvement.

PERFORMANCE DASHBOARD TEMPLATE	
POPULATION MEASURE #1	POPULATION MEASURE #2
CLINICAL OUTCOME MEASURE	EXPERIENCE OUTCOME MEASURE

PROCESS MEASURE #1	PROCESS MEASURE #2

A basic dashboard template can be used to structure measures of population, outcome (clinical and experience of care), and process measures that can be extracted from the initial 5P assessment.

A data wall can be created in an agreed upon space to display the dashboard along with PDSA cycle measured results to keep mesosystem staff and people informed on how the mesosystem is performing. Also, recall the "Big Room" section as an example of data displays including digital displays.

Reference

Nelson, E.C., Batalden, P.B., Godfrey, M.M., and Lazar, J.S. (2011). Using Measurement to Improve Health Care Value. In: *Value by Design*, 129–160. San Francisco, CA: Jossey-Bass.

PERFORMANCE DASHBOARD Example	
POPULATION MEASURE #1	**POPULATION MEASURE #2**
DH-Family Medicine by age category % Females: 52 Est # (unique) patients in practice: 12438	Percentage of patients transferring by season
CLINICAL OUTCOME MEASURE	**EXPERIENCE OUTCOME MEASURE**
Registry Outcome Data	Satisfaction Survey Scores
PROCESS MEASURE #1	**PROCESS MEASURE #2**
Patients with transfer problems by season	Percentage of eligible patients transitioned within 90 days by quarter (pChart)

(*Source:* University Texas Southwestern ll Children's Medical Center Dallas and Plano, Pediatric Program OneCF Center and B.J. Oliver, PhD.)

STEP 5: Sustaining Improvement (Nelson, et al., 2007, Scoville et al., 2016)

"Holding the Gains of Improvement"

For decades, healthcare organizations have invested valuable time and resources to improve systems of care and outcomes. The challenge continues to be how to sustain the improvement gains made and not reverting to old performance levels.

Why Mesosystem Leadership Matters for Sustaining Improvement:
- **Connecting the Dots:** Microsystems (individual units or teams) often focus on their own specific areas. Mesosystem leaders help them see how their work contributes to the bigger picture of patient care across the organization. This shared understanding fosters a sense of purpose and encourages collaboration.
- **Breaking Down Silos:** Health care can easily become siloed, with different departments or units operating independently. Mesosystem leaders bridge these gaps, promoting communication and partnership between microsystems. This helps to spread best practices, reduce duplication of effort, and ensure consistent care.
- **Creating a Culture of Improvement:** Mesosystem leaders champion a culture where continuous improvement is valued and expected. They provide resources, remove barriers, and celebrate successes, making it easier for microsystems to sustain their efforts.
- **Role Modeling:** When leaders actively participate in improvement initiatives and demonstrate their commitment to quality, it sets a powerful example for others to follow.

How Mesosystem Leaders Can Support Sustained Improvement:
- **Establish Shared Goals:** Clearly communicate the organization's vision for improvement and how the mesosystem contributes to it.
- **Facilitate Communication:** Create opportunities for microsystems to share their work, learn from each other, and collaborate on projects.
- **Provide Resources and Support:** Ensure microsystems/mesosystems have the training, tools, resources and time they need to implement and sustain improvements.
- **Recognize and Reward Success:** Celebrate achievements and acknowledge the efforts of individuals and teams involved in the mesosystem improvement work.
- **Promote Continuous Learning:** Encourage ongoing evaluation and reflection to identify areas for further improvement.

By taking these steps, mesosystem leaders can create an environment where improvement is not just a one-time event, but an ongoing process that benefits both patients and healthcare providers.

References

Nelson, E.C., Batalden, P.B., and Godfrey, M.M. (2007). *Quality by Design.* San Francisco, CA: Jossey-Bass.

Scoville, R., Little, K., Rakover, J., Luther, K., and Mate, K. *Sustaining Improvement.* IHI White Paper. Cambridge, MA: Institute for Healthcare Improvement, 2016. (Available at ihi.org).

Follow-Up: Improvement in Healthcare Mesosystems Is a Continuous Journey

Sustaining improvement in healthcare mesosystems is a continuous journey, not a destination. It requires ongoing effort and attention to ensure positive changes become embedded in daily practice.

Monitoring and Reinforcement:

- **New processes and habits need constant monitoring:** It's not enough to just implement changes; you need to track their impact and make adjustments as needed. This helps identify any slippage or areas where further support is required.
- **"Huddles" are vital for reinforcement:** Regular, brief huddles provide opportunities to review progress, address challenges, and keep improvement at the forefront of everyone's minds. They foster a sense of accountability and shared responsibility.
- **Mesosystem Improvement Team meetings provide ongoing focus:** These meetings allow for broader discussion of progress, identification of emerging challenges, and coordination of efforts across microsystems.

Embedding New Habits:

- **Repetition and reminders are key:** Consistent use of tools like data walls, storyboards, and regular meetings helps to reinforce new ways of thinking and acting. They make improvement a visible and integral part of the organizational culture.
- **"Big Room" sessions foster collaboration and learning:** These dedicated sessions bring together diverse stakeholders to brainstorm ideas, share best practices, and generate solutions.
- **Involving patients and families is essential:** Including patient/family as partners in meetings ensures that improvement efforts result in coproduced care and services.

Continuous Improvement:

- **Regular assessments are crucial:** Ongoing evaluation of outcomes and performance metrics helps to identify new areas for improvement and refine existing processes.

- **The Mesosystem Improvement Team plays a vital role:** They should continuously analyze data, identify emerging themes, and guide the next cycle of improvement efforts.

By embracing these strategies, healthcare organizations can create a sustainable culture of improvement that leads to better patient care and outcomes. It's about constantly learning, adapting, and striving for excellence.

Improvement Tracking Worksheet			
What	**When**	**Who**	**Where**
Huddles			
Weekly Meetings – Microsystem Improvement Team			
Monthly Meetings-Mesosystem			
Quarterly Reports on Outcomes and Progress to Mesosystem and Senior Leaders			
Annual Retreat for Review and Reflection			
Data Wall/"Big Room"			
Storyboards			
Annual Professional Meetings			

Patient and Family Partnership

There are countless ways that patients and families can partner in improving care. They can serve as full members of improvement teams, help with orientation of staff, education, quality improvement, and in making connections with others. Some are formal and ongoing, others are time-limited and informal. At other times, it may be important to seek patients' and families' input on one specific issue. All are necessary to ensure that health care is truly responsive to the needs, priorities, goals, and values of patients and their families. Below is a list of some of the ways that patients and families can be involved.

EDUCATION

- Have patients and families involved in planning, developing, and/or revising educational materials.
- Involve patients and families in the development of the program website.
- Ask patients and families to assist in translating patient information materials (e.g., into another language or making information understandable for others).
- Have families and patients involved in planning, developing, and presenting to staff and patients.

QUALITY IMPROVEMENT

- Include patient and family in benchmarking visits to other programs.
- Develop a consumer satisfaction survey with patients and families and involve them in developing the responses to issues and problems identified (i.e., start with the satisfaction survey in "Assess Your Program" [pg.18]).
- Keep suggestion forms readily available so patients and families can record their ideas. Allow opportunities for suggestions to be submitted anonymously either in person or by mail if desired.

ORIENTATION

- Invite patients or families to present at staff orientation and in-service programs. Include residents, fellows, health professional students. Topics such as:
  - Care needs of the patient/family.
  - Specifics about the mesosystem of care.
- Have patient or families orient new patients and families when appropriate.

MAKING CONNECTIONS

- Develop a newsletter about mesosystem happenings – written and produced by health professionals, patients/families.
- Hold a quarterly/regular family/staff gathering.
- Create peer mentor or family liaison positions.
- Create regular opportunities for patients and families to talk with the mesosystem team and senior leaders.
- Conduct follow-up phone calls with patients and families after discharge.
- Set up "exit interviews" with administrators when patients and families are leaving the mesosystem.

ADVISORY COUNCIL

- Create an advisory council with patients and families to provide input and direction to mesosystem work (e.g., QI activities, educational materials, support network).
- Have a patient/family task force that reviews suggestions or is a contact for others for suggestions/issues/comments. This task force works closely with the professional care providers to make change happen.
- Appoint patients and families to task forces and work groups related to mesosystem flow, quality improvement, infection control processes, renovations when occurring, admitting procedures, discharge planning, patient safety, pain management, and other *continuous quality improvement* endeavors.
- Convene focus groups of patients and families as specific issues arise.

References

Adapted from Jeppson, E. and Thomas, J. *Essential Allies: Families as Advisors.* Bethesda, MD: Institute for Patient- and Family-Centered Care, 1994. Revised 2005.

Additional resources are available through the CF Foundation (CFF.org) or the Institute for Patient- and Family-Centered (ipfcc.org):

Webster, P. D. and Johnson, B. H. *Developing and Sustaining a Patient and Family Advisory Council.* Bethesda, MD: Institute for Patient- and Family-Centered Care, 2000.

Blaylock, B., Ahmann, E., and Johnson, B. H. *Creating Patient and Family Faculty Programs.* Bethesda, MD: Institute for Patient- and Family-Centered Care, 2002.

Onboarding Patient/Family Partners (PFP)

1. Develop a plan to invite practice patient and family partners (PFP) including clear expectations of being a PFP.
2. Take the time to consider the families that are cared for and what they bring to the mesosystem. The inclusion should emphasize a variety of races, ethnicities, incomes levels, sexual orientation, socio-cultural aspects, etc.
3. Schedule a time to meet with those who express interest to discuss and co-design their partnership and involvement
   a. Discuss how they want to be involved, e.g., improvement meetings, learning sessions, regional and national meetings.
   b. Identify interests and skills the PFP would like to contribute.
   c. Assure the PFP that there is flexibility in participating with the improvement team depending on their situation and ability.
   d. Discuss with the PFP the frequency of joining the improvement meetings e.g., weekly, every other week, monthly. PFPs do not need to attend all improvement meetings and by communicating what is convenient for them

will help the improvement team focus on specific PFP interests at the meetings they can attend.

   e. Discuss days/times that work best for the PFP to participate in the meetings. Emphasize there is flexibility for the improvement team to adjust meeting day/time to meet their needs and availability.

   f. Discuss length of involvement. Several months, 6 months, one year depending on their availability including periodic evaluations and feedback based on their experience as a PFP and their own life situation.

   g. Identify what the most convenient method is for the PFP to join the meeting e.g., in person, Zoom, telephone, etc. and if they have the equipment, infrastructure (internet) to join easily. It is important to share the sessions can be recorded if they are unable to join.

   h. Identify communication preferences with the PFP including frequency and type of communication. Do they want to be included in all QI Team correspondence or only topics they are interested in?

4. If a patient or family member agrees to participate, discuss mutual expectations of the PFP with the improvement team and leaders. Document the expectations.

5. Identify an improvement team "buddy" who can meet with the new PFP in advance of the first meeting and between meetings, as needed, to support the PFP by answering questions and providing clarifications.

6. Ensure improvement meeting agendas are sent in advance (follow the 7-step meeting process with advance agendas set at the end of each meeting) and include partner interests and topics in the agendas they want to attend - confirm partner interest and comfort with agenda topics.

   a. Be mindful of sensitive information discussed in team meetings (especially around outcomes, life expectancy and mortality) and alert the PFPs if these topics are on the agenda to help them decide if they want to participate or not. Communicate with improvement team members the need to be mindful about these topics.

   b. The PFP is an active member of the Quality Improvement Team. Include them in all aspects of the meeting including meeting roles, action items, and other activities that they express an interest in.

7. During the meetings, seek PFP feedback and be receptive to their suggestions and comments. Their unique perspective adds value and important considerations to the quality improvement work.

8. Provide clarification, information and invite the PFP to review the improvement resources, e.g., "Microsystems at a Glance," textbooks, worksheets and other content specific to the improvement collaborative.

9. Identify which team member will respond to PFP emails in a timely manner to build trust and communicate that their time to participate in the work is valued. (Consider the "buddy" in this role).

10. Plan time every other month to review partner participation, what is working and what can be improved and other ideas.

11. Include PFP as interested in national meeting preparations. As applicable, the partner (if a family member) may be able to attend in person depending on location and situation. Encourage virtual attendance if attending in person is not possible or if the PFP is a patient who cannot attend due to infection control practices.

12. Encourage the PFP to communicate with, convene and include other patients and family members.

References

Further information about patient and family engagement can be found at the Institute for Patient and Family Centered Care ipfcc.org.

Adapted from Cystic Fibrosis Foundation CF Learning Network Patient and Family Partner Collection of Tools and Success with Therapies Research Consortium (STRC) Steering Committee, 2023.

Adapted from 2nd Edition Action Guide for Accelerating Improvement in Cystic Fibrosis Care. Cystic Fibrosis Foundation, October 2017.

The M3 framework

Clinical microsystem awareness and development
Micro-meso-macro framework
Microsystems developmental journey: the stages

1. Create awareness of our clinical unit as an interdependent group of people with capacity to make change
2. Connect our routine daily work to the high purpose of benefiting patients: see ourselves as a system
3. Respond successfully to a strategic challenge
4. Measure the performance of our system as a system
5. Successfully juggle multiple improvements while taking care of patients…and continue to develop sense of ourselves as a system

Microsystem level "inside out"	Specific activities	Meso/macro system level "outside in" and "creating the conditions"
0-6 months *		
• Dartmouth microsystem improvement curriculum	• Ground rules/mission statement	• Develop clear vision for meso/microsystems
• Interdisciplinary lead team	• How will decisions be made	• Link strategy, operations and people - "Make it Happen"
• Rehearsing within studio course format	• Learning to work together utilizing effective meeting skills	• Support meso/microsystems protected time to reflect and learn
• Practicing in clinical practice	• Daily huddles, weekly lead team meetings, monthly all staff meetings	• Identify resources to support meso-micro development including information technology and performance measure resources
• Learning sessions (monthly)	• Microsystem Assessment Tool and Workforce Survey	• Develop measures of microsystem performance
• Conference calls (between sessions)	• Dartmouth microsystem toolkit	• Design meso/microsystem manager and leadership professional development strategy
	• PDSA-SDSA aim/improvements	
6-12 months		
• Staff reinforcement by leadership	• Aims/Practice improvement fundamentals	• Expect improvement science and measured results from meso/microsystems
• Colleague reinforcement	• PDSA-SDSA	• Develop whole system measures and targets/goals
• New habit development through repetition	• Measures/dashboards/data walls	• Convene meso/microsystems to work on linkages and "handoffs"
• Improvement science in action	• Playbooks and Storyboards	• Attract cooperation across health professional discrepancy traditions
• Add more improvement cycles	• Relationships between microsystems (linkages)	• Design review and accountability quarterly meetings for senior leaders
• Build measurement practice	• Best Practice using Value Stream Mapping/LEAN design principles	• Track and tell stories about improvement results and lessons learned at meso/micro levels
	• Link with electronic medical records	
	• Link Business initiatives/Strategic plan to microsystem level	
12-18 months		
• Continue "new way of providing care, continuously improving and working together"	• Daily "operations" huddles	• Develop professional development strategies across all professionals
• Actively engage more staff involvement	• Weekly "improvement" meetings	• Design HR selection and orientation process linked to identified needs of macro/microsystems
• Multiple improvements occuring	• Monthly "all staff" meetings	• Link performance management to daily work and results
• Network with other microsystems to support efforts	• Annual review, reflect, and plan retreats	• Consider incentive programs for reaching target/goals
• Coach network and development	• Playbooks and Storyboards	• Create system to link measurement and accountability at micro/meso/macro level
• Leadership development	• Data Walls and Dashboards	• Develop "Quality College" for ongoing support and capability building throughout organization
	• Quarterly system review and accountability meetings to meso-macro leadership	

*Pre-work: Visit www.clinicalmicrosystem.org/Read Part 1, 8, 9 of series/Watch Batalden streaming video

Adapted from Godfrey et al., 2005.

Case Study: Mesosystem (Advanced Lung Disease (ALD) Referring to Lung Transplant Program), Anywhere, USA

Context

Mesosystem members of the referral to lung transplant programs did not have shared consistent information about the ALD patient referral to transplant processes. Information sharing with ALD was often confusing and frequently with mixed information from the microsystems providing care. All mesosystem members not knowing the details of the "process" and the unknowns only further complicated a frightening time for patients and families. Referral for lung transplant is a complicated process that requires (1) **Patient education and preparation,** (2) **Timely referral** with **adequate information,** (3) Referring and transplant center **coordination,** and (4) **Patient co-management** before and after transplant. Improved communication, formal tracking, and co-management of the patient can be improved to ensure improved patient outcomes, patient preparedness, and comprehensive management of the CF and transplant patient.

Global Aim

We aim to improve the referring to lung transplant process in the Anywhere mesosystem.

The process begins with identifying a person with advanced lung disease in a referring program **The process ends** with referral to the lung transplant program

By working on this process, we expect to improve patient and staff education, patient preparation, ensure timely referral with accurate information, increase referring and lung transplant coordination of care and enhance co-management of the patient before and after transplant and improve mesosystem communication, formal tracking of the patient through the mesosystem.

It's important to work on this now because referrals have not been timely, the transition from the referral to the transplant programs do not always include important patient information, the referral and lung transplant programs may not consistently education patients and families in a standard way, and we realize the referral and transplant programs are not familiar with the interprofessional members and do not have current contact information.

FLOWCHART

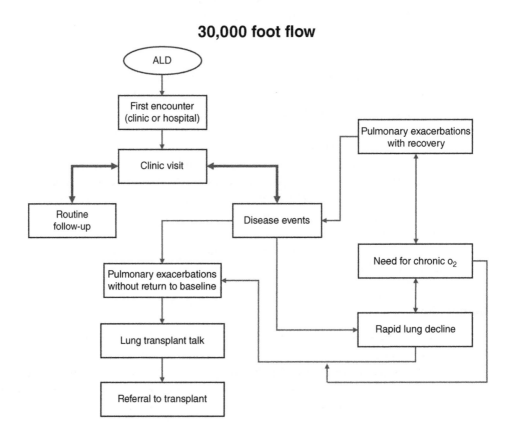

30,000 foot flow

Specific Aim

We aim to increase referring and transplant programs insight and understanding about each other's processes and roles in the referral to transplant programs for people with advanced lung disease.

We will have 100% participation of all roles in educational programs about the referral to lung transplant mesosystem **by January 2023.**

FISHBONE

ALD

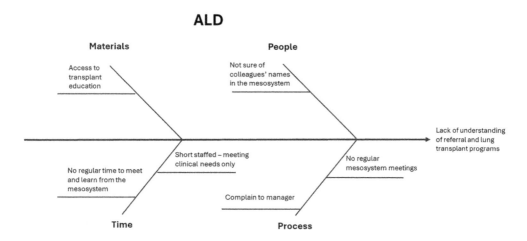

Change Idea: Conduct a one-day on-site visit to the transplant program, where members of the referring center participate in an education session that reviews the transplant phases for patients, from referral to transplant and get to know each other. An 11-question evaluation with a 5-point scale to rank knowledge from 0 (no knowledge) to 5 (complete knowledge) will be completed by each participant both pre-education and post-education.

RESULTS:

The pre-education and post-education 11-question evaluation showed significant improvement because of the site visit.

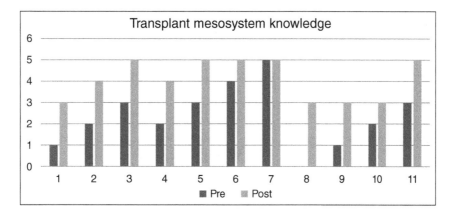

As a result of the "exchange" site visits between the referring and lung transplant programs, the mesosystem care team has improved communications regarding ALD patients by sustaining a weekly meeting, increasing the identification of patients and standardizing education.

1. Implemented patient education about ALD and lung transplant to give to people with ALD that was co-created by the referring and lung transplant programs.
2. Created a process flow to identify ALD patients.
3. Implemented weekly mesosystem meetings to discuss ALD patients in addition to patients scheduled for clinical care.
4. Improved communication among mesosystem care team members with weekly mesosystem team meetings and a standardized report template.
5. Improved mesosystem care team coordination of care with the addition of a standardized weekly meeting including care center leadership.
6. Standardized patient referrals process and handoffs to transplant program.

LESSONS LEARNED:

- What, when, and how we share health related information about our patients saves time, improves the quality of mesosystem communication, and reduces cost of care, while improving patient and healthcare provider engagement.
- On-going communication between the microsystems in the mesosystem improved timely scheduling, testing, and interventions for patients
- Mesosystem team collaboration and communication makes identification of ALD patients timely, and referrals made more easily.
- Having a mesosystem agreed upon standard process for all the patients has helped ensure that no patients are slipping through the cracks in the mesosystem, and allows all patients to receive equal treatment and attention.
- Weekly mesosystem discussions regarding ALD patients allowed for focused and expedited referrals, mitigating personal decision-making of individuals.

Glossary

5P Framework Puts improvement themes into context and is a great place from which to start your improvement work. Use global aim template.

Action Plan Detailed "next steps" and "to do" with clearly identified and accountable people and timeline.

Agenda Meeting process that includes meeting roles to result in productive meetings with timed segments and clear objectives.

Aim (Global) Puts improvement themes into context and is a great place from which to start your improvement work. Use global aim template.

Aim (Specific) Detailed focus and includes measurable outcomes with specific dates. Use specific aim template.

Algorithm A sequence of specified actions to reach a goal.

Benchmarking To search for best practices that consistently produce best in-the-world results. A systematic process of continuously measuring an organization's critical business processes and results against leaders anywhere in the world to gain information that will help the organization take action to improve its performance.

Best Practices A process that is generally accepted as preferred to any alternatives.

Clinical Mesosystem Two or more microsystems: e.g., A patient pathway.

Change Concepts Stimulants for developing and designing detailed and specific change ideas to test.

Change Ideas Generated from literature review, best practices, benchmarking, and change concepts to select a change idea to test.

Checklist Comprehensive list of items and actions to be taken in a specific order.

Chronic Care Model (CCM) Comprised of six interrelated systems meant to make patient-centered, evidence-based care easier to accomplish.

Clinical Mesosystem Two or more microsystems: A patient pathway.

Clinical Microsystem The place where patients, families, and care teams meet. A small group of people who work together on a regular basis to provide care to discrete subpopulations of patients. Frontline clinical units including patients, families, professionals, data, and information with common purpose with shared business and clinical aims. It produces performance outcomes.

Co-design Users as "experts" of their own experience become central to the design and improvement process.

Communication Plan Clear actions to share improvement progress.

Conceptual Definition The conceptual definition tells what will be measured (e.g., patient waiting for clinic visit).

Continuous Quality Improvement A management philosophy that is a preventive, proactive process to continuously improve and learn how current processes and systems are performing.

Contributing Units Clinical units (microsystems) a patient travels through for an episode of care.

Control Chart Graphic format for displaying information that show data points in the order in which they occurred with statistically calculated upper and lower natural process limits.

Coproduction Effective participation of patients, their families, and healthcare providers in the design and improvement of care.

Core and Supporting Processes Core processes are the routine activities that are essential to functioning within a system of care. Supporting processes intermittently provide care and services to support the process of care.

Cycle Time Total time from the beginning to the end of a process.

Dartmouth Microsystem Improvement Ramp A disciplined and organized improvement process including PDSA to guide improvement.

Data Owner Accountable person to oversee specific data collection and display.

Data Transparency Full public disclosure of performance and outcomes that can be a driver of accountability.

Data Wall Designated space to display measures and improvement progress over time. Utilized daily and weekly to review current values and target values to assess progress toward aims.

Decision-Making Criteria A set of criteria to help individuals select an improvement idea to test. Usually includes: don't need permission to work on, can start right away, doesn't cost money, and will have the biggest impact on needed improvement.

Driver Diagram A tool to organize and track multiple improvements to achieve the "Global Aim" of the "Theme" of improvement. It also shows the relationships among the theme, global aim, specific aims, measures, and PDSA cycles in a quick, visual way.

Facilitator Person with training, skill, and expertise in both clinical improvement and group process.

Fishbone Diagram An analysis tool that depicts the possible causes that contribute to a single effect. Also called a "cause and effect" or Ishikawa diagram

Flowchart Graphic representation of a process using symbols and arrows.

Gantt Chart A chart in which a series of horizontal lines shows the amount of work done or production completed in certain periods of time in relation to the amount planned for those periods.

Hold the Gains System improvement over time and assurance that new habits are embedded in daily practice.

Huddle Short meeting, no longer than 10 minutes, of a clinical team to review clinical care, anticipate needs, and review any improvement progress.

IHI Institute for Healthcare Improvement (IHI), an independent not-for-profit organization based in Cambridge, MA, that is a leading innovator in health and healthcare improvement worldwide.

Improvement Model Developed by Associates in Process Improvement, is a simple yet powerful tool for accelerating improvement with two parts: three fundamental questions and the Plan-Do-Study-Act (PDSA) cycle.

Improvement Sciences An emerging concept that focuses on exploring how to undertake quality improvement well. It inhabits the sphere between research and quality improvement by applying research methods to help understand what impacts quality improvement.

Lead Improvement Team Interdisciplinary team of a microsystem leading improvement actions and strategy.

Measurement and Monitoring (Ticks and Tallies) Observational data tracking through documenting frequency with a "Tick" or hash mark and then a total "Tally" of the individual hash marks.

Measurement Triangle The model of disciplined improvement measurement linked to The Dartmouth Microsystem Improvement Ramp.

Metrics that Matter (MTM) Key measures specific to diagnostic group or system of care. Can include organizational goals, professional standards, and national benchmarks (e.g., outcome measures of BMI, FEV1).

Microsystems Front-line units that provide day-to-day health care. A small group of people who work together on a regular basis to provide care to discrete populations of patients. It has clinical and business aims, linked processes, and a shared information environment and it produces performance outcomes.

Operational Definition Defines how metrics will be measured (e.g., time elapsed from patient appointment time until time patient enters exam room in minutes).

Outcomes Short- and long-term changes that occur as a direct result of "processes" on inputs.

Owner Person with the responsibility and authority to lead the improvement of a process. Also, the person with responsibility for a given process.

Pace of Improvement Consideration of operational and seasonal impacts that affect the pace of improvement like vacations, snowstorms, The Joint Commission.

Patient and Family Advisory Group Group to assist in planning, implementing, and evaluating improvement projects and needed improvement of the program.

Patient Experience Maps The lived care experience of patients and families as experienced through their own visit. What did the experience feel like? How does the experience compare to the "mechanical" process map of the clinic?

Patient Registry An organized system to collect uniform data (clinical or other) to evaluate specified outcomes for a population defined by a particular diagnoses and serves a predetermined scientific, clinical, or policy purpose.

Patient Satisfaction Survey Patient evaluation of care to provide opportunities for improvement, monitor healthcare performance, and provide benchmarking information.

Patients One of the 5Ps, patients are at the core of quality improvement work in a microsystem. Their top diagnoses, age distribution, and satisfaction with current care are a few measures.

Patterns One of the 5Ps, patterns are repeating predictable cycles and behaviors that can be observed and articulated (e.g., meeting frequency, communication and relationships, social activities, financial performance).

PDSA (Plan-Do-Study-Act Cycle) Schema for continuous quality improvement originally developed by Walter Andrew Shewhart and made popular by W. Edwards Deming, who ascribed inherent variation in processes to chance and intermittent variation to assignable causes. The PDSA cycle is a four-part method for discovering and correcting assignable causes to improve the quality of processes.

Performance Dashboards Provide at-a-glance view of the microsystem key performance, process, and clinical outcomes to create actionable information environments to facilitate continuous improvement.

Personal Skills Assessment Tool Documents strengths and development topics to determine quality improvement education and training needs.

Pilot Test Small-scale test of a proposed solution.

Playbook Collection of process maps to standardize care and processes that all staff are aware of and accountable for.

Point of Service Exact real time of interacting with patients to deliver care or services.

Process Maps Chronological graphical displays of steps in a process. Different types of process maps include flowcharts, deployment charts, and value stream mapping.

Processes One of the 5Ps, a process is any activity that is a series of steps with a beginning and end resulting in products or outcomes.

Professionals One of the 5Ps, professionals are members of the frontline team including anyone who has the privilege to provide care and services. administrative staff, lead MDs, nurses, therapists, social workers, dietitians, etc.

Purpose One of the 5Ps, this is the common aim and reason to come together to strive and be accountable for achieving.

QI Learning and Leadership Collaboratives (QI LLC) Contribute to creating cultures of improvement at the front line of care through a blend of face-to-face and virtual learning sessions to increase improvement capabilities.

Reaccreditation Site Visit The accreditation site visit is typically conducted by Accreditation Committees who review standards.

Redesign Methodical process of opening insight into current states, exploring best knowledge practices, systems, and creating a new process.

Rework Work to redo or correct what was not done right the first time.

Rhythm of Improving Disciplined improvement supported by regular meetings, monthly all-staff meetings, and annual retreats to plan and execute improvement.

Scatter Plot Display Used to plot data points on a horizontal and a vertical axis in the attempt to show how one variable is affected by another.

SDSA (Standardize-Do-Study-Act Cycle) Steps taken when PDSA Cycle has been successfully done to achieve the original aim. The purpose is to hold the gains that were made using PDSA cycles and standardize process in daily work.

Self-Management Individual control and management of health care.

Senior Leaders The C Suite: Chief Executive Officer, Chief Nursing Officer, Chief Operating Officer, Chief Quality Officer.

Shadowing Following a patient/family through their care experience to inform improvement and redesign of care processes and systems.

Small Pilots Small-scale preliminary study conducted in order to evaluate feasibility, time, cost, adverse events, and impact to improve upon the study design prior to performance of a full-scale research project.

Smart Change Ideas Best practices.

Snapshot of the Data Small sample in a set time rather than an exhaustive collection of data.

SPC (Statistical Process Control) Developed by Dr. Walter Shewhart and further expanded upon by Dr. W. Edwards Deming to monitor process variation to improve quality.

Staff Satisfaction Survey Employee affective and cognitive satisfaction with the workplace.

Standard Operating Procedures (SOP) See Playbooks.

Storyboards Visual display used to document and communicate a team's improvement journey. Includes aims, PDSAs, team members, measured outcomes, and next steps.

Subpopulations of Patients A specific group of individuals with common patient characteristics (e.g., race/ethnicity, age, risk factors).

Sustaining Improvement Utilizing SDSA and playbooks to sustain improvement while creating conditions in the microsystem to continue to provide care and improve care.

Systems Within Systems Bertalanffy, the founder of the scientific, mathematical "Theory of Systems," defined a system as a set of interacting, interrelated, or interdependent elements that work together in a particular environment to perform the functions that are required to achieve the system's aim.

Target Value The measured output of the desired process results.

Tests of Change See PDSA.

Theme Focus of improvement after reviewing information and data of a clinical microsystem.

Through the Eyes of the Patients Direct real-time observation of patients in their care experience – process and interactions.

Transition and Transfer Process Specific to transition from pediatric to adult care with all processes to ensure smooth seamless transfer from pediatric care, services, and staff to adult care, services, and staff.

Trend Charts (Run Charts) Used to show trends in data over time.

Unplanned Activity Interruptions, waits, and delays in the processes of providing smooth and uninterrupted patient care.

GLOSSARY

Chapter 1

Clinical microsystem: A small group of people (including health professionals and care-receiving patients and their families as well as information and information technology) who work together in a defined setting on a regular basis (or as needed) to create care for discrete subpopulations of patients.

Complex adaptive system: A complex adaptive system includes autonomous but interdependent agents that are capable of adaptation.

Information technology: Tools used to move and share information. This can be as sophisticated as an electronic health record, or as simple as pen and paper.

Interdisciplinary: Involving more than one academic field of study.

Interprofessional: Involving more than one profession (for example, nurses, pharmacists, physicians).

Macrosystem: The larger organization in which mesosystems are embedded, such as a hospital, multispecialty group, or health system.

Quality by Design: A Clinical Microsystems Approach, Second Edition. Edited by Marjorie M. Godfrey, Tina C. Foster, Julie K. Johnson, Eugene C. Nelson and Paul B. Batalden.
© 2025 John Wiley & Sons, Inc. Published 2025 by John Wiley & Sons, Inc.

Mesosystem: Two or more microsystems providing healthcare services for a specified population and context that are linked in some way.

Metasystem: System about other systems, which links concepts of a system with an overarching system.

Microsystem: See **Clinical microsystem**.

Model for improvement: A framework developed by Associates in Process Improvement and popularized by the Institute for Healthcare Improvement to guide improvement work. It includes three questions: What are we trying to accomplish? How will we know if a change is an improvement? What change can we make that will result in improvement? which are then addressed through a series of small experiments or Plan-Do-Study-Act cycles.

Sensemaking: The process by which people understand or give meaning to experiences.

Sharp end: The place where activity (and problems) can occur; in health care this often refers to actual interactions with patients and families.

Team coaching model: A framework based in Team Coaching Theory using 4 phases: "work before the work," pre-phase, action phase, and transition phase for developing improvement capabilities and socio-behavioral skills of interprofessional frontline teams to develop a culture of improvement.

Value: Value in health care is often thought of as $\dfrac{Quality + Outcomes}{Costs}$.

Chapter 2

5Ps: The 5Ps framework is a tested and useful method for microsystem members to begin to see their microsystem from a system perspective using Donabedian "structure, process, and outcomes." Purpose, patients/population, professionals, processes, and patterns.

Action-learning theory: An experiential learning method in which participants learn by doing and then reflecting on what they have done.

Balancing measures: Looking at a system from different directions or dimensions and asking if the changes are designed to improve one part of the system and cause new problems in other parts of the system.

Clinical value compass: To manage and improve the value of healthcare services, providers will need to measure the value of care for similar patient populations, analyze the internal delivery processes, run tests of changed delivery processes, and determine if these changes lead to better outcomes and lower costs. A clinical value compass has four cardinal points: (1) functional status, risk status, and well-being; (2) costs; (3) satisfaction with health care and perceived benefit; and (4) clinical outcomes.

Data wall: Designated areas in the clinical microsystem where data over time specific to the microsystem are displayed for all members of the microsystem to review and take action on. Data walls typically include data over time from organization-strategic measures, service line data, and clinical microsystem data that reflect current performance such as cycle time or length of stay.

Multidisciplinary team (MDT): A team of healthcare professionals who are members of different disciplines (**for example**, Psychiatrists, Social Workers, Pharmacists, Nurses, etc.), each providing specific services to the patient that work together towards a specific set of goals.

Parking lot: A list of tangential topics or issues that arise in a meeting that should be dealt with later.

PDSA (Plan-Do-Study-Act): Schema for continuous quality improvement originally developed by Walter Andrew Shewhart and made popular by W. Edwards Deming, who ascribed inherent variation in processes to chance and intermittent variation to assignable causes. The PDSA cycle is a four-part method for discovering and correcting assignable causes to improve the quality of processes.

SDSA (Standardize-Do-Study-Act): Steps taken when PDSA cycle has been successfully done to achieve the original aim. Purpose is to hold the gains that were made using PDSA cycles and standardize process in daily work.

Value compass: See **Clinical value compass**.

Chapter 3

Accountable care organization (ACO): Groups of doctors, hospitals, and other healthcare professionals that work together to give patients high-quality, coordinated service, and health care, improve health outcomes, and manage costs. ACOs may be in a specific geographic area and/or focused on patients who have a specific condition, like chronic kidney disease.

Balanced metrics: Refer to a set of measures that assess the impact of a change or intervention from multiple perspectives, ensuring that improvements in one area do not inadvertently cause negative consequences in another. This approach recognizes the interconnectedness of healthcare systems and the potential for unintended consequences when focusing on a single outcome.

Bend the cost curve: To drive down medical costs.

Care coordination: The deliberate organization of patient care activities between two or more participants (including the patients) involved in a patient's care to facilitate the appropriate delivery of healthcare services.

Community-based interventions: Refers to multicomponent interventions that generally combine individual and environmental change strategies across multiple settings aiming to prevent dysfunction and to promote well-being among population groups in a defined local community.

Coproduction: The interdependent work of users and professionals to design, create, develop, deliver, assess, and improve the relationships and actions that contribute to the health of individuals and populations.

Fee for service: A payment model where services are unbundled and paid for separately. In health care, it gives an incentive for providers to provide more treatments because payment is based on the quantity of care, rather than the quality of care.

"Feed forward": The collection of patient-reported outcomes (PROs) in routine clinical practice provides opportunities to "feed-forward" the patient's perspective to his/her clinical team to inform planning and management.

"Feedback": Patient-reported outcomes (PROs) data can also be aggregated to "feedback" population-level analytics that can inform treatment decision-making, predictive modeling, population-based care, and system-level quality improvement efforts.

Globally capitated (Global capitation): A payment model specifically for integrated healthcare delivery. By accepting a defined fixed payment to provide contracted services, providers assume the financial risk for their patients, usually including both insurance risk and technical risk.

Handoffs: Transfer of information, responsibility, and authority regarding patient care from one healthcare provider or team to another.

Health continuum: Describes the delivery of health care over a period of time and refers to an integrated system of health care that follows a patient through time or through a range of services. The goal of a health continuum is to offer more comprehensive patient care.

Huddles: Brief, typically 10–15 minutes, interdisciplinary team member stand-up meeting that involves discussion about patient safety, review of previous shift, and proactively identifies potential concerns for the day.

Multispecialty group practice: Healthcare organization comprised of physicians and healthcare professionals from various medical specialties who work together to provide comprehensive care to patients.

Physician "compact": Popularized by Dr. Jack Silversin, founder of Amicus Consulting, a physician compact is where the healthcare organization and their physicians choose to engage with each other to understand their respective perspectives of the changing healthcare landscape, and to negotiate a new set of mutual expectations (Silversin, 2000).

Population health: Refers to the health outcomes of a group of individuals, including the distribution of such outcomes within the group. It is an approach to health that aims to improve the health of an entire population consisting of health outcomes, health determinants, interventions, and policies using non-traditional partnerships among different sectors in the community – public health, industry, academia, health care, local governments, etc.

Reflection: Process of thinking deeply or carefully about something that involves examining one's thoughts, feelings, experiences, or actions to gain a better understanding or learn from them.

Relative value units (RVUs): Originally developed as a physician payment mechanism, RVUs have expanded into a valuable practice management tool that allows common denominator analyses and per-unit comparisons for both clinical productivity and expense data. Use of RVUs in practice management falls into three broad categories: productivity, cost, and benchmarking (Glass, 2002).

Root cause analysis: Systematic problem-solving method used to identify the underlying causes of an adverse event or problem. It aims to dig deeper than the surface-level symptoms to uncover the fundamental issues that contribute to the occurrence of the problem. The primary goal of RCA is to identify and address the root causes so that similar problems can be prevented in the future. By understanding the underlying causes, organizations can implement effective corrective actions that target the root of the problem rather than just treating the symptoms.

Team-based care model: A delivery model where patient care needs are addressed as coordinated efforts among multiple healthcare providers and across settings of care (Schottenfeld, 2016).

Value-based care: Healthcare delivery model that focuses on improving patient outcomes while reducing costs. It differs from the traditional fee-for-service model, where providers are paid for each service they provide, regardless of the outcome.

White space: In the context of healthcare transitions, "white space" refers to gaps or inefficiencies in the processes and communication during patient handoffs between different healthcare providers or settings. It represents the areas where information may be lost, overlooked, or misinterpreted.

Chapter 4

Distributed decision-making models of leadership: Involves leadership practices that are more collaborative, open, and decentralized – designed to mesh more effectively with new forms of work and new technologies. It is a kind of leadership that blends top-down, and bottom-up decision-making. And while it is difficult to leave behind models of the pyramid with the omniscient, omnipotent leader at the top, organizations are beginning to view leadership not as an individual characteristic, but as a system involving networks of leaders – some formal and others informal – operating at all levels of an organization and often across organizational boundaries. The result is that organizations can more effectively mobilize the collective intelligence, motivation, and creative talent of their employees, partners, and customers (Ancona, 2017).

Doctor of nursing practice (DNP): The Doctorate of Nursing Practice (DNP) is a terminal degree in nursing. DNPs possess the highest level of nursing expertise to influence healthcare outcomes through organizational leadership, health policy implementation, and direct patient care and work either in a clinical setting or leadership role upon obtaining the required credentials. The DNP differs from the PhD in Nursing, which is a research-focused degree. DNP graduates are prepared to lead and implement change in clinical practice.

Early adopters of change: These individuals have the highest degree of opinion leadership among the adopter categories (early adopter, early majority, late majority, and laggards). Early adopters are respected by peers and are the embodiment of successful, discrete use of new ideas. The early adopter decreases uncertainty about a new idea by adopting it, and then conveying a subjective evaluation of the innovation to near-peers through interpersonal networks (Rogers, 1995).

Experiential learning: Experiential learning involves learning from experience. The theory was proposed by psychologist David Kolb who was influenced by the work of other theorists including John Dewey, Kurt Lewin, and Jean Piaget (Kolb, 1984).

Focus group: A qualitative research method in which a trained moderator conducts a collective interview of typically six to eight participants from similar backgrounds, similar demographic characteristics, or both. Focus groups create open lines of communication across individuals and rely on the dynamic interaction between participants to yield data that would be impossible to gather via other approaches, such as one-on-one interviewing. When done well, focus groups offer powerful insights into people's feelings and thoughts and thus a more detailed, nuanced, and richer understanding of their perspectives on ideas, products, and policies (Lavrakas, 2008).

Hospital acquired conditions (HACs): A medical condition or complication that a patient develops during a hospital stay, which was not present at admission.

Mixed methods research: An approach to inquiry that combines or integrates both qualitative and quantitative forms of research. It involves philosophical assumptions, the use of qualitative and quantitative approaches, and the mixing or integrating of both approaches in a study (Creswell, 2018).

Qualitative research: A means for exploring and understanding the meaning individuals or groups ascribe to a social or human problem. The process of research involves emerging questions and procedures collecting data in the participants' setting, analyzing the data inductively, building from particulars to general themes, and making interpretations of the meaning of the data (Creswell, 2018).

Quantitative research: A means for testing objective theories by examining the relationship among variables. These variables can be measured, typically on instruments, so that numbered data can be analyzed using statistical procedures (Creswell, 2018).

Shared governance: A decentralized approach that gives nurses greater authority and control over their practice and work environment, engenders a sense of responsibility and accountability, and allows active participation in the decision-making process, particularly in administrative areas from which they were excluded previously. The primary aim is to support the relationship between the service provider (nurse) and patient (client). It is not a one-time implementation process, with a concrete, fixed set of rules, but rather an ongoing and fluid process, which requires continual assessment and revaluation to be flexible and adaptive to the environment (O'May, 1999).

Success characteristics of high-performing clinical microsystems: Robert Wood Johnson supported research conducted at Dartmouth identified nine success characteristics related to high performance in healthcare systems: leadership, culture, macro-organizational support of microsystems, patient focus, staff focus, interdependence of care team, information and information technology, process improvement, and performance patterns. These success factors were interrelated and together contributed to the microsystem's ability to provide superior, cost-effective care and at the same time create a positive and attractive working environment.

Team coaching: Direct interaction with a team intended to help members make coordinated and task-appropriate use of their collective resources in accomplishing the team's work (Hackman, 2005).

Tipping point: The tipping point is that magic moment when an idea, trend, or social behavior crosses a threshold, tips, and spreads like wildfire.

"Walk the talk": To do what one said one could do, or would do, not just making empty promises (YourDictionary, n.d.).

Chapter 5

Clinical pathways (CPWs): A common component in the quest to improve the quality of health. CPWs are used to reduce variation, improve quality of care, and maximize the outcomes for specific groups of patients (Lawal, 2016).

Context: The complex set of factors that surround and influence a patient's health, care, and outcomes. It encompasses both internal and external elements that shape the patient's experience and the healthcare system's ability to provide effective care.

Functional outcomes: One of the four clinical value compass measures (clinical, functional, cost, and satisfaction) including physical function, emotional status, social/role function, and health risk status.

Gantt chart: A horizontal bar chart developed by Henry L. Gantt, frequently used to manage overall improvement work. A Gantt chart provides a graphical illustration of the improvement activity schedule, helping to plan, coordinate, and track specific tasks.

Geographic cohorting: Also known as co-location or regionalization, refers to the practice of assigning a hospitalist team or group of healthcare providers to a specific inpatient unit or geographic location within a hospital. This means that the majority of the team's patients are admitted to the same unit, allowing for closer proximity between the providers, nurses, and patients.

National Committee for Quality Assurance (NCQA): Is an independent 501(c) (3) nonprofit organization in the United States that works to improve healthcare quality through the administration of evidence-based standards, measures, programs, and accreditation.

Pathways: See **Clinical pathways.**

Patient and family experience: The patient [and family] experience encompasses the range of interactions that patients have with the health care system, including their care from health plans, and from doctors, nurses, and staff in hospitals, physician practices, and other healthcare facilities. As an integral component of healthcare quality, patient [and family] experience includes several aspects of healthcare delivery that patients value highly when they seek and receive care, such as getting timely appointments, easy access to information, and good communication with healthcare providers (AHRQ, 2017).

Patient-centered medical home (PCMH): A care delivery model that focuses on providing comprehensive, coordinated, and patient-centered primary care. The goal of PCMH is to improve the quality, accessibility, and affordability of health care while enhancing the patient experience.

Playbooks: A collection of core and supporting processes used routinely by the microsystem including flowcharts and diagrams of processes that have been tested using improvement science and represent the way the microsystem wants things done.

Relational coordination: Is a mutually reinforcing process of communicating and relating for the purpose of task integration. It captures the relational dynamics of coordinating work.

Shared decision-making: An approach where clinicians and patients share the best available evidence when faced with the task of making decisions, and where patients are supported to consider options to achieve informed preferences (Elwyn, 2012).

Chapter 6

Appreciative inquiry (AI): A change management approach that focuses on identifying what is working well, analyzing why it is working well, and then doing more of it. The basic tenet of AI is that an organization will grow in whichever direction that people in the organization focus their attention.

Change concept: A stimulant for developing and designing detailed and specific change ideas to test.

Digital interfaces: The mediums by which humans interact with computers. Interfaces represent an amalgamation of visual, auditory, and functional components that people see, hear, touch, or talk to as they interact with computers.

Evaluation: A reflection on how well the project was executed (process) and whether it met its objectives (outcomes) after project completion.

Hospital Consumer Assessment of Healthcare Providers and Systems (HCAHPS): A survey instrument and data collection methodology for measuring patients' perceptions of their hospital experience. It is the first national, standardized, publicly reported survey of patients' perspectives of hospital care.

Implementation: The process of putting a plan, idea, or system into action. It involves translating a concept into a tangible outcome by taking the necessary steps to make it a reality.

Initiation: The selection of a problem, the commissioning of a solution, and the designation of the necessary problem-solving resources within a larger system.

Patient-reported outcome measures (PROMs): Tools used to collect and assess information directly from patients about their health status, quality of life, and perception of their treatment or care. PROMs are typically questionnaires or surveys that ask patients to report on their symptoms, functional status, well-being.

Pay-for-performance (P4P): A healthcare payment model that rewards healthcare providers for meeting specific performance measures related to quality, efficiency, and patient satisfaction. It contrasts with the traditional fee-for-service model, where providers are paid based on the quantity of services rendered regardless of outcomes. Also known as "value-based purchasing."

Planning: Determining what will be done, by whom, by when.

Speak Up campaign: The Joint Commission's award-winning Speak Up™ program urges patients to take an active role in preventing health care errors by becoming involved and informed participants on their health care team.

Chapter 7

Active errors: Errors or mistakes that occur at the point of contact between a healthcare provider and a patient, or between a human and a specific part of a larger healthcare system. These errors are typically immediately apparent and often involve frontline healthcare workers.

Catheter-Associated Urinary Tract Infection (CAUTI): A urinary tract infection (UTI) is an infection involving any part of the urinary system, including urethra, bladder, ureters, and kidney. UTIs are the most common type of healthcare-associated infection. Among UTIs acquired in the hospital, approximately 75 percent are associated with a urinary catheter, which is a tube inserted into the bladder through the urethra to drain urine. Between 15 to 25 percent of hospitalized patients receive urinary catheters during their hospital stay. The most important risk factor for developing a catheter-associated UTI (CAUTI) is prolonged use of the urinary catheter. Therefore, catheters should only be used for appropriate indications and should be removed as soon as they are no longer needed (Source: CDC, NCEZID, DHQP).

Central Line-Associated Blood Stream Infection (CLABSI): A central line (also known as a central venous catheter) is a catheter (tube) placed in a large vein in the neck, chest, or groin to give medication or fluids or to collect blood for medical tests. A central line-associated bloodstream infection (CLABSI) is a serious infection that occurs when germs (usually bacteria or viruses) enter the bloodstream through the central line. Central line-associated bloodstream infections (CLABSIs) result in thousands of deaths each year and billions of dollars in added costs to the U.S. healthcare system (Source: CDC, NCEZID, DHQP).

Countermeasures: An action taken to counteract a danger or threat designed to mitigate the negative effects of a problem and prevent its recurrence or escalation.

Diagnostic error: A diagnosis that is missed, wrong, or delayed, as detected by some subsequent definitive test or finding.

Haddon matrix: The most commonly used paradigm in the injury prevention field. Developed by William Haddon in 1970, the matrix looks at factors related to personal attributes, vector or agent attributes, and environmental attributes; before, during, and after an injury or death.

Hindsight bias: Refers to the common tendency for people to perceive events that have already occurred as having been more predictable than they actually were before the events took place.

Human factors: A science at the intersection of psychology and engineering – is dedicated to designing all aspects of a work system to support human performance and safety. Human factors, also known as ergonomics, uses scientific methods to improve system performance and prevent accidental harm. The goals of human factors in health care are twofold: (1) support the cognitive and physical work of healthcare professionals; and (2) promote high-quality, safe care for patients (Russ, 2013).

Latent factors: The systems approach focuses on working conditions rather than on errors of individuals, as the likelihood of specific errors increases with unfavorable conditions. Since the factors that promote errors are not directly visible in the working environment, they are described as latent risk factors (van Beuzekom, 2010).

Near miss: An unplanned event that has the potential to cause, but does not actually result in human injury, environmental or equipment damage, or an interruption to normal operation.

Psychological safety: Psychological safety is the belief that one will not be punished or humiliated for speaking up with ideas, questions, concerns, or mistakes. It is a shared belief held by members of a team that the environment is safe for interpersonal risk-taking. In psychologically safe teams, team members feel accepted and respected.

Public reporting: Data, publicly available or available to a broad audience free of charge or at a nominal cost, about a healthcare structure, process, or outcome at any provider level (individual clinician, group, organization).

Socio-technical: An approach to complex organizational work design that recognizes the interaction between people and technology in workplaces.

Chapter 8

Balanced scorecard: The balanced scorecard was originally developed by Dr. Robert Kaplan and Dr. David Norton in the early 1990s. It has since become a widely adopted tool in various industries and sectors, including healthcare as a strategic management tool that helps organizations measure and improve their performance by considering a balanced set of perspectives beyond just financial metrics. It translates an organization's mission and vision into specific, measurable goals and provides a clear plan of action.

Benchmarking: A systematic process of searching to identify best practices.

Cascading measures: A method that allows for simultaneous and linked analysis and visualization of data at increasing levels of aggregation, including individual, system, and population levels.

Clinical decision support (CDS): Timely information, usually at the point of care, to help inform decisions about a patient's care. CDS tools and systems help clinical teams by taking over some routine tasks, warning of potential problems, or providing suggestions for the clinical team and patient to consider.

Data dashboard: A visual display that features the most important information needed to achieve specific goals captured on a single screen. Effective dashboards should be designed as monitoring tools that are understood at a glance. Dashboards are useful tools because they can leverage visual perception to communicate dense amounts of data clearly and concisely.

Decision support: A decision support system is an information system that supports decision-making activities.

Dummy display: A make-believe figure or table showing the results you might get. Helps you find relationships between data, discover what variables you will need to answer your questions, and decide how you will analyze data and display results (Nelson, 2011b, p. 77).

Feed-forward/feedback: Describes the use of clinical and patient-reported data in learning health systems: (1) "*feed-forward*" refers to the use of data to predict needs of patients ahead of clinical visits or to inform clinical encounters at the point of care; (2) "*feedback*" refers to the transmission of data to health systems describing the outcomes of care for use in monitoring and improving system performance, healthcare outcomes, and related research.

Feed in/feed out: Refers to data flow pathways used in learning health systems that use patient-reported data to inform coproduction, comparative effectiveness research, and/or predictive analytics. Patient-generated clinical data can be "*fed in*" to health systems to inform care coproduction, including decision support, shared decision-making, self-monitoring, and patient-facilitated networks. Data can also be "*fed out*" to registries that can be used to inform research about effectiveness and can be used to inform predictive analytics and precision healthcare approaches.

Feed up/feed down: Refers to the application of cascading measurement in multi-center learning health system or collaborative improvement contexts in which short-term measures are used at micro- and mesosystem levels to inform frontline improvement efforts, and aggregated into or linked to longitudinal outcome measures used at the macrosystem or population level to inform collaborative improvement efforts and research.

Informatics: Informatics is a broad field that deals with the study, design, and development of information technology systems for the purpose of storing, processing, and communicating information. It often focuses on the interaction between humans and information systems, as well as the design of interfaces that make these systems easy to use. Health Informatics field applies informatics principles to healthcare, focusing on the use of technology to improve patient care, research, and public health. This includes electronic health records (EHRs), telemedicine, and data analytics for disease prevention and management.

Learning health system: A healthcare system that is designed to continuously learn and improve by using data and evidence to inform clinical decision-making and patient care. LHSs integrate research and clinical practice, aiming to create a feedback loop where new knowledge is generated and applied to enhance the quality, safety, and efficiency of healthcare delivery.

Patient portals: A secure online website that gives patients convenient, 24-hour access to personal health information from anywhere with an internet connection. Using a secure username and password, patients can view health information.

Patient-reported outcome (PRO): A health outcome directly reported by the patient who experienced it. It stands in contrast to an outcome reported by someone else, such as a physician-reported outcome, a nurse-reported outcome, and so on.

Performance dashboard: Provides consolidated, real-time displays of patient- and clinician-generated information, including well-being, needs, goals, and interventions. The impact of using dashboards to improve knowledge, health, and care delivery has been demonstrated: outcomes are optimized when patients, families, and clinicians have information they need at point-of-care, over time, and in a supportive delivery system capable of making and sustaining improvements (VanCitters, 2020).

Registry: An organized data repository that houses data gathered for use in research and improvement for a specified population or clinical condition, such as the SRQ registry for adults with rheumatoid arthritis in Sweden or the Cystic Fibrosis registry.

Run chart: A time plot (line graph) of data plotted over time, which also includes a measure of central tendency (usually the median). By collecting and charting data over time, you can find trends or patterns in the process. Because they do not include control limits, run charts are not as sophisticated as statistical process control (SPC) charts. However, run charts are very simple and easy to use, can be constructed manually, and can accurately detect common signals of non-random (special cause) variation, including shifts and trends.

Statistical process control (SPC): Refers to a body of measurement, analytical, and statistical approaches focusing on the study of performance variation. SPC is commonly used in quality control and quality improvement to monitor, analyze, improve, and control process performance.

Chapter 9

Clinical nurse leader (CNL): A graduate-level nursing role that was developed in the United States to prepare registered nurses focused on the improvement and leadership of quality and safety outcomes for patients or patient populations.

Competency-based education: *Competency-based education* refers to systems of *instruction*, assessment, grading, and academic reporting that are *based* on students demonstrating that they have learned the knowledge and skills they are expected to learn as they progress through their *education* (Gruppen, 2012).

Interprofessional education: Refers to occasions when students from two or more professions in health and social care learn together during all or part of their professional training with the object of cultivating collaborative practice for providing client- or patient-centered health care (Gilbert, 2010).

SQUIRE (Standards for QUality Improvement Reporting Excellence): Guidelines that provide a framework for reporting new knowledge about how to improve health care. They are intended for reports that describe system-level work to improve the quality, safety, and value of health care.

Team competencies: Competencies needed to enable good team function. The term may also refer to competencies that teams (as opposed to individuals) demonstrate.

Chapter 10

5Ps: An assessment process that evaluates the anatomy and current performance of the clinical microsystem, for example, primary care practice. Donabedian's structure, process, and outcome framework provides the foundation to the microsystem purpose, patients/population, professionals, processes, and patterns evaluation (Donabedian, 1966).

5Vs: (Value, Vision, inVolve, eVidence, Visualization): A modified conceptual model of the 5Ps utilized by the Sheffield Flow Academy to assess a mesosystem.

A3 method: Also known as A3 thinking or A3 reporting, is a structured problem-solving and continuous improvement approach originating from Toyota and commonly used in lean management practices. It involves summarizing a problem, analysis, corrective actions, and action plan on a single A3-sized sheet of paper (11×17 inches).

A3 problem-solving: See **A3 method**.

Advanced Cystic Fibrosis Lung Disease (ACFLD): A person with Cystic Fibrosis who has a lung function of forced expiratory volume (FEV1) <40%, other severity markers who may be referred for lung transplant evaluation.

"Big room": Definition of Obeya. Bringing a multidisciplinary team (including patients/families) together in one large room for collaboration and problem-solving using visual representations of data and processes of a mesosystem.

Care map: Also known as a care pathway or clinical pathway, is a visual representation of a patient's planned course of treatment and care for a specific condition or procedure. It outlines the expected timeline and sequence of interventions, assessments, and outcomes, serving as a guide for healthcare providers and patients throughout the care journey.

Care pathway: See **care map**.

Cause and effect diagram: A term used interchangeably with fishbone diagram, often called an Ishikawa diagram. Used to identify the causes of an effect that the microsystem is interested in.

Change ideas: Generated from literature review, best practices, benchmarking, and change concepts to select a change idea to test.

Clinical pathway: See **care map**.

Co-coaching methodology: A structured model of coaching an improvement team where two individual coaches form a co-coaching relationship with the team being coached. Identification of strengths and interests of each coach to partner contributes to customizing technique and behavioral processes to support improvement success.

Complex adaptive system: Dynamic networks made up of many individual components, which all interact and influence one another in non-linear ways.

Critical pathway: See **care map**.

Cystic Fibrosis Transplant Consortium (CFLTC): A network of **10** academic lung transplant programs whose mission is to advance outcomes in cystic fibrosis patients who may need or have received a lung transplant.

Dartmouth Microsystem Improvement Ramp: A systematic approach which helps guide improvement teams gain an understanding of their core and supporting processes, identify global and specific aims, generate change ideas, and conduct rapid tests of change (PDSA cycles) involving assessment, flowcharts, global aim, specific aims, fishbones, change ideas, PDSA, SDSA cycles, and measures.

Discharge to assess (D2A): A care process to assess patient's needs after discharge in the patient's own home rather than in the hospital.

Effective meeting skills: Organized and structured meeting process consisting of timed agenda, meeting roles, for example, meeting leader, recorder, facilitator, and timekeeper to ensure all members equally participate by creating and using ground rules, practice communication skills, and increase productive and value of meetings.

Exchange program: Clinical microsystems who belong to a "mesosystem" of care visit each other's microsystem, to observe work and delivery of care processes while developing improved relationships, communication, and new perspectives.

Flow coaching academy (FCA): Developed within the National Health Service (NHS) in the UK based on the Dartmouth Institute Microsystem Academy model and processes. The academy exists to provide a learning and development academy for healthcare professionals to increase improvement capabilities and successful improvement of processes and systems of care.

Flow coaching methodology: A model of replicable training in team coaching and technical improvement skills that equips staff at all levels to make sustained improvements to health and care outcomes, experience, and cost-effectiveness.

Frail people: A person who meets three or more criteria developed by Johns Hopkins: unintentional loss of 10 or more pounds in the past year, weakness, exhaustion, trouble standing without assistance or reduced grip strength.

Frailty assessment unit: Frail patients and elderly that present to an emergency department are comprehensively assessed by a multidisciplinary team to perform a comprehensive geriatric assessment in order to reduce unnecessary hospital admissions and reduce length of stay.

High-level process maps: Graphic representation using standard symbols to depict high-level steps in a selected process to assess and improve.

High-performing frontline teams: A multidisciplinary group of individuals who care for patients who have shared vision, defined roles and responsibilities, clear and respectful communication with mutual trust and respect in an environment of continuous learning and improvement (see Quality by Design, Chapter 1).

Improvement breakthrough series (BTS): A collaborative quality improvement methodology developed by the Institute for Healthcare Improvement (IHI). It aims to help organizations achieve significant and sustainable improvements in health-care outcomes.

Institute for Healthcare Improvement (IHI): Founded in 1991, with a commitment to redesigning health care into a system without errors, waste, delays, and unsustainable costs, which has evolved to meet current and future health care challenges.

Integrated care pathway (ICP): A structured, multidisciplinary care plan designed to guide the management of a specific patient population with a particular condition or set of conditions. It outlines the optimal sequence and timing of interventions, from diagnosis and treatment to rehabilitation and follow-up care. ICPs aim to improve patient outcomes.

Mesosystem: Two or more microsystems – **for example**, a patient pathway.

Microsystem improvement curriculum: See **Dartmouth Microsystem Improvement Curriculum**.

Mindfulness: The practice of paying non-judgmental attention to the present moment. It involves being aware of your thoughts, feelings, and bodily sensations without getting caught up in them or reacting to them.

Obeya methodology: Originating from Toyota's Lean management system, a visual management and collaboration tool designed to improve communication, alignment, and problem-solving within organizations. In Japanese, "Obeya" translates to "big room."

"Ownership" of the workplace: The sense of personal responsibility and accountability that employees have for their work, which involves taking the initiative to make a difference.

Plan-Do-Study-Act (PDSA): A model of continuous quality improvement that uses scientific approach, plan-do-study-act. Originally developed by Walter Shewhart and made popular by W. Edwards Deming, who ascribed inherent variation in processes to chance and intermittent variation to assignable causes. The PDSA cycle is a four-part method for discovering and correcting assignable causes to improve the quality of processes.

Playbook: The "how we do things" book. Written directions or "plays" for how different activities (usually standardized best practices) are completed on the unit. Consists of primarily a collection of best practice process maps to standardize care and processes that all staff are aware of and accountable for.

Principles of systems engineering: Design, integration, and management of complex systems over their life cycle utilizing systems thinking principles.

Quality improvement assessment tool (QIA): A validated instrument that assesses individual and aggregate team changes in quality improvement skill growth QI Importance and Confidence, QI Tools and Skills, Improvement Measurement, Communication and Team Dynamics, and Organizational Context and Leadership.

Relational coordination (RC): Mutually reinforcing process of communicating and relating for the purpose of task integration.

Standardize-Do-Study-Act (SDSA): A model for standardizing improvement, standardize-do-study-act. The steps taken when PDSA cycle has been successfully done to achieve the original aim consistently – "best it can be" now. The purpose is to hold the gains that were made using PDSA cycles and standardize the process in daily work.

Structure, process, and outcome: A conceptual model by Donabedian (1980) for evaluating the quality of health care.

Vertically integrated provider: Providers fulfilling different functions along the care continuum.

NAME INDEX

SUBJECT INDEX

Quality by Design: A Clinical Microsystems Approach, Second Edition. Edited by Marjorie M. Godfrey, Tina C. Foster, Julie K. Johnson, Eugene C. Nelson and Paul B. Batalden.
© 2025 John Wiley & Sons, Inc. Published 2025 by John Wiley & Sons, Inc.